D1233817

APHASIA, APRAXIA AND AGNOSIA

APHASIA, APRAXIA AND AGNOSIA

Clinical and Theoretical Aspects

By

JASON W. BROWN, M.D.

Director
Department of Neurology
St. Barnabas Hospital
Assistant Clinical Professor of Neurology
Columbia University
New York, New York

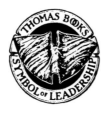

CHARLES C THOMAS • PUBLISHER

Springfield • Illinois • U.S.A.

c.1

Published and Distributed Throughout the World by
CHARLES C THOMAS • PUBLISHER
BANNERSTONE HOUSE
301-327 East Lawrence Avenue, Springfield, Illinois, U.S.A.
NATCHEZ PLANTATION HOUSE
735 North Atlantic Boulevard, Fort Lauderdale, Florida, U.S.A.

© 1972, by CHARLES C THOMAS • PUBLISHER
ISBN 0-398-02211-9
Library of Congress Catalog Card Number: 70-169873

With THOMAS BOOKS *careful attention is given to all details of manu-*
facturing and design. It is the Publisher's desire to present books that
are satisfactory as to their physical qualities and artistic possibilities and
appropriate for their particular use. THOMAS BOOKS *will be true to*
those laws of quality that assure a good name and good will.

Printed in the United States of America
EE-11

For my father,
Samuel
and mother,
Sylvia

PREFACE

THIS MONOGRAPH is an effort toward a new interpretation of aphasic and related phenomena. Specifically, a theory is presented in which the various aphasic disorders are viewed as interruptions at successive planes in the process of language formulation. This process is conceived as a productive activity which consists in an hierarchic unfolding of levels in a path from memory and cognition to articulated speech. The agnosias and apraxias are also discussed in this light.

As it has proved necessary to cover a vast amount of specialized and relatively unfamiliar literature, the chapters are arranged so as to provide both an historical perspective and an introduction to testing procedures. Where advisable, personal cases are included as illustrations. The chapters covering aphasic and apraxic disorders are ordered so as to complement the advancing theoretical design, and may be taken to represent the sequence of (arbitrary) stages which occur with language breakdown. Though the classification employs a traditional nomenclature (the author wishing to avoid yet another terminology), the ordering of the syndromes reflects a distinct theoretical bias. Deviation from this pattern occurs only to the extent that insufficient data exist to maintain uniformity of style.

In preparing this work for publication, I have been fortunate to receive the advice and support of many friends. In particular, I would like to express my deepest appreciation to the staff of the Aphasia Research Center, Boston, for the opportunity to spend with them an enjoyable and fruitful year, and to the National Institutes of Health for the necessary support. I owe a great personal debt to Dr. D. Frank Benson for many enjoyable conversations and permission to publish a number of cases seen on the Aphasia Unit, and to Drs. Edith Kaplan, Harold Goodglass and Norman Geschwind for many hours of stimulating discussion. My gratitude goes also to Dr. Richard Masland, for his always friendly advice and encouragement, and to the directors of St. Barnabas Hospital and, in particular, Dr. Daniel Larson, for making available to me the facilities with which to realize and continue this work. I would also like to acknowledge the invaluable assistance of my secretary, Mrs. Marie Zito, who has cheerfully typed the manuscript. My wife, Jo-Ann, has patiently watched this book grow over the years and has given greatly of herself towards its completion. Lastly, whatever of value there is in this work I owe to the example and guidance of my father and mother, to whom I offer it in modest dedication.

J.W.B.

CONTENTS

APHASIA, APRAXIA AND AGNOSIA

Chapter 1

INTRODUCTION

IF WE LOOK over the 150 years since the contributions of Gall and Bouillaud, one of the major issues in "higher function" study has been that of holistic versus atomistic organization. The controversy among adherents of either doctrine has, in fact, been so characteristic of the field as to serve almost as a yardstick of its progress. At the core of this debate is the relationship between part and whole, a problem which has been discussed, in one form or another, in every thoughtful presentation.

One interpretation of the part:whole relationship which is most familiar to modern workers is that advanced by Wernicke in 1874, and supported by many neurologists thereafter. This begins with the isolation, then the localization, of various symptoms or symptom-complexes, and leads eventually to a redefinition of these in terms of deficits in real functions. Ordinarily, the isolation process proceeds so far that holistic considerations no longer appear relevant. For example, the component features of Gerstmann's syndrome were initially defined, then correlated with dominant angular gyrus, and then judged to reflect the disruption of some more or less unitary function concerned with finger gnosis. The relationships between different symptom groupings, or between symptom and other aspects of behavior are, in this account, relegated to an associational pathway. This pathway is then conceived as a marker for the relational process, which itself remains unspecified. In its favor, the approach offers a simplification which may be didactically useful, and the attempt at clarity is always to be recommended. Yet, there is a certain deficiency in associationist logic, for the autonomy of any syndrome depends, ultimately, upon an acceptance of its associative relationships, and these in turn are inferred from the "autonomous" character of the symptomatology. One unfortunate consequence of this reasoning is that the whole dynamism of the system is reduced to an otherwise inert and often nonexistent connection, and the syndrome itself, for the sake of the anatomy, becomes more rigidly defined and considerably more substantial an entity than clinical study would warrant.

Other workers, noting common elements within the various language and perceptual disorders, have judged these elements to be in the nature of *fundamental* disturbances to which the diversity of clinical observation can be reduced. Examples are Marie's "intellectual defects," von Monakow's "diaschisis," and in a manner perhaps not altogether intended by the author, Goldstein's "abstract attitude." However, principles of such wide application generally do not have a great usefulness, for either irreconcilable contradictions will appear in the case which does not conform, or the application will be so universal that the principle will be considered extrinsic to the problem under study.

A third and equally successful strategy is, in reality, little more than a compromise of the other two, and for that reason is more deceptive in its appeal. In this approach, complex functions are isolated and interaction postulated between these functions and other psychopathological states. For example, some writers now argue that visual agnosia is a combination of low-level visual defects, disturbed intelligence and dysphasia; that conduction aphasia is only a mild word-deafness plus dysphasia; word-deafness, a low-level auditory defect with intellectual reduction, and so on.

One might illustrate these different views in the following way. In the first, A, B and C are independent entities connected by otherwise functionless pathways; in the second, A, B and C are manifestations of a single defect, let us say *x*, which is itself irreducible; and in the third, A is in reality *x* plus B. Set in this light, such roundabout ways of brain study will appear to be highly nonproductive.

There is to be considered another, and I think, preferred school of thought, that of hierarchical organization, of which Pick (1931) and Schilder (1951) are most representative. This is not Jacksonian hierarchy, which emphasizes higher control and release of lower centers, but rather bears a relation to the Würzberg account of thinking, and to modern cognitive theory. One might schematize this as A→ B→C, where A, B and C represent planes in cognitive development from the earliest stage to the final form. The advantage here is that connection, combination and interaction do not play a significant part, for all of the properties of mentation are subsumed in the simplest intellectual performance. Further, the system is defined in terms of process, not static groupings, and thus the possibility is opened of *rapprochement* with related fields of physiological investigation. Drawbacks have been the indefinite anatomical correlation, the fluidity of syndrome boundary, the strong emphasis on introspective data and perhaps most importantly, the inability of some theorists to adjust their speculations to the less visionary attitudes of their readers. The contribution of hierarchy to aphasia theory will be assessed more fully in the chapters to follow. For the present, however, it will be helpful to review briefly some aspects of this approach.

THEORETICAL BACKGROUND

Generally, we may say that in the formative or microgenetic process through which concepts develop, there is a progression toward states of increasing clarity. This is true of both productive and reproductive thinking, and applies to both images and words. In the experiments of the Würzburg group, the pre-history of this development was searched for in the imageless background of thought (see Humphrey, 1963). In the initial studies, subjects were presented with a variety of simple questions or calculations and were tested as to their subjective experiences on arriving at a solution. Later investigations emphasized such parameters as response to single word presentations or the interpretation of an aphorism of Nietzsche. The many experiments that were carried out all pointed toward the presence, at the earliest stage of thought production, of non-sensory (imageless) contents in awareness as the first sign of the developing thought. This vague and intuitive early stage, which Marbe designated as *Bewusstseinslagen*, is only an intimation of the thought, a feeling of its dynamism or at most some apprehension of its general character without qualitative elements. From here the thought passed into a stage of some structure and determination, the *Bewusstheit* of Ach. Here there is awareness of direction, the thought is committed, and a pattern and some organization can be discerned.

In 1913, Pick, who was familiar with this work, described four stages in the transition of thought to speech: an early stage (1) in which thought is formulated with increasing clarity out of memory in such a way that its partial contents are combined to a type of schematic or structural whole; this stage (2) that of structural thought, is prior to linguistic formulation; there is a preparation toward a predicative arrangement, and elements of tone, tempo and grammar come into play; the next stage (3), that of the sentence pattern develops under the influence of an (imprecisely defined) emotional factor, and leads to (4) the automatic choice of words. Pick's work, which will be discussed more fully later on, was continued by Schilder (1935), von Woerkom (1925), Bouman and

Grunbaum (1925) and others. According to the latter authors, the fundamental defect in aphasia was an arrest, at an earlier stage, in the development of a process which proceeds from an amorphous total reaction to more differentiated and definite forms. A common effort of these studies was the attempt to demonstrate, at an early prelinguistic level, spatial defects referable to a structural stage in thought development. Head's semantic aphasia, for example, and Lashley's (1951) insistence on the importance of spatial-serial trans- formations in the progress of thought to speech, were outgrowths of this formulation. Lashley, moreover, commented that the memory trace was probably integrated in the space-coordinate system.

The view that gradually emerged from these and other writings may be expressed in the following way. Thought develops from a deeper structure into an experiential form. At the earliest stage, that of imageless thought, there is little more than a vague intuition of the idea to be expressed. This may be a feeling of the presentation of the thought rather than an apprehension of its nature. This is a transitional zone, a preparatory phase not yet at the level of the idea, the concept. Subsequently, a structural phase can be recognized, that of the concept, where cognition has a directedness and a commitment, though not necessarily to one mode of expression. The concept as- sumes its structurality by virtue of an increasing delimitation. The stage is designated by our first ability to perceive its "sensory" char- acter. In the course of this development, there are (multiple) transi- tions from patterns of spatial simultaneity to the patterns of temporal succession which they prefigurate, as in the sequencing of words out of a sentence pattern. The process achieves its orientation and intensity through both intrinsic (e.g. affectual, motivational) and extrinsic (e.g. Aufgabe) factors. The two early stages are the *Bewusstseinsla- gen* and *Bewusstheit* of the Würzburg school, intuitive and structural thought of Pick and van Woerkom, and the sphere and concept of Schilder.

While much of this early work led naturally into modern cognitive theory, its influence on aphasia study was restricted to but a few authors. Among these, Conrad (1947) has extended the microgenesis work to gestalt theory, and accounts for aphasia as an arrest of a formative process at a pregestalt (Vorgestalt) stage. The views of Bay (1964), though incompletely expounded, give the impression of sympathy with theories of concept formation, and Werner (1956) has contributed to the subject a small but valuable paper. Luria (1964, 1966) has been critical of the notion of imageless thought and appears to favor the view that all thought depends on verbal mechanisms. However, the hierarchic approach figures importantly in his work. Thus, speaking of language organization, he writes that the system of semantic codes ". . . possesses a complex hierarchical structure. It begins with the system of words, behind each of which there stands not only a unitary image, but a complex system of generalizations of those things which the word signifies."

PERCEPTION

While the view that speech and volitional action are creative products of cognition is not particularly heretical, there is some resistance to a similar account of perception. Few contemporary authors are as insightful as Luria in his treatment of this subject. Thus, perception is studied not as a simple receptive function but as ". . . an active investigatory activity" which comprises ". . . the recognition of the dominant signs of an object, the creation of a series of visual hypotheses or alternatives, the choice of the most probable of these hypotheses, and the final determination of the required image. . . ." This sequence is identical to that characterizing the stages of problem-solving behavior, i.e. thinking. This formulation is not, however, without philosophical precedence. Thus, Bergson (1911) held that "the *actuality* of our perception . . . lies in its activity . . . (and that perception) consists in detaching from the totality of objects the possible action of my body upon them. Perception appears, then, as only a choice." A somewhat similar argument has been advanced by Cassirer (1953). "If we reflect," he says, "that 'things' and 'states,' 'attributes' and 'activities' are not given contents of consciousness, but modalities and directions of its formation, then it becomes apparent that none of them is immediately perceived, and expressed by language according to this perception; what takes place is rather that an undifferentiated diversity of sensory impressions is *defined* in accordance with one or another form of thought and language. It is this fixation into an object or *activity*, not the mere naming of the object or activity, that is expressed in the spiritual operation of language as in the logical operation of cognition." The situation has also been clearly expressed by Bertalanffy (1968). In the old view, he says, ". . . the organism is a passive receiver of stimuli; sense data, information—whatever you call it—coming from outside objects; and these are—in a rather mysterious way—reprojected into space to form perceptions which more or less truly mirror the ex-

ternal world. In many ways . . . this is not so. In a very real sense, the
organism *creates* the world around it . . ."; and further on he writes,
"the principle of the active psychophysical organism thus pertains
not only to the motoric or 'output' part of behavior, but also to
'input,' to cognitive processes." All of this work rests on the recognition of one inescapable fact, that the object of perception does not
come to us as a given, but rather, that it must actively be sought after
and constructed through cognitive processes.

In dealing with perception in this way, disorders of auditory comprehension and the visual agnosias come to refer not only to defects
of the in-processing of information (hereafter, sensation), but as
symptom-complexes reflecting an impairment at corresponding levels
in the construction of perceptual images out of thought (hereafter,
perception). Since the major emphasis is on aphasic disorders, a brief
review of some work in auditory perception may help to clarify the
point.

It would appear self-evident that the perception of a phonemic
sequence is a step introductory to an understanding of the word. After
all, we "hear" phonemes in a certain order and it only seems reasonable to think they are decoded in the manner of their presentation.
Yet we can scarcely be so sure of this. In the first awareness of a word
there is no hint of the building-up process that goes into its final
form, nor of the relation to memory through which word recognition
is achieved. According to the old view, speech sounds are separated
from a diffuse acoustic background and reassembled through a kind
of additive process, into a sequence identical to that received. After
the auditory perception (word) has been formed, a relationship is
established to verbal memory, and recognition occurs. There is a good
deal of evidence to suggest that this view of auditory perception is
incorrect, that in certain respects recognition is a stage preparatory
to perception.

Proof of this assertion can be found in the everyday perception of
one's own language, for to truly *hear* the language, is to bring to
bear an action by memory upon the sensory material itself. Speech
perception is both discriminative and predictive. A word or sentence
is grasped before it is fully perceived, the meaning of the sentence is
apprehended often after only a word or two. Not only do we leap
ahead when listening to our own language, but we may fall behind
if the rate of speaking is too fast. Thus, Americans may find difficulty
understanding the speech of Englishmen because of the rapid rate of
speaking. This failure to perceive one's own language can hardly be

explained by a "passive" or sensory theory of speech perception. The inability to understand relates to the failure to anticipate or predict sounds in advance of their perception. Music is also learned in this way. On the other hand, when we listen to a foreign language or a new musical work, we do not really perceive the individual tones or speech sounds at all.

Another source of evidence comes from experiments by Liberman and co-workers (1952), Chistovich (1963), Halle and Stevens (1962) and others. These authors share the view that in auditory decodage, the acoustic signal is first transformed into a "representation" corresponding to that in an abstract store of the lexical units of the language. The decoded signal is then matched, according to certain rules governing the production of speech out of that lexical store, these rules being to a degree independent of the articulatory movements to which they lead. The acoustic signal is thus recognized, i.e. matched, at the same time or before it is perceived. Warren (1970) has recently demonstrated that if a phoneme in a recorded sentence is replaced by an extraneous sound, listeners are unaware of the substitution, even if informed of the actual stimulus. There is, the author notes, an ". . . illusory perception of the speaker's utterance rather than the stimulus actually reaching our ears." This suggests that the perception is a product of the matching process. In its present form, this account, the so-called "motor theory," gives the productive element in perception to a kind of sublimated articulatory act, though recognizing that perception is itself also an active process. In this respect, it is compromise toward the more extreme position taken here.

It is of interest that one worker in the field (Fant, 1967) has suggested that it may not be possible to prove whether the motor theory is or is not correct. Personally, I suspect this is very likely the case, for the passive and active theories of perception, far from differing with respect to data interpretation alone, look at each other from opposite sides of the mind-body problem.

Perhaps the strongest evidence for this dynamic view of perception comes from the study of aphasia. This material, which will be discussed in the pages to follow, brings us to the following preliminary formulation. It is maintained that the acoustic signal first undergoes a process of "structuralization" on its way to "memory." The resultant *abstract* representation of the signal then becomes a part of the spatially-distributed trace system where matching (recognition) of signal to store takes place. The perceptual phase concerns the emergence of the matched signal complex into private or mental space and awareness. In the auditory system, the sensory stage involves, at the minimum, processes of temporal summation and the localization of the signal in acoustic space, the perceptual stage concerns the re-sequentialization of the signal-complex into private space. As visual perception develops out of a level common to action, so auditory perception issues out of a level common to speech. The central point about auditory perception is that the same deep organization elabo-rates both speech-production and speech-understanding.

This discussion is by no means exhaustive (see Neisser, 1967) and is intended only to indicate to the reader a novel approach to cer-tain recurrent problems in language study. One consequence of this new orientation in thinking, however, is that many tacitly accepted principles of brain action now need to be reconsidered.

GENERAL PRINCIPLES

Firstly, the common view that syndromes result from the combina-tion of two or more similar defects must be treated with great caution. This is not to say that hemiparesis and alexia cannot coexist as discrete impairments. These involve disparate systems. Rather, syn-dromes which relate to disturbance in a single sphere, such as lan-guage function, are not a compilation of units disorganized within that sphere, but represent a molar level of function to which that sphere has been reduced. Thus, Wernicke's aphasia is not word-deafness *plus* verbal paraphasia *plus* anosognosia *plus* euphoria but a defect in language formulation at some level where processes under-lying these functions are coextensive. Moreover, a syndrome in isola-tion does not reappear unaltered in combined form, but is then an entirely new syndrome. The degree to which this holds is not certain, for the determination as to which systems are disparate is not a simple matter. Probably the relation to cognitive organization is the crucial factor.

Related to this is the question of mildness and severity. It is exceptional that one sees in mild form an attenuation of the same disorder as when severe. Not only does the defect change, but its accompaniments often differ according to the degree of severity. Thus in conduction aphasia, as repetition improves there is also recovery of naming, comprehension and conversational speech. There may be alteration in the response to questions in series speech, in the character of phonemic and verbal paraphasia, and in the ability to self-correct. Those symptoms which accompany the principle disorder under study, as in this example repetition, are often understood as a reflection of the extent or multifocality of the lesion. However, since these changes occur with some degree of internal consistency, they have to be viewed as of molar character, rather than secondary to the disparate recovery of partial functions. Severity will, therefore, often entail a difference of kind as well as degree. Further, a distinction between anatomical and clinical severity must be drawn. The problem of severity in an hierarchical system has been clarified greatly by Conrad (1947), who points out that the lower (i.e. more thought-distant) the lesion, the more severe, but the more restricted, the local effect. Higher (i.e. thought-close) defects, on the other hand, produce slight impairment in more widespread functions, and involve more of the patient's native personality.

A misunderstanding also exists as to the independence of functional and instrumentality change. For Conrad (1947), aphasia is intermediate between disturbance of instrumentality (e.g. hemiplegia) and disturbance of function (e.g. dementia), and varies closer to one or the other depending on aphasia type. Thus, to use the analogy of a tree, impairment of the more resistant trunk will affect all branches but mildly, while distant involvements will severely affect the solitary branch and minimally influence the trunk. As there is no true distinction between trunk and branch, there is none between conceptual and effector organization. Finally, as in the organic form of a tree, principles of hierarchic construction are repeated at many stages. The variety of symptoms which are observed in aphasia do not require a diversity of underlying processes, but often reflect only a change in level where reiteration of the process occurs.

With regard to localization, the correlation of symptom-groupings with specific brain regions has suggested that local functions are nodal and discontinuous with those of distant regions. But there is no evidence that anatomical discontinuity precludes functional relatedness. There is the possibility of temporal interdependence among processes lacking anatomical contiguity. Certainly, one should at least withhold judgment on this point until more information is available.

Concerning emotional changes which accompany the various disorders under consideration, these also are not *added to* the "higher-level" defect but represent, at least in part, a subjective component attached to each level in the hierarchy. There have been prior suggestions along these lines. Schilder wondered whether the apathy

(Willenlosigkeit) or depression of Broca's aphasia and the euphoria of Wernicke's aphasia were intrinsic to the speech disturbance rather than a secondary reaction. Scheerer (1954) and Hillman
(1961) have also discussed the cognitive aspect to emotion. While it
is not our aim to explore this question, the difference in approach has
to be emphasized. In other formulations, emotion is usually external
to cognition. In the present work, each level in cognitive development can be characterized by some intrinsic affectual state. Strong
evidence for this contention comes from important studies by Sander
and Wohlfahrt (see discussion in Conrad, 1947). In these studies,
subjects were given tachystoscopic exposures of figures at varying
stages of clarity. They were noted to undergo extreme anxiety at
stages of low resolution (vorgestalt), which gave way gradually to a
condition of relief and relaxation on final definition of the figural
gestalt (endgestalt). The vorgestalt stage was also characterized by a
greater passivity. The inference is that these affective states which
accompany levels in the perception of tachystoscopic forms correspond to affective states associated with levels in normal thinking; that
is, that the emotions represent, or are another aspect of, different
stages in the cognitive process.

IMAGERY

With respect to auditory and visual perception, it is necessary to
call attention to imaginal phenomena which may occur in aphasic
and agnosic conditions, for these are of great theoretical interest. By
visual imagery is meant simply the emergence of some unbound
visual content in the imagination. Here especially belong hallucinatory and dream images, eidetic and related phenomena. Some evidence will be presented to suggest that imagery forms the substrate
of perception. In fact, perception appears to have the nature of a
dream image which lacks external (sensory) control. Thus, we find
that disorders of sensory cortex often entail a deficiency or heightening of image activity. There may be loss of waking or dream imagery,
nightmares and/or vivid hallucinatory experiences, usually limited
to that perceptual sphere affected in the aphasic or agnosic state.
However, more than just the sensation is needed to attain a veridical
perception, for real objects may take on imaginal features. Whether
the perception is imaginary or real seems to depend also on certain
aspects of the formative process itself. Thus, each disorder of perception and language has a subjective and an objective character.

An important part of the process of perceptual formation concerns the passive or receptive attitude in the individual towards the image produced (Rapaport, 1951). This attitude develops as an accompaniment to the perception. In its fullest form, this passivity leads to the "exteriorization" of the perception as a real object in the external world. It is in this way that objects achieve autonomy in extrapersonal space. In imagery this passive relationship is less pronounced, and the object does not fully separate out of the intrapersonal sphere. In this respect, there is no clear border between image, perception and sensation. This is particularly evident in the case of visual phenomena, but is also true for other sensory systems and for the imaginal side of movements. Russell (1921), for example, has written:

> I am by no means confident that the distinction between images and sensations is ultimately valid . . . I think it is clear, however, that, at any rate in the case of auditory and visual images, they do differ from auditory and visual sensations, and therefore, form a recognizable class of occurrence, even if it should prove that they can be regarded as a sub-class of sensations.

Hughlings Jackson (1932) believed that ". . . the only difference between seeing (e.g. a brick) and thinking of it is a difference of degree (and) . . . an idea (or image) is only a faint external perception (percept) and an external perception is only a vivid idea."

Verbal imagery concerns what has come to be known as inner-speech (Vygotsky, 1962; Goldstein, 1948). This is a dynamic process including both the pre-verbitum and the auditory image. Recent studies (e.g. Inouye and Shimizu, 1970) suggest that the acoustic component, which comes into prominence mainly in dream and pathological states, is of great importance. However, here the verbal image has a passive quality and seems detached from the personality (Anastasoupolous, 1967). This may not be true of the verbal imagery of waking thought, which has a more active character. Luria (1964), for example, writes that it has to do with the relationship between the propositional context of a word and the expression of the word itself. Visual and verbal imagery come to the fore particularly when the perceptual and expressive avenues are obstructed. This should not be interpreted to mean that images play a secondary role, either as aids to thought or as intermediate stages. The image is as much the goal of thought as the perception or the action.

CLASSIFICATION OF APHASIA

It has been implied in our discussion of auditory perception that the disorders of speech comprehension which complicate the expressive aphasias are not to be viewed as ancillary disturbances brought on by an ever-widening pathology, but are inherent features of each aphasic form. It follows, therefore, that all disorders of speech understanding, even those with the most limited pathology, are likely to have an expressive element, while some defect in speech comprehension should be a constant feature of the motor aphasias. The importance of this finding has certainly not received proper attention in the literature. One need only point to the fact that there is not one careful study of speech comprehension in restricted cases of Broca's aphasia, nor a comparable study, of the much rarer word-deafness, of the true state of expressive speech. Disinterest in this problem has no doubt been the result of initial success in aphasia classification, or at least in the isolation of specific symptom groups. If, however, instead of looking for artificial differences between the aphasias we search for functional bonds among the different forms, a wholly different picture of the neurological organization and breakdown of speech emerges: namely, that with pathology in a common language system, the expressive-receptive as a unit undergoes a harmonious and predictable decay. Lesions interfering with the normal operation of this system will have, according to their location in the speech development sequence, both an expressive and a receptive effect. Thus, with pathological involvement of the deeper structure, a disorder akin to semantic aphasia occurs. Impairment at some intermediate level results in the Wernicke aphasia complex (sensory, and transcortical sensory aphasia) and conduction aphasia, while surface defects produce word-deafness and Broca's aphasia. The deeper the level of involvement, the more "diffuse" the symptomatology, and the less intense the impairment of speech and speech perception. On the other hand, surface lesions produce more severe and more discrete impairments, and tend to spare cognitive mechanisms. Expressive defects are interruptions at successive stages in a process which leads from word-finding to articulation. These range from the anomias, through verbal and phonemic paraphasia to agrammatism and dysarthria. Conjointly with these difficulties on the productive side appear defects at successive levels in the process of speech understanding. Though these are not as well studied, still a progression occurs from deeper impairments of contextual and combinatory functions (sen-

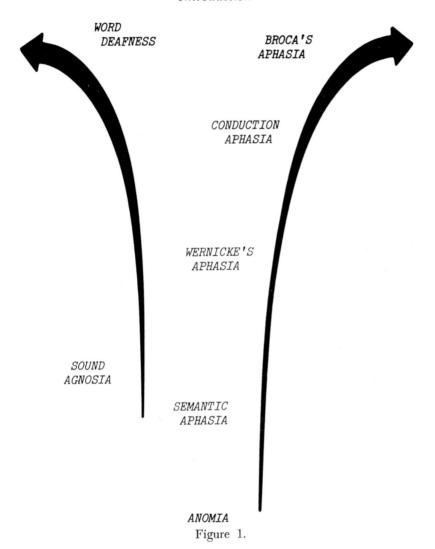

WORD
DEAFNESS

BROCA'S
APHASIA

CONDUCTION
APHASIA

WERNICKE'S
APHASIA

SOUND
AGNOSIA

SEMANTIC
APHASIA

ANOMIA

Figure 1.

sory agrammatism) through intermediate stages (Wernicke's aphasia)
to what might be termed the "sensory dysarthria" of the word-deaf,
i.e. a failure to "articulate" specific speech sounds.

With this bare outline, then, we can proceed to a discussion of
the clinical forms. The anomias are taken up first, and are held to
represent an impairment at a stage of lexical entry. The substantive
or content words of the phrase, which are selectively affected in this
disorder, are the starting point of sentence formation. This leads

through a form of aphasia which we have designated semantic aphasia, to the verbal paraphasia and comprehension defects of Wernicke's aphasia. Accentuation of the comprehension defect in Wernicke's aphasia permits the appearance of echolalia (transcortical sensory aphasia), while an advancement of the defect on the expressive side leads to conduction aphasia. Word-deafness and Broca's aphasia are the end-stage of each limb of the process (Fig. 1).

TERMINOLOGY

By *aphasia* is meant simply an acquired disorder of language, apparent in speech, writing (*agraphia*) and reading (*alexia*). Although aphasia is generally due to pathology of the brain, aphasic states can occur under normal conditions, e.g. sleep and fatigue, and possibly with the psychoses. *Agnosia* refers to an acquired cortical sensory ("apperceptive") or perceptual ("associative") disorder, regardless of the modality concerned, and *apraxia* to an impairment of voluntary movement, without obvious sensorimotor deficits. Semantic (verbal) paraphasia is the substitution of one word for another, phonemic (literal) paraphasia, the distortion of one or more phonemic constituents within an otherwise correct word, and neologism, the use of nonsense words. The definition of other terms used in this monograph will become evident in the individual sections where those terms appear. In all cases, however, usage is conventional and does not differ from that in standard reference works (e.g. Weisenberg and McBride, 1935; Goldstein, 1948).

I. APHASIA

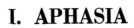

Chapter 2

ANOMIA

THE CONCEPT OF verbal amnesia as a defect in the mental evocation of words was an early development in aphasia study. As a distinction was made between internal and external speech, verbal amnesia came to be set against Broca's aphasia, the latter being considered largely a motor disturbance. Wernicke's (1874) notion of internal speech as the revival of acoustic images tended to obscure the anomias under the new description of sensory aphasia. Thus, Marie (1906) and Marie and Foix (1917) held that anomia was a residual of sensory aphasia, though Wernicke himself maintained that anomia was a form of transcortical motor aphasia. Subsequent workers fragmented the anomic state into visual, auditory and motor components, each corresponding to a separate aphasic form, and for this reason it was rather late that an isolated anomia came to be recognized. The paper of Pitres (1898) was especially important in this regard and still makes valuable reading, but the modern conception certainly must be traced from the studies of Kurt Goldstein (1924, 1948).

According to Goldstein, the difficulty in object naming, as well as the companion disorders of reading, writing, and calculation, all stemmed from a common underlying defect, an inability to assume an "abstract attitude" with regard to the item being tested. With respect to naming, the central problem in such patients, words which could not be produced as names, or which could be produced but not brought into relation with the object designated, may appear spontaneously in conversation. This indicates that word memory is unimpaired, and that it is rather the condition under which the word is evoked that is altered. Goldstein concluded that it was the ability to apply words as symbols for objects, i.e. as word concepts, which was lost, a difficulty which became even more apparent if the patient was asked to sort objects according to various attributes such as color, size or shape. Here the inability to give the name of a single object, reflecting a disturbance of the word concept of that object, is exaggerated by the requirement that diverse objects be categorized

19

according to shared attributes, the latter designated by a single word concept. Goldstein held that the abstract attitude was necessary for the following potentialities: assuming and shifting set; apprehending multiple contents simultaneously; combining parts into a whole and isolating out essential contents; abstracting common properties of different stituations; and detaching the ego from the outer world. Goldstein was not explicit in the relation of amnesic aphasia to other aphasic forms, but his remarks concerning central (conduction) aphasia are worth quoting in full: "A combination of amnesic aphasia with symptoms of central aphasia is frequent. There arises the question of whether we are dealing with an accidental combination due to similar locality of the underlying lesion, or whether there is an inner relationship between both defects. As little as we are able to say now, the latter possibility is worth pondering in respect to the closeness of the phenomenon of inner speech to the nonspeech mental processes."

Goldstein's description of amnesic aphasia (anomia) certainly achieved wider acceptance than did his psychological account. It was pointed out that abstraction was frequently impaired in the absence of anomia, and that anomia occurred with categorical behavior that was not strikingly abnormal, or if so, no different from that seen in other aphasic syndromes. Also to be included in this period are works by Heilbronner (1908) and Lotmar (1919), particularly as concerns verbal paraphasia. Lotmar especially discussed the spheric nature of word substitution, and attempted to show how apparently random substitutions occurred through intermediate links.

For Head (1926), nominal aphasia was characterized by diminished power to use or understand names. The patient therefore not only fails to name objects but has difficulty pointing to objects named for him. Repetition is excellent, reading and writing are poor and spelling is impaired. Patients have difficulty in taking dictation, and transliteration is poor. There is considerable trouble with single numbers or letters, a finding which is discussed more fully under agraphic alexia (Chap. 27), often an accompaniment of anomia. Head also listed defects in constructional tasks similar to those in his semantic aphasia, and which in any case appear outside the language disorder. This description is generally conceded to be rather close to the classical account, though the defect in comprehending names is not stressed by most authors, with the singular exception of Kleist.

There has been little attention to this disorder since Goldstein's summary work. Most authors have treated anomia as something apart from aphasia proper, as in Weisenburg's (1935) classification where amnesic aphasia seems almost tagged on to the expressive-receptive forms. Among modern workers, there has been interest in the relation of anomia to impaired verbal memory. Ajuriaguerra and Hecaen (1964) insist on a defective memory for words, though little proof for this is forthcoming. Luria (1966) speaks of a temporal form secondary to memory disorder, which does not respond to cueing, and a parietal form which does, a distinction which, however appealing, has not yet been substantiated.

CLINICAL DESCRIPTION

The modern approach to anomia is directed toward a (presumed) impairment in processes through which lexical entry occurs, an impairment which results in defective word finding in all modalities of object presentation, difficulty in naming to description and, usually, emptiness and circumlocution in conversational speech. In the restricted case, speech is fluent without marked disturbance of comprehension, repetition or reading. Usually the most recently learned language is first affected. Periphrasis is common, and in what seems at times to be a form of self-cueing, patients will describe the function or structure of an object rather than its name. The disorder affects substantives first, especially proper names and abstract nouns, with some relation to word-frequency, then verbs and adjectives, usually sparing prepositions and articles. Cases have been described with inability to name verbs and preservation of nouns (Heilbronner, quoted by Pitres, 1898) but this is unusual.

Ongoing speech is generally empty, vague and cliché-ridden, though in exceptional cases it may be normal (Pick, 1931). The sentence pattern is preserved, and articulation is intact. In most cases, speech is maintained by stereotypes, e.g. "probably," "rather," "you know," and strings of grammatical words with indefinite nouns, "It's a gismo for the . . . ," "One of the things in the. . . ." Word lists are affected, but are a poor indication of anomia in that they may be impaired in the presence of superior naming. In some cases, speech is so limited it actually becomes nonfluent. This is not uncommon in the acute stage, but may persist for many months. In this state, grammatical as well as content words are lost, and the picture then resembles a Broca's aphasia, a point of considerable theoretical interest.

Patients should be studied carefully for any difference in the ability

to name within or across modalities. Color naming appears particularly sensitive to posterior lesions, and when so affected appears as
a bridge to the alexias. Some patients will show a difference in their
ability to name objects and body parts. At times, body parts, both on
the patient himself and the examiner, may be named quite well,
while objects are uniformly failed. Certainly, we cannot readily accept Nielsen's (1940) explanation of selective damage to an association between temporal lobe and the occipital area concerned with
animate and inanimate object concepts. Nor is it a function of word
frequency, as has been suggested by other authors. Possibly, the combination of visual and kinesthetic information, and the fact that the
body part is, as it were, embedded in context, i.e. the body itself,
whereas the object often is presented in isolation, accounts for this
discrepancy. Further study of this phenomenon is certainly needed.

Word finding in speech often parallels the degree of improvement
with phonemic cueing. Both tend to follow the same course, since
cueing is an index of the patency of the entry mechanism. The test of
having the patient select the desired word from a group is a variation
of phonemic cueing, and in general has the same significance. This
does not hold as clearly for sentence completion. Barton *et al.* (1969)
have shown that naming to open-ended sentences, e.g. "One shaves
with a _____," is an easier task for the great majority of aphasics. Goodglass (1967) has emphasized the greater redundancy and
automatic nature of sentence completion as compared to confrontation naming, noting that a noun in a sentence context may have less
nominal quality than when standing alone. Sentence completion may
also serve rather to facilitate articulation of the word, as in the
anterior aphasic, than to help in its evocation. Further, even in cases
of so-called isolation syndrome, where the patient has primarily echolalic speech remaining (Stengel, 1947), sentence completion may be
possible. Other forms of cueing include synonyms, antonyms, category
hints, rhymes and spelling part of the word. Weisenberg has described an unusual case where words could be spelled which could
not be pronounced.

Performance may also vary considerably from one test category to
another. Thus, at times patients may produce names of objects poorly
but name actions correctly, or the reverse; or misname actions but
name those demonstrated quite well. Naming to description will depend on whether functional or descriptive terms are used, or whether
the target word is cued or implicit in any element of the description,
or to be inferred from an interpretation of all elements, each in itself

insufficient to reach a correct choice. The more limiting the task, the more likely an accurate response. Naming to rhymes given within generic groups may be well preserved. Word association tests in which only the function of a noun (e.g. sweep-broom) is given may also be done well. Analogies such as red:cherry, _____:banana may either facilitate or impair choices depending on the anomic form.

With regard to response patterns, the anomic characteristically fails to produce the word, generally without phonemic paraphasia. At times speech is greatly reduced because of consciousness of error. Most patients will be able to give a circumlocution relating to the demanded name. According to Kaplan (1970, personal communication) temporal anomics tend to simply not answer or say they do not know. Occasionally verbal paraphasia is seen, this occurring in both the temporal and the parietal form. The paraphasias respect the appropriate semantic field, and are accepted or rejected by the patient according to their closeness to the target word. It is my impression that the closer the paraphasia to the target word, the less is the awareness of error. If, however, a verbal paraphasia is represented to the patient among a set of semantically related words, he can generally select the word most appropriate to the test object. This suggests that word-meanings are intact, but that the semantic control of speech is tenuous. The occurrence of semantic paraphasia is an example of a momentary speech form which, when more constant, and less categorical, leads to Wernicke's aphasia. Kaplan's observation that the verbal paraphasias of the anomic tend to be closer to the word-concept than those of the Wernicke's aphasic, indicates that the paraphasia of the latter involves more than just logorrhea and an increase in frequency.

The localization is generally placed in T2 for the temporal form, and parietal area of dominant hemisphere, especially angular and supramarginal gyri, for the classical form, though it has been shown that frontal and diffuse lesions, pressure effects, fatigue and exhaustion can also produce an anomic state. The fact that lesions remote from the speech area can produce anomia has been a particular difficulty toward its theoretical understanding. Recent studies indicate that much of this confusion may resolve around the question of word frequency. It has been shown, for example, in normals, in dysphasics (Howes and Geschwind, 1964; Rochford and Williams, 1962) and in patients with organic dementia (Barker and Lawson, 1968) that word-finding difficulties relate very closely to the word frequency of the object or action to be named. In fact, the demonstration of anomia in many otherwise nonaphasic patients requires close attention to the word-frequency variable. With regard to the anomia of dementia, it is of interest that such patients do not initially show circumlocutory speech though naming may be impaired. Circumlocution will appear later, at which stage it cannot readily be distinguished from the accompanying memory loss. Facilitation by phonemic cueing is common, while contextual cues, rhymes and first letters are of little help. No constant correlation between the severity of memory loss and degree of anomia has been established, though in one form of dementia, progressive supranuclear palsy, where the pathology appears to spare cortex, some memory loss with word-finding difficulty commonly occurs. Concerning the word-frequency effect in the anomia of dementia, it should be noted that misnamings do not at all follow this pattern. Often patients will have difficulty with quite common words, and substitute words of very low frequency, as in "fuschia" for red, or "microscope" for glasses.

Deriving from the work on naming and word frequencies, an experiment by Wingfield (1966) is of some interest. In this study, subjects were presented first the name or the picture of an object and then a (another) picture of an object, and required to give a yes (same) or no (different) response. The finding that the reaction time for common and uncommon objects did not show a word frequency effect induced Oldfield (1966) to propose a two-stage model of naming. The first stage, perceptual identification of the object, is independent of the frequency of the object name, while the second stage, word finding, is frequency dependent. This model, which is in agreement with enlightened clinical work, suggests that modality-specific naming disorders (*q.v.*) should not show the effect of word frequency, a fact which in my experience is true.

MODALITY-SPECIFIC ANOMIAS

A second form of anomia occurs as a disturbance in the elicitation of words through one or more modalities. This form is marked by naming difficulty in restricted perceptual spheres, and heightened threshold for modality-dependent naming in the face of normal word production in conversational speech. Usually, such patients can name to functional description what cannot be named perceptually. Thus, failing to name a razor on visual or tactile presentation, they will succeed with a description of its use, i.e. "What you shave with in the morning." This points to a relatively intact lexical entry mechanism. Further, the impairment in modality naming is to some extent a matter of threshold, for there is a spectrum from inability to identify objects in one perceptual class to a mildly uneven performance across modalities. In some cases, clues to the perceived object, such as descriptive hints, rhyming words or phonemic cues, will facilitate naming though one must be careful not to circumvent the modality altogether. Other patients with involvement of one or more modalities may be able to describe the structure or use of the object which they are unable to name. Such cases indicate that the disorder does not lie with the object as "elicitor," but rather with a disturbance in the process of elicitation. This disturbance appears to affect the more specific response first, i.e. naming, and only in severe cases the general or descriptive response.

In the more severe cases, confined to one modality, there is inability to give any stimulus-related response at all. Patients will often confabulate the name of the object and will not be helped by linguistic aids if the latter provide only minimal cues. It is interesting that such patients, once having confabulated a name, will usually not accept the correct name, nor will they self-correct on exploring the object through another modality. This group of patients probably falls into the category designated by Geschwind (1965) as "disconnexion syndromes." This category, however, is only an extreme instance of what is seen in the partial case, and must be explained in a comparable manner. One feature of these cases which has been emphasized is the "two-way" naming defect. Thus, patients not only fail to name objects, but cannot point to objects on command. This has been attributed to disconnexion of the perceptual zone from speech cortex. This would suggest that a "one-way" defect, failure to name with correct pointing, if limited to one modality or one class of items, should result from interruption of the modality→language pathway leaving the reverse pathway intact. Clearly such reasoning is inadmissible. Yet it is an obligatory consequence of the two-way explanation when having to deal with intermediate disorders, viz.: impaired visual naming with good tactile or auditory naming, and good ability to point to objects on command. If we consider this problem, it is obvious that the ability to point to objects named is better in normal subjects than object naming, to the extent that word comprehension is superior to word finding. Matching a given name to one of three or four objects is less demanding than matching an object to a dictionary of names. Also, in naming only one term (the object) is given, whereas in pointing, both terms (the name and an object choice) are given, a condition which places a further disadvantage on the former test. The disparity between these two performances, characteristic of most amnesic aphasics, will be affected by obscuration of the object. This hinders naming in the anomic patient (Lotmar, 1933; Bisiach, 1966). In the perceptually disadvantaged patient it could be expected to interfere with object pointing. As the perceptual impairment becomes more limiting, the "two-way" symptomatology is achieved, though clinical observation reveals all intervening stages in this transition.

One form of modality-specific naming disorder is for colors. Some patients will show a severe defect for colors within a general anomia, and as the anomia clears, a milder color-naming defect may persist, giving the impression of a restricted color anomia. Such patients can usually produce color names fairly well on spontaneous lists, can sort and match accurately, and can indicate colors to command, but have considerable difficulty with naming to description (e.g. "the color of a banana?"). This establishes the nonperceptual nature of the disturbance. This is further brought out by the ability of patients to cue on the color name, and the occurrence of descriptive paralexias, e.g. "the Irish color" for green, "blood" for red. A difficulty with written material and proper names, which may accompany this condition, can simulate an alexia with color agnosia. This disorder is clearly related to the original anomia, however, since color names have extremely narrow relationships with the things they designate, and therefore, may be affected in an apparently selective fashion. Nevertheless, the condition can be understood as a form of the "one-way" defect discussed above, which an appropriate lesion distribution can deteriorate to the "disconnexion" picture. Other aspects of color as well as optic naming are discussed with the agnosias.

Disorders in tactile identification have been thoroughly discussed by Critchley (1953), who recounts the complexities of this problem, as well as the variety of defects which can occur. The special instance of tactile aphasia was first introduced, in a case inappropriate to its demonstration, by Raymond and Egger (1906), and was subsequently discussed critically by Dejerine (1906, 1907). Geschwind (1965) has aligned the disorder with his general callosal theory. Clearly there appears to be a wide range of physiological disturbance and a great variety of clinical forms. Impaired object identification in the hand contralateral to cerebral lesion, with minimal sensory impairment in that hand, can probably be attributed to agnosia (astereognosia) of the apperceptive type. If occurring in the left hand only, and if obvious sensory defects can be discounted through careful nonverbal testing, a callosal lesion should be considered. If the disturbance is bilateral, without significant sensory or other aphasic symptoms, and with good naming in other modalities, then it is possible to speak of tactile aphasia. All patients, however, in addition to thorough sensory examination as outlined by Critchley (1953), should be tested both verbally and nonverbally and should be given matching and cross-matching tests. Ability to describe the object or its function, draw it, demonstrate its use, or sort it categorically, should be tested. Unfortunately, insufficient case material is available to allow for a systematic classification, though it is unlikely that such a classification would differ greatly from that proposed for the visual object agnosias.

Finally, it has been shown by Spreen *et al.* (1966) and Goodglass *et al.* (1968) that sense modalities may differ in their ability to arouse concepts, a reduction of informational content within a modality lowering the level of concept arousal through that modality. Clinical evidence suggests that, in unusual cases, the lexical entry mechanism may be subject to the modality nonspecific effects which influence arousal thresholds for all modalities, leaving spontaneous evocatory processes intact. In cases of this type, with naming affected on all confrontation tests but good ongoing speech, we are evidently in a transition zone to involvement of the process of lexical entry.

DISCUSSION

In the patient with a naming disorder of the modality-specific type, naming is facilitated, in mild cases, by augmenting sensory information within a single modality or by circumventing the modality altogether. Within this group are seen patients with inability to name objects through one modality (e.g. visual) but intact pointing to command; patients with inability to name or point, but preserved matching across modalities; and patients with an anomic aphasia in which the anomic element is accentuated for one modality. There is a transition to the patient with all modalities affected and normal ongoing speech. Here, because the disorder is closer to the lexical entry stage, naming is not greatly aided by sensory (nonphonemic) cues. This disorder may have affinities with "nonaphasic" misnaming (*q.v.*). Next, there is a stage of moderately limited but fluent speech, consisting of strings of grammatical words and indefinite nouns (anomic aphasia). Phonemic cueing, and especially repetition, are able to elicit the desired word. Errors will be recognized and the correct word can be selected from a group. This gradual transition between the perceptual and the linguistic is evident on careful case study.

Within the anomic aphasias, it is possible to distinguish a variety of pathological states which are, presumably, referable to stages in normal speech production. As an indication of the stage involved, one may rely on the ability of the anomic patient to respond to such cues as the following, arranged in a tentative ascending order of efficacy for classical anomic aphasia: 1) Responsive: functional— ("It is for shaving"); descriptive—("a metal blade," etc.). 2) Embedding: ("Use a _____ for shaving"). 3) Synonyms; antonyms. 4) Rhyming: ("lazor"). 5) Spelling the word: ("r, a, z . . ."). 6) Open-ended sentences: ("one shaves with a _____"). 7) Automatic completions: ("A straight-edge _____"). 8) Phonemic cues: ("ra, raz . . ."). 9) Repetition: ("razor").

Also to be noted here is the "tip-of-the-tongue" phenomenon (Brown and McNeill, 1966). This refers to the fact that individuals who are searching for a "known" word, can often supply the initial letter or syllable length. In a series of aphasic patients, Barton (1970, personal communication) has shown that a significant number are able to supply the initial letter (62%), or syllable length (72%) of unevoked nouns, suggesting the presence of the word in some abstract form even though it cannot be articulated. It would be useful to attempt a distinction of temporal and parietal anomics on this test.

With regard to cues toward naming, at least some of these appear to have facilitatory effect in a graded, or hierarchical way. Thus, some anomics respond to sentence completion and phonemic cues, and repeat well. Those who facilitate only with phonemic cues, will also repeat at the single word level, while many patients will respond to repetition only. The anomic who neither cues nor repeats (i.e. does not cue with the whole word) is the conduction aphasic. This sequence in reverse is the characteristic pattern of recovery out of a conduction aphasia to a mild anomia, as well as the pattern of anomic deterioration. It is accompanied by verbal and then literal paraphasia. At the level of conduction aphasia, the word has "come up" farther than in the other conditions, such that deformations in the "programming" of the word now come to the fore. Substantives are no longer selectively impaired, the disorder affecting all forms. This is an intermediate step toward Broca's aphasia, where the grammatical words will be selectively blocked. This pattern, anomia, to verbal and then to literal paraphasia, is then repeated, in mirror-like fashion more anteriorly for grammatical words. There is a kind of staggered effect. The nouns which first come up are affected earlier, while rostrally, the same pathology affects the grammatical words. Thus, with anterior lesions the noun is already "fully formed," so to say, while the grammatical words are still "on the way up." One might say that the concept is to the noun (in anomia) as the noun is to its function words (Broca's aphasia). Each disorder, anomia and Broca's aphasia, is characterized by a more or less automatic production of more anterior stages, grammatical words in the anomic, and stereotypes in the Broca's aphasic. The grammatical words are accompanied by awareness, since they undergo a development in the speech system, whereas there is no awareness for the residual stereotypies of the Broca's aphasic, for these pass only through the final phase.

The selectivity for nouns in anomia has to be interpreted as indicating a noun priority in the sequence of lexical entry. Even if one discounts the act of naming as an artificial performance, the lack of nouns in ongoing speech is sufficient to support this contention. This priority, however, is only a partial explanation, for there is no obvious reason, apart from word-frequency, why abstract nouns should fall out sooner than concrete nouns, nor is the variable cueing response in different anomics readily explained. While there are some anomics who appear to have totally lost the noun, more commonly patients give definitions or functional descriptions of the needed word, and select it from a group. This indicates a certain intactness of the semantic field of the given word. Moreover, the circumlocutions arising from this field take the place of the noun itself. With defects at a more advanced level, the noun is available but its semantic base is uncertain. The relation between noun and meaning is less evident to the listener. At this stage, naming may still be intact in the presence of circumlocutory speech (semantic aphasia). Here, the "naming" situation helps to stabilize the word-meaning. This stage is also accompanied by logorrhea, reduced speech awareness and a tendency for euphoria. As the relationship between word and meaning (i.e. verbal paraphasia) becomes even more indefinite, the picture approaches Wernicke's aphasia. Anomic aphasia, therefore, leads in two directions: 1) to semantic and Wer-

nicke's aphasia, with breakdown in word-meanings and speech comprehension defect, and 2) to conduction aphasia, with preservation
of word-meanings, and an accentuation of the disturbance on the
side of speech production.

Chapter 3

SEMANTIC APHASIA

IN THE LAST SECTION we considered anomic aphasia as an impairment surrounding the process of lexical entry in which there is a relative alignment between the noun, though unrealized, and its meaning. The closeness of this alignment is seen in the circumlocutions and verbal paraphasias within sphere which characterize this form. The deeper and more general nature of this stage in language is reflected in the frequency of its impairment, and its predilection for diffuse, nonlocalizing pathology. Less common is the condition where the lexical entry process is reasonably intact, but the semantic disalignment more severe. Here, the patient names fairly well, but the relation between word and meaning is unstable. Because of this instability, and the prominence of paralogical formations, these patients are often spoken of as impaired at the "thought-speech transition." While there is much to be said for this formulation, it should be recognized that the defect appears to represent a stage in advance of that affected in anomia, i.e. midway between the anomic and Wernicke's state. A continuity seems to exist from relatively preserved logical thinking with anomia through paralogia and verbal paraphasia to Wernicke's aphasia with semantic jargon. In such a progression, paralogia appears as a disturbance within a language system, and not an impairment of language-independent cognitive mechanisms. This view has relevance for those conditions, not in the strict sense aphasic, in which paralogia is of fundamental importance, for example, schizophrenia.

The syndrome which is of first importance in any discussion of impaired word-meaning relationships is the semantic aphasia of Head (1926). This disorder, held to reflect an interruption at a prelinguistic phase in the thought-speech transition, is characterized by a want of recognition of the full significance of words and phrases apart from their verbal meaning, failure to comprehend the final aim or goal of an action, and inability to clearly formulate a general conception of what has been heard, read or seen in a picture, although many of the details can be enumerated. Memory and intelli-

31

gence are relatively intact, counting is possible, but calculations are affected, and there is a failure to understand jokes, games and puzzles.

It must be admitted that in Head's descriptions the recorded statements and short letters of his cases do not always convey to the reader the full flavor of the defect as emphasized in the commentary. These statements were, for the most part, brief two or three sentence responses, or extracts from written samples that do not readily gain the reader's confidence. Nor did many of the tests which Head employed clearly illustrate the specific nature of the disorder, consisting as they did of right-left orientation, picture interpretation, clock-setting and free drawing, all of which, especially at the level of severity as in Head's cases, would now be included in the testing battery for spatioconstructive rather than aphasic disorders. Yet in spite of these deficiencies, there has remained, at least on the theoretical grounds, a strong attraction about this disorder, concerning as it does one of the central issues in aphasia theory, the relation of speech to thought. Though Head never postulated explicitly a continuity between the semantic and the syntactical functions, he has often been interpreted in this way, and indeed, his classification implies such a progression. Moreover, most of his cases of semantic aphasia demonstrated some grammatical disturbance.

Thus, Head's (1926) Case #5, for example, wrote:

Just a few lines to let you know that I am getting on all right and I shall will be home again. I must tell you that Uncle George and Aunt Ann cane (came) and see me yesterday and more so Bob Higgins so I am very Lucky for getting friends.

On another occasion, this patient remarked, "I was worked for. . . ." Case #8 wrote, ". . . one could spend one's time in a more profitably . . . ," and case #18 said, "If I pay too much attention I get wrong with what I've got to do." Case #24 said, "My son is just home from Ireland. He is a flying man. Takes the ship about to carry the police, to give information, to carry the letters of the police."

Between Head's semantic and his syntactical (or Wernicke's) aphasia, lie processes which have scarcely been alluded to in the neurological literature. Of the few workers who have concerned themselves with these processes, Pick's (1931) account is perhaps the best known. For him, aphasic disorders began at the thought-speech interface, where grammatical rules governing the structure of the sentence first came into play. Upon application of these rules, the developing sentence pattern first receives meaning-laden words, then the small (form) words, and then it undergoes "grammatization" of the content words. The accentuation pattern of the sentence appears even before the sentence pattern itself, determining whether a question, a command etc., will be produced. The sentence pattern is decisive in determining the order of words, while the process of grammatization is applied to the words themselves as they come up. A disorder at this deep level, at a stage close to that of word choice, produces the condition of paragrammatism. Pick argued that this disorder would involve both thought and speech formulation, and for this reason considered that it might arise from conditions not directly involving the speech field, or secondary to disorders affecting other levels of the thought-speech transition. For example, an impaired verbal memory might derange the syntactical structure, since a word substituted for the correct one may have a damaging effect on the sentence construction. In the primary case, at any rate, the pathology would involve that stage of the thought-speech transition where grammatization matches what is to be said to the sentence pattern. Pick also pointed out that at this level other relationships come into play; relationships between thoughts themselves, relationships to the task at hand and to other current tasks, and relationships of speaker to content. If these are impaired, there is loss in unity and control, i.e. the "thread" of the thought is lost.

PARAGRAMMATISM

This was originally described by Pick (1913) as an "expressive form of sensory agrammatism" in contrast to the motor form, i.e. telegrammatism or agrammatism. Later renamed by Kleist, it is characterized by fluent logorrheic speech, disturbances in grammatical usage, and some awareness of errors. These errors, in both speech and writing, consist of impaired use of auxiliary words, tenses and articles, and confusion of pronouns. In some languages other than English, there is confusion in the use of formal and familiar pronouns. In addition, prefixes and suffixes are mistakenly employed, and word inflections are either dropped or used in an abnormal way. The overall sentence pattern and intonation are usually intact, and patients may be able to distinguish between grammatical and ungrammatical sentences, though unable to put the sentence into correct grammatical form. This discrepancy is explained as due to defective "feeling for speech" (Sprachgefuhl), which is insufficient to guide spontaneous speaking but can be evoked in speech perception. The disorder is closely related to amnesic aphasia and paraphasia, and when associated with these to a severe degree, results in an unintelligible semantic jargon. Localization is in T2 and T3 of dominant hemisphere. Further, Pick noted that paragrammatism induced by left-sided lesions reappears or is intensified by secondary lesions in right hemisphere. In regard to localization, Kleist (1934; 1962) placed the pathology in posterior T1.

Paragrammatism was also the subject of a scholarly analysis by Isserlin (1936). This author accepted Pick's formulation, adding that the sentence pattern may occasionally be impaired for complex sentences, that the sentence melody may often be exaggerated and unnatural, and that younger patients tend to be more word impoverished, older patients more paraphasic. His localization was posterior superior left temporal convolution. Isserlin emphasized that although the condition is close to thought mechanisms, a primary thought disorder is not present. At times there may be defects in the expression of meaning, which suggest a thinking disorder, but these can arise from uncertainty over the utterance and erroneous and circumlocutory productions. The basis of the syndrome lies in the realm of the "acoustic-mnemic (sensory) sphere." This relates to the digressions in speaking, the paraphasia and the word-finding difficulty. But, Isserlin insists, paragrammatism is *not* the result of a normal sentence that is deformed by paraphasic errors. The defect lies at the level of the grammatical organization of the sentence prior to word selection.

SENSORY AGRAMMATISM

Along with these disturbances in expressive language, there are, as in all aphasic states, matching levels of impairment in the comprehension of spoken speech. These "receptive" defects have not been studied to a great extent, for the obvious reason that they merge imperceptibly with cognitive or aphasic speech disturbances, and are therefore, not readily separable from the latter in the test situation. One such disturbance, however, which was described in the earlier literature and which to a greater or lesser extent accompanies the picture of "expressive" paragrammatism, is that of sensory or impressive agrammatism.

According to Pick (1931), this has to do with stages in the understanding of a sentence which correspond to stages in its grammatization, and affects the relationships between words in the sentence. It appears mainly in mistaken subject-object relationships, but relationships between sentences or terms, as in puns, jokes, syllogisms and formulae may also be defective, and there is poor performance on proverb interpretation. In addition, the patient exhibits difficulty in following the line of thought, diminished retention and a constriction of the attention over all elements in the sentence. For Pick the problem referred to disordered combination of acoustic sequences heard into a single whole, and contrasted with the preserved ability, noted in other patients, to combine the sense of the sentence on the basis of partially understood words. The pathology was thought to be in central and posterior T1. This formulation was accepted by Salomon (1914), and Isserlin (1936), who emphasized the normal understanding at a simple level, and the difficulty in distinguishing between correct and incorrect grammatical sentences as the principle feature of the disorder.

There are, in addition to the above, other tests that can be used to bring out this deficit. Goodglass has shown the value of genitive constructions such as "my brother's sister"; passive and active voice, on command (e.g. "with A touch B"), or single word response (e.g. "Bob was hit by John. Who was hit?"). Patients may fail on tests of grammatical and directional prepositions (Goodglass); they may have difficulty following a rapid conversation, or sudden shifts in the subject. There may be difficulty with English spoken in a foreign accent. To some extent, this syndrome may be said to constitute the minimal speech comprehension deficit, for Broca's aphasics will also fail on many of these tests, and patients with dementia also do poorly.

SEMANTIC JARGON

When paragrammatism combines with verbal paraphasia, or when the verbal substitution alone is very marked, the patient is said to have semantic jargon. According to Alajouanine *et al.* (1952), the picture is one of verbal paraphasia linked by subtle categorical or conceptual bonds to the correct words, with similar disturbances in comprehension. An example of such jargon is the patient of Alajouanine who, asked to define the word fork, said: "Ah, fork, that's the need for a schedule." The disorder is held to lie at a deeper level than Wernicke's aphasia for patients may recover to a Wernicke's stage. It is postulated to result from damage, at the thought-speech transition, to mechanisms through which the semantic value of language is derived.

Cases similar to those of the French workers were reported by
Kinsbourne and Warrington (1963). One of their patients, asked to
explain the proverb: Strike while the iron is hot, said: "Ambition is
very very and determined. Better to be good and to Post Office and
to Pillar Box and to distribution and to mail and survey and head-
master. . . ." Here the verbal paraphasia is quite marked and even
in this brief sample one can see how the discourse is derailed by word
substitutions. The disturbance in speech, however, need not be so
severe. A case of Cohn and Neumann (1958, #3) responded to a question concerning his daily activity with: "We work on the dairy
farm and my younger sister going to school so I try to be up early,
along accordingly. So that we have more than enough to rush or
anything like that." Isserlin (1936) quotes a patient of Heilbronner
as saying, to a question about his health: "Yes, I think that I am now
so safe, that I now much with others, to some extent directly." A patient of Weinstein *et al.* (1966), asked the name of the hospital, replied: "Uh . . . patients or etimology, one of the two, I'm not sure, sir.
I've been in part where you had the majority of them on the floor and
some of them were not." A similar picture is also seen in confusional
states. A case of Clarke *et al.* (1958) with Korsakoff syndrome responded to the proverb: Safety first, with "It's rather a lateral term
which means it could apply to a host of things. A road for one thing."
These authors point out the similarity to jargonaphasia and quote
Kleist (1934) in accounting for the disorder as a confabulation within the language sphere (paralogia) at the origins of the thought-
speech transition. The occurrence of jargon in confusional states is
well known, but deserves still closer attention. A patient of Pick in a
manic state said, "I had been deathly bronchial catarrh." Another
patient showing paragrammatism in Czech and German said, "I want
to wish you and is they have locked me in." A personal case in
delirium tremens, read the line: The barn swallow captured the
plump worm, as: "A barn swallow charged the plumber six dollars
and work eight millions dollars." This subject is also discussed in the
next chapter.

SCHIZOPHRENIC SPEECH

Similar disturbances have also been described in schizophrenic
patients. Kleist (1914) noted the similarity of aphasic and schizophrenic paraphasia, and suggested the term paralogia. More recently,
Domarus (1964) has defined paralogical thinking as being of the
form: "Certain Indians are swift. Stags are swift. Therefore, certain

Indians are stags." This difficulty in the isolation of a specific item in a phrase, or the isolation of a common element in a set of two phrases, has been discussed also by Kasanin (1964), who commented on the ". . . inability to abstract one principle of the given material while (the patient) neglects the others. He takes all the possibilities into simultaneous consideration. . . ." Examples from Cameron (1964), such as "A boy threw a stone at me to make an understanding between myself and the purpose of wrong doing," are very similar to the aphasic disorder under consideration.

Arieti (1948, 1955) accepted the principle of von Domarus, and summarized the schizophrenic language disorder as caused by an identification based upon an identity of predicates, not as in the normal person, an identity of subjects. This predicative fusion is the basis for word-association responses, but is uncharacteristic of normal speech. " (In schizophrenia) each fragment of a context is equivalent to any other fragment or to the whole. What in a normal person is only an associative link, becomes in the schizophrenic an identifying link." There is also a shift in word use from connotation to denotation, i.e. from contextual to referential meaning, which may lead to extreme concreteness in response. With severe regression, word-salad appears, e.g. "The house burnt the cow horrendendously always," which is only an extreme example of associative bonding. Arieti suggested that in the regressed schizophrenic, comprehension of spoken language takes place in only a very approximate way. Regarding self-awareness, Arieti speculated that the patient has only ". . . a vague idea of what he wants to say, but he cannot focus very well, cannot isolate concepts."

In a similar vein, Goldstein (1943) discussed the similarity between schizophrenic and organic regression, and attempted to draw both conditions together as defects in the abstract attitude, although in the organic case the disintegration leads to "a more simplified and inane form." Several examples were given of word misuse in schizophrenia, e.g. "the song" for a bird, "kiss" for mouth, in which the obvious predicative nature of the misnaming suggests a relation with other organic states, i.e. with semantic aphasia and semantic jargon. Schilder was particularly interested in this problem (Schilder and Sugar, 1926; Curran and Schilder, 1935), and concluded that ". . . a slight sensory aphasia due to a particular lesion of the brain can lead to speech disturbances, in which the stilting of expressions, mannerisms and perseverations play the outstanding parts. Instead of the full-blown paraphasia (there is) the use of unusual words which may lead to unusual thoughts." Schilder believed there was an inner relationship between the two disorders, which pointed to the possibility of an "organic nucleus" for schizophrenic speech disturbances. In this connection, it is worth noting that the "word-salad" seen in some schizophrenics is not easily differentiated from certain cases of jargonaphasia. The possibility exists that paralogia and word salad, given the personality of the schizophrenic, bear the same inner relationship as semantic aphasia and semantic jargon (see Critchley, 1964 and Alajouanine, 1968). In this respect it would be of interest to establish speech perceptual norms in the psychiatric groups.

SLEEP SPEECH AND APHASIA

There are scattered references in the literature to the occasional aphasic nature of utterances which occur during the sleep of normal subjects. Kraepelin (1910) and Curran and Schilder (1935) have made observations of this kind. Arkin (1967) has described some of the qualitative features of sleep-speech, noting the variability in both length and clarity of utterances, and the tendency for syntax and inflection to be preserved in REMP, and defective in NREM speech. In a recent study (Arkin and Brown, 1971), defective sleep utterances have been shown to bear a striking correspondence to certain of the above-discussed forms of aphasia. The following categories were observed:

1. *Phonemic (literal) paraphasia.*
   "David, I day (?say) David . . . that's you that day dated day dravid Dave dravid about 25 or 30 noked naked day dreams."
   ". . . sneak to go, reek you reek to, steak, stoke . . . to find some theft."
2. *Semantic (verbal) paraphasia*
   ". . . very funny fishes, flashes . . . funny red, yellow and bigger and yellow."
   ". . . six books (?blocks) home."
3. *Neologistic paraphasia*
   "Gundrum is the word for hundred."
   ". . . it goes drench more about Ronnie."
4. *Semantic jargon*
   ". . . you kept bouncing them on and on as if you had a regular meter . . . as if you had a regular dream . . . as if you were continuing on to the next paragraph."
5. *Mixed jargon*
   ". . . she shad hero sher, sher sheril shaw (spelled) takes part, loses but lost, invincible is you as usual."

In addition, paragrammatic errors were noted, as in ". . . the most respect and . . . revered of all the ladies," or ". . . it might break is the only one." There was frequent use of cliché expressions, as "I don't know," "I mean . . ." etc., although "emptiness" of speech was not seen, and vocabulary did not appear to be reduced. Phonemic paraphasias were notable for the attempts at self-correction, though the propagatory nature of the paraphasia, and the frequent clang associations were more prominent than is usually seen in aphasic states. Self-correction was less common for sleep-speech showing the characteristics of semantic paraphasia and semantic jargon, similar to what is observed in the corresponding aphasic conditions. Word-stress, prosodic values and the affective quality of speech were not markedly defective. Speech disturbances were more common during NREM than REMP sleep. No clear relation of "aphasic" type to stage of sleep was observed, though recall appeared better at Stage 2 than Stages 3 or 4. Though it is possible to communicate with sleep-talking subjects, it has not been etablished whether disorders of speech comprehension accompany the above-described forms. However, Berger (1963) has described the modification of dream content by verbal stimuli (names), in the direction of assonantal or clang associations (Robert-"rabbit"). The responses of his subjects bear a resemblance to those of aphasics with speech comprehension disorders.

Also to be mentioned in this regard are studies of transitional phenomena. Schjelderup-Ebbe (in Mintz, 1948) recorded some of his own utterances on falling asleep, which bear a resemblance to aphasic speech, viz., "He is good as cake double," "Conceit is not often being named a phantabilit," and "The pencil holds well. To the sidewalk with Tell too." Froeschels (1946) gave some interesting samples of speech in the hypnagogic state, and compared these to the speech of aphasia and schizophrenia, viz., nonsensical utterances ("amarande es tifiercia"), semantic jargon ("They are exposed to verbally inter-lection"), and paraphasias ("One is hol stitched chin lengthened against the other"). Froeschels also (1953) demonstrated that in transitional fragments where analysis of the meaning is possible, the major factor at work was the fusion of two separate thoughts based on a category of similarity. The thoughts were identified in the fusion according to a single shared attribute. This would seem to correspond quite well with the definition of paralogia given above.

NONAPHASIC MISNAMING

Weinstein and co-workers (1964) have described a disorder of naming, distinct from anomic aphasia, which occurs in certain patients in the presence of diffuse disease, drowsiness or confusion. The picture is that of failure on naming simple objects, often with success on difficult names, and selective difficulty for illness-related stimuli. Thus, patients may name everyday objects correctly, but misname such objects as a thermometer or medicine dropper. Paraphasic responses have a pretentious, jocular quality, as in a patient who called a syringe a "hydrometer to measure fluids," or one who referred to doctors as "butchers," and the hospital as a "butcher shop," in an elaboration on the doctor's white coat. The term "ludic" which is applied to this speech behavior has affinities, as Geschwind (1967) has pointed out, with the classical moria or Witzelsucht. Geschwind has also commented that in contrast to aphasic anomia, patients with "nonaphasic misnaming" generally have normal spontaneous speech, and that the condition is associated with bilateral involvements of the nervous system, as in post-traumatic cases, toxic or acute encephalopathic states, increased intracranial pressure, etc. In some patients, there may be a relation to anosognosia and/or a Korsakoff syndrome with confabulatory tendencies.

There are several problems with the description of this syndrome which need clarification. Firstly, the misnaming of hospital or illness-related material has not been adequately differentiated from a deficit in recent memory, of which the patient's illness would form the major part. Secondly, the word-frequency effect of objects in a medical surrounding has not been taken into thorough consideration. Finally, the fact that a patient demonstrates ludic behavior with the physician may not reflect a specific denial, but rather may indicate that it is the interview situation, not the illness *per se,* that determines which material will be denied. Thus, the patient who describes a recent football game in careful detail and confabulates when questioned on his surgery, might show the reverse tendency if interviewed in a gymnasium.

With regard to the interpretation of this disorder, Weinstein and Keller (1964) have stressed the motivational aspect and have tried to align the syndrome with symbolic factors related to denial of illness. Moreover, Weinstein has discussed the anosognosic component in nonaphasic misnaming in relation to certain of the jargonaphasias to illustrate the importance of denial as a factor in the appearance of jargon. However, this very relationship argues against Weinstein's conclusion. The bulk of evidence suggests rather that nonaphasic misnaming is a form of aphasia, linked to the semantic or jargon aphasias. This is evident in the reduced speech awareness, the euphoric tendency and the heightened impulse to speak. The misnaming reflects a loosening of the semantic constraints which determine proper discourse, whereas the denial is an epiphenomenon of this aphasic level rather than its central point. The "paralogical" naming disturbance without anomic or circumlocutory features in spontaneous speech sets this disorder slightly apart from semantic aphasia. Both conditions appear to represent defects transitional between classical anomia and Wernicke's aphasia, one affecting primarily expository, the other referential speech, and both indicative of mechanisms operant at this level. Further, the syndrome points again to the existence of an inner relationship between the semantic aphasia on the one hand and the Korsakoff syndrome on the other. Certainly, the anosognosia and confabulation of the latter are often confined to verbal material, and the boundaries between confabulation of a verbal concept (Korsakoff syndrome) and verbal paraphasia are by no means clear.

These instances of disturbance at a level intermediate between anomia and Wernicke's aphasia, and the companion defects in speech understanding, appear to be interrelated in some subtle fashion, though the exact mechanisms which come into play are not known. The problem has been touched on by Hecaen and Angelergues (1965) who, under the term dyslogia (after Seglas), attempted to bring together the language disorders of dements and psychotics, with the semantic aphasia of Head. One of the problems with this interpretation has been the seemingly disparate nature of these different states. But we must recall from the introductory discussion that one inference from the hierarchical approach is that disorders at a deeper level should concern more of the patients premorbid personality. This fact is of help in understanding the interrelationships between these conditions. The dream or transitional state is an accomplishment of imaginal mechanisms which have not achieved the full differentiation of waking speech and perception; the aphasic condition is characterized by a pathological limitation of this process of differentiation in an otherwise normal personality; the schizophrenic, a less tangible organic state, but a personality acquired through a biased nervous system in which normality represents the unachieved goal; and the dement, a broad deterioration affecting many systems. At this level of pathology, therefore, it is more important to delineate some of the rules which govern symptomatology, than to simply describe the symptoms. For this purpose, the aphasic represents the most satisfactory case study.

Case 1

A thirty-year-old left-handed man was admitted to the Aphasia Unit in December, 1969 for evaluation. Two years previously he was in an automobile accident, suffering a fracture of the right temporal bone, resultant acute subdural hematoma and coma. At craniotomy, the hematoma was evacuated and the *right* temporal lobe noted to be lacerated. Following surgery, he was described as having difficulty in word finding, and also some impairment of comprehension. Over the following months, there was gradual and complete recovery, to the point where he could return to work. A plate was put over the right temporal defect one year later, and he remained in excellent health until November, 1969, when he had another automobile accident, this time with *left* temporal injury. He was unconscious for a day or so, and on arousing was said to be markedly aphasic with "unintelligible speech" consisting of well-articulated speech sounds but no comprehensible words, and severe impairment of speech understanding. The description is consistent with a jargon-type aphasia. Because of this, a bilateral carotid angiogram was performed, demonstrating a large left subdural hematoma. This was evacuated through left temporal burr hole, with rapid improvement in speech following surgery. He was seen for the first time in aphasia evaluation in December, 1969, from which point his condition remained relatively stable.

The patient was a high school graduate, left-handed, with no family history of sinistrality. He had worked as a highly-skilled mechanic for jet engines. Neurological testing was normal, apart from the evidence of previous craniotomy and trephination. Examination revealed excellent remote and recent memory. WAIS verbal IQ was 93, performance IQ 84. Performance was in the 75th percentile on Ravens matrices. Verbal memory and verbal learning were fairly good; digit span was 5–6 forward, 3–4 reversed.

Conversational speech was fluent, with some verbal paraphasia, circumlocution and an excess of stereotypic filler words and clichés (see examples). Inflection and articulation were normal, but sentence intonation was somewhat disorganized. There were no literal paraphasias. There was a tendency toward pedantic and pretentious forms, some euphoria, and frequent self-repetition without correction of errors. Series speech and singing were normal.

Naming was extremely well preserved, for objects, pictures, body parts, and colors, even for very low-frequency items. Visual, tactile and auditory naming were intact, as was naming for attributive and functional descriptions, word associations and analogies (e.g. houses/people = nests/_____). Word lists were normal. He supplied the names of fifteen cars in thirty seconds, including, indeed emphasizing, the most obscure models. Similarly, he provided fourteen animal names in thirty seconds, listing mainly the most exotic and little-known forms. Naming actions performed before him was good, though some difficulty occurred in action-picture naming.

Repetition and reproduction of tapped or spoken rhythms was entirely normal.

Comprehension was excellent for yes/no questions, pointing to objects and body parts, object series to five items, and pointing to objects described. He was able to perform perfectly on a directional preposition test* in which he was required to match pictures to twenty-four sentences such as "Show me the girl (above, behind, against, etc.) the car," as well as on a test of grammatical prepositions, as in "Be home (in/by) lunchtime." Possessives were done well. He was able to determine which of a group of sentences presented him was grammatical. Sentences containing constructions such as, "Do you put your shoes on before your socks?" and "Do you have lunch after supper?" were done well. He could understand the elements of formulae. Identification of sounds such as tearing paper and pouring water was flawless, and musical recognition was intact. In contrast to these performances, he did show some evidence of impaired comprehension. At times, he would make no response to the simplest question or command, as if he did not hear it at all. This proved to be mainly a problem of set, for once grasping the trend of the questioning, he had no difficulty. In addition, he occasionally showed a questioning repetition of the examiner's questions or commands, always, however, substituting the appropriate pronoun. There was considerable difficulty with more complex material; a simple syllogism such as, "Mary is a girl/All girls are pretty/Therefore, Mary is _____," was interpreted as, "Well, Mary must be the

*Courtesy of Dr. H. Goodglass.

prettiest. . . ." His response to a story read to him was piecemeal and vague, much as in the sample of reading comprehension. There was also some difficulty with active/passive transformations, and with genitive constructions. It is of interest that he complained of difficulty in understanding rapid speech, or English spoken with a foreign accent. This also emphasizes the moderate recognition of the comprehension defect in the face of anosognosia for speech production.

Spelling and comprehension of words spelled was good. *Reading* aloud was excellent; he could match written names to spoken words or objects, and carry out written commands quite well. Comprehension of more complex written material such as a story or multiple choice sentence completion tests showed vagueness and error respectively, increasing with the complexity of the task. With the story test, however (see sample), it was not possible to clearly separate the reading and the expressive components.

Writing was normal as to form and spelling. In longer samples (*quod vide*), defects similar to those of spoken speech were seen. He was unable to correct his grammatical errors on reviewing his writing some weeks after. When given a written story with many grammatical mistakes, he corrected most of the errors but in the process of correction, added his own.

Calculations were done well mentally and on paper. *Drawing*, three-dimensional constructive tasks, map-drawing and clock setting were excellent. He was able to draw complex plans to scale. *Praxis* was normal. He was able to play tic-tac-toe and put together rapidly a jigsaw puzzle, but had difficulty with simple card games such as black jack. Performance on a mechanical aptitude test was poor, and there was difficulty in learning complex motor activities such as running a movie projector. There was also some impairment in playing the guitar, with which he was quite proficient prior to injury. This concerned his inability to make the proper chords or play the desired melody. However, there was no receptive or expressive amusia.

A Wada Test at the time of left carotid arteriography produced right hemiparesis and marked increase in verbal paraphasia after titration of 35 mg sodium amytal. This test was interpreted as showing significant left-sided representation, which would go along with the history of aphasia following left temporal lobe damage. Presumably, the right hemisphere has some speech function in this patient, as mild aphasia followed right temporal injury in the initial episode of trauma. A brain scan revealed uptake over both temporal regions superficially, secondary to contusion and surgery.

In summary, a thirty-year-old man, left-handed, with bilateral temporal lobe damage from subdural hematomas and contusion, and residual language difficulty. There was logorrhea, circumlocution, some verbal paraphasia and paragrammatism. Comprehension was mildly impaired for complex tests only, reading was excellent, though reading comprehension and writing were impaired at a level comparable to auditory comprehension and speech. Spelling, calculations, praxis and constructional performances were unaffected.

Example 1

The following is a written description of speech difficulty:*

The speech Problem with me honestly can *some* what be a complete Problem but cannot Be easily Discovered.

Speech that could be found as a Type of speed I believe. *I* (the) possible mood of my own *maybe because* (Possibly be) of misunderstanding.

Possibly because of my own thought In a certain way. a friend of mine told myself. I had a "cast Iron Fact" *especially* during a conversation.

Also the Loss of a Vocabulary and a grammar in its conversation or speech, also possibly the subject causing excitement may also damage grammar and speech, meaning the subject causing my *own* Excitement.

Example 2 (Written)

Life of England

I arrived in England 28 Sept 1957 landing by Air in R.A.F. Burtonwood.

Burtonwoods Station was Based in the town of Warrington in the County of Lancaster Which is rather close to the Well known Liverpool town.

There are certain incidence which unfolded from my last living time in England Therefore I would rather not Inform people of the last month of my Last England Life.

My Station was stationed in the R.A.F. Sculthorpe a damned cold Bleak station, rather crude in Barracks, Hanger, Flight shacks, Lord knows what about as now its deactivated.

R.A.F. Sculthorpe was station in the County of Norfolk. Approximately 135 North East from London. 135 meaning in miles, approximately.

Italicized words are those crossed out two weeks later on rereading sample. The words in parentheses are those inserted at that time. The punctuation, spelling and capitals are those of the patient. The capitalized words tend to correspond to those given emphasis in the writing, and illustrate the defect in sentence intonation and word stress.

In the first night, in the time around about 11:30–12:00 midnight, At our first Arrival to Sculthorpe, we went to the Dining Hall.

After about 20–30 minutes we all walked in to "Chow Hall" There was a riot. the reason Being on the riot, I would not rather not discuss. There were only one Enlisted men "chow hall" After the riot—Hall, one Hall was shutdown for approximately as I remember, 4–6 months oh Gee What a Gazoo party we had after that mess

Sculthorpe was the largest Base in Europe, quite a many a man Liked to starve, I swear they even Issued Coffins, for mess kit repair squadron after a short while. This first sentence is only a Joke really.

Fights and riots did a rather good Job in such as designation on a friday night, as usual, we had a good "war". at this situation, we lost all heat, this was in the month of, I Believe in December, the Window froze inside in each room. every one had to go to bed in Heavy scale clothing for both drunk & sober at that time, one particular fellow came in Barracks dead drunk, unknown of no heating in Barracks. He rolled in a 55 gallon drum, known popularly as garbage can, into in barracks emptying most of refuse, tore his door apart in his room, Broke up the Pieces of the door, contain the pieces in the Can & lit them off for a ridiculous reason for heat. He lit off door to Fire which had been painted but the smell & remaining trash at approximately 2:00–3:00 turned the Barracks unstandable.

Example 3

The patient was given the following written story (from Talland, 1965).

Story:

A cowboy went to San Francisco with his dog which he left at a friend's while he went to buy a new suit of clothes. Dressed in his brand new suit of clothes, he came back to the dog, called it by name and patted it. But the dog would have nothing to do with him in his brand new coat and hat and gave a mournful howl. Coaxing was of no avail, so the cowboy went away and put on his old suit, and the dog immediately showed its wild joy on seeing its master as it thought he ought to be.

Patient's Interpretation (spoken, from tape):

As far as a dog which left at a friends, well now this is, this possibly, this possible, this is possibly, this could possibly be a situation so we'll just kind of override that. Basically, I've had dogs, quite a few dogs actually but just because of the owner comes up to the dog after a brand new set of clothes, it doesn't say the exact age of the dog. Now if it was an older dog usually they can pretty well identify by they can smell the owner of the dog. Of course, this is quite obvious as to why, but if it was just a young puppy, no that of course they have, they have to get something in the way of knowledge, just like a human being. So that basically is the only, of course there are, you know, well anyway they're supposed to be. . . .

Comment: Both speech and writing show similar and about equally severe deficits. The general sentence pattern is normal, and word order is fairly well preserved. The defect in grammatization is quite striking. Even in the title of the written sample, the preposition is inaccurate, and in the first sentence the last *in* seems to be a perseverative substitute for *at.* Tense is applied mistakenly as in, "There are certain incidence," and "There were only one," or the tense is dropped as in "was station (ed)." Pronoun usage is also disturbed, as in such written sentences as, "I possible mood of my own maybe because of misunderstanding," and "a friend of mine told myself." Articles are usually normal, but occasionally they are dropped, substituted or reduplicated, as in "into in Barracks" for "into the Barracks," and "He lit off door" for "He lit the door." There are abnormal constructions which defy exact analysis, such as (written) ". . . unknown of no heating in Barracks," presumably a substitution for "unaware" or "not knowing" that there was no heat in the Barracks. The capital letters in the written sample probably correspond to words emphasized during the writing, for on other occasions, when he was asked to write in the examiner's presence, the capitals tended to show this correspondence. This illustrates the abnormal pattern of word emphasis and intonation, stressing inappropriate words at abnormal moments in the sentence, and at times dropping capitals on words that should ordinarily be capitalized. (A review of some of his letters written prior to the head injuries showed no abnormalities.)

In spite of the errors, it is generally possible to follow the meaning of the utterance. Thus, in the story interpretation, each component of the story is treated in proper sequence, the dog, the friend, the new clothes, the failure of identification and the relation of smell, but a synthetic narrative is not achieved. To further evaluate story interpretation, he was asked to produce a series of illustrative drawings depicting only the *essential* elements in the story. The written cowboy story was left in his possession over a few weeks and he produced three drawings, each descriptive of a major episode. However, the drawings were definitely abnormal, and comparable in some respects to his verbal interpretations. Representative of this performance is Figure 2.

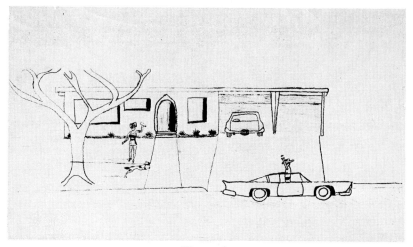

Figure 2.

In this drawing, which is typical of the three, the patient has shown the critical point, the cowboy's departure, but has substituted the cowboy's wife for his friend, and a car for a horse. There is considerable attention to detail. The plants, the license plate, the paper in the woman's hand, the whole background in fact, all inessential to the drawing, are depicted in spite of repeated admonitions to leave out all but the barest necessities. In spite of a tangential and exaggerated style, in all of the drawings the content to be communicated is retained. Shown each of the drawings immediately, and a few weeks after completion, and asked to cross out all but those items essential to conveying the sense of the story to an uninformed viewer, he was unable to eliminate any item, and in fact, pointed out the deficiencies in the drawing, the incompleteness of the house, the poverty of trees and so on. The lack of self-correction in drawing compares with the failure to correct written or spoken speech, and as in speech, correction is not for what is produced, but for the incompleteness of the account. Following this test, he was given the T.A.T., and demonstrated similar, though less severe, defects in interpretation. Also, shown a series of 7–9 cards, each picturing a stage in a simple action (e.g. the blossoming of a tree and the gradual ripening of fruit), he was able to arrange the cards in proper sequence. If two separate action sequences were incorporated in one set of pictures, he was able to arrange the cards to fit one sequence only.

In other tests he was given indicative forms of a verb in a simple sentence (such as, "The boy rides the bike") and asked to adjust the sentence to past, present, and future tenses. This was performed well. He was also able to match the pronoun appropriate to first, second and third person singular of the indicative form, as well as match singular and plural pronouns to appropriate singular or plural verbs. He could construct simple sentences in both declarative and interrogative form out of a set of randomly arranged constituent words but had difficulty with sentences of greater length or complexity, particularly if the sentence required the assimilation of two separate terms, e.g. "tigers cat in lions the family and are." Proverb interpretation revealed difficulty with the multiple elements of a standard proverb, though one item of the proverb could be interpreted fairly well, i.e. partial abstraction of one term, but failure with the whole proverb. Interpretation of idioms and metaphors was correct.

Cloze Test

In this test, the patient was given a set of passages with words of various categories deleted and was asked to supply the required word. The following sample is representative of his performance.

I LIVE IN THE COUNTRY   and   MY HOBBY IS MY GARDEN.   I   HAVE COLLECTED ALMOST   all   DIFFERENT KINDS OF PLANTS. ON SATURDAY MORNINGS   it   IS MY DUTY TO LOOK   at   MY BABY BROTHER JOE. I USUALLY PLACE THE YOUNGSTER ON A BLANKET IN THE   bedroom   OF THE HOUSE. WHILE JOE   works   I WORK IN MY GARDEN. TODAY I AM SO   busy   THAT I FORGET   to   KEEP AN EYE ON JOE. I HEAR SOME LOUD YELLS WHICH REMIND ME   what   I WAS SUPPOSED TO BE DOING. THE BABY   was   SOMETHING THAT HE HAD   been   DONE BEFORE. HE HAD CRAWLED INTO THE GARDEN AND   put   HIS ARMS ON SHARP BRANCHES OF A BUSH. JOE WAS MORE FRIGHTENED   and   HURT. SO I   kissed   JOE'S FEARS AND HELD HIM   on   MY LAP.

It is apparent that many of the insertions are inadequate to the context of the phrase, even though a match is often achieved with the preceding or succeeding segment.

Word-Concept Test

The Kaplan-Werner (1952) test of concept formation was administered by Dr. Edith Kaplan. In this test, the patient is required to build up a concept of a nonsense word through a series of phrases which contain the word in different usages. The sentences are presented successively on cards, and aloud, the cards remaining in the order of presentation in front of the patient, while the examiner moves on to the next phrase. Ten series of nonsense words were used. The patient's performance on this test was so unusual and so informative that a sample of one of the shorter responses is reproduced, the circumlocutions having been deleted.

1. A corplum may be used for support: "a type of . . . a tool (Now make it fit in the sentence. A tool may be used for support. Is that ok?) yes, in my definitive version of it."

2. A corplum may be used to close off an open place: "Well, that would be moreso . . . as a gate, a gate would be used to close off (How does that fit in the first sentence?) Well, for one thing . . . the word corplum, I've never seen the word before . . . It could be considered as a tool even as a gate because it's usable. Anything that you use can be considered as a tool. (So what would you substitute for corplum here?) You could say for support . . . you could use it as . . . a sawhorse. (Does that fit here?) a gate . . . a gate may be used to close off again (How does that fit?) It could be . . . used as such, it would be. As to support for holding up a sign . . . such that you can't go in the open place anymore."

3. A corplum may be long or short, thick or thin, strong or weak; "Sure . . . it can be so in such as in a sawhorse."

4. A wet corplum does not burn: "If you have a sawhorse that's made of aluminum, it wouldn't burn."

5. You can make a corplum smooth with sandpaper: "That's, I'm using the one I was using previously. Well, if I'm considering it as being a sawhorse, you understand that? Well, for one thing, if your sawhorse of which there are many, they are made of just plain pine, so of course being of pine, it's very easily."

6. The painter used a corplum to mix his paints: "If you use it and set it on top of the sawhorse, so he wouldn't have to reach down sort of a bend down so to speak, is not to mention mix his paint, well, you use the . . . paint barrel or paint bucket, whatever it may be, put it up on side on top of a corplum."

The patient's method of analysis on all sets is identical. There is a stabilization of one possible interpretation (e.g. sawhorse) and an adjustment of successive contexts to fit the initial interpretation (e.g. a sawhorse of aluminum not burning). Flexibility is limited to either the noun concept or more often, the changing contexts, but in no instance are both assimilated. Clearly what is required is comparable to that in the cloze test, the fixation of one term (e.g. the noun concept) so as to match two or more attributes, or contexts.

Discussion

There are some inferences that we may draw from this case. Firstly, there is evidence from the defect in drawing that the basic disturbance goes beyond language. This is supported by the poor performance on tests of mechanical aptitude, as well as the impairment in complex motor performance, these occurring in the presence of excellent spatial, constructive and motor function. A second point concerns the marked discrepancy between (intact) naming on confrontation testing, word-lists and word-association, and the lack of substantives in open discourse. Study of this problem indicates that the impairment of referential (or associative) speech, and of creative, expository speech may occur in selective fashion. This is consistent with the work of Miller (1967), who has argued for such a distinction.* In this patient, expository speech is empty and circumlocutory, characteristic of anomic aphasia but without naming difficulties. This difference is an occasional observation in aphasic patients, but has not yet received close attention.

The Word-Concept, Cloze and Proverb tests are of help in exploring the word-finding disorder. In the first of these, there is a fixation on either the nonsense word or the context, with inability to assimilate both. At times, a given context is stabilized so as to achieve some trial word. However, in contrast to the normal approach, the subsequent phrase is then interpreted according to the preceding trial. Similarly, a Cloze test demonstrates ability to combine only the initial or the following segment of a phrase with the inserted word. The latter is assimilated to either the first or second segment, but ordinarily not both at the same time. Proverb interpretation generally requires the combination of at least two separate terms into a common denominator. Thus, in the proverb, "The early bird gets the worm" both "early bird" and "worm" must be interpreted to some extent independently, the final analysis resting on shared attributes

---

*I am indebted to Dr. Eugene Green for pointing this out to me.

of each term. It it, therefore, not surprising that performance on proverbs was consistent with that on other tests, namely a tendency to interpret proverbs with respect to one term only. As would be expected, the response to one-dimensional idioms, such as "swell headed" or "cold shoulder" was much better.

As noted, analysis of speech production revealed frequent misuse of prepositions, misapplication or dropping of tense, and abnormal pronoun usage. Articles were usually normal but at times were deleted or substituted. There was occasional verbal paraphasia and very rarely, literal paraphasia. The great difficulty with those grammatical words which serve to link up phrase segments, such as prepositions, may relate to performance on word-concept, cloze and proverb tests. These tests, in addition to spontaneous speech and writing, all seem to reflect the same underlying disorder. We will return to this point shortly.

In speech, the patient's verbal paraphasia is dependent on the sentence structure, in contrast to the verbal substitutions which characterize anomia. In the former, the verbal paraphasia generally embodies only one attribute of the target word, and is not apprehended as an approximation. The paraphasic word is accepted as fulfilling the intended meaning, and plays a role in determining the subsequent discourse. In anomia, the paraphasia is ordinarily in categorical relation to the desired word, and is recognized by the patient as imprecise. Moreover, anomic paraphasia does not greatly determine either the sentence within which it is embedded or the utterance to follow. In the present case, each substantive is accepted as correct, and conditions its immediate grammatical relationships. These latter will also play a role in governing subsequent noun choice. If the choice is not readily made, the expression will break off into stereotypies until a new start can be initiated.

Performance in ongoing speech, therefore, parallels that in Cloze testing. In both, no more than a single component of the sentence is satisfactorily linked with another at any one time. It is for this reason that relational words such as prepositions are among the most severely affected. The patient cannot integrate more than two dominant elements in a phrase at a time. Thus, topic and action, or action and object, are securely bonded but not all three. Similarly, in proverbs only one term is analyzed and the other is adjusted to this analysis. Idiomatic or metaphoric expressions require a one-dimensional analysis for a correct interpretation and therefore are performed more or less normally. A similiar argument can be advanced to explain deficient word-finding in conversation in the presence of excellent confrontation and associative naming. Thus, referential speech is distinguished by a relative freedom from syntactical constraints which would reduce the likelihood of paralogical substitutions, and limit their propagatory nature. On the other hand, naming in conversation is a direct outgrowth of the sentence pattern, which we have seen to have a reciprocal influence on word-finding. The nature of the naming difficulty is clearly illustrated by the failure to name action-pictures. Here the desired word, e.g. jumping or kicking, is an interpretation of object-relationships in a picture, and as such is a performance similar to the Cloze test. This contrasts with the success in naming identical actions performed by the examiner. Along the same lines, tests of descriptive naming indicate a better performance when multiple attributes of one object are given (the response being to name the object), than when multiple objects are given, the response being to determine the shared attribute.

In many ways, therefore, this patient appears transitional between anomic and Wernicke's aphasia. This is also evident in the logorrhea, euphoria and the lack of speech awareness. A relation to the verbal paraphasia of Wernicke's aphasia could be seen in the tangential use of words and paragrammatism. The misapplication of words in conversation, particularly substantives, is midway between the category errors of anomia and the seemingly random substitutions of Wernicke's aphasia. From these findings, one might speculate the (pathological) stages in word production to be the following: (1) inability to produce the correct word in expositional or referential speech, with or without spheric paraphasia; (2) good referential use of words with difficulty in word-finding restricted to expositional speech; paraphasia is no longer noun-for-noun, but is dependent on sentence structure; the substitutions condition the subsequent discourse and are not fully perceived as approximations to the correct word; the substitution embodies only one aspect of the desired noun or phrase, but is treated as if it fully expressed its entire meaning; and (3) paraphasia having a less perceptible relationship between the substituted and the correct word, and affecting both expositional and, to perhaps a lesser extent, referential speech. It is of interest that the second stage, with intact referential speech, may have its correlate in the syndrome of "nonaphasic misnaming" (*quod vide*), where expositional speech is often quite good in the presence of paralogical naming defects. This opens up the possibility that independ-

ent involvements of the referential and expositional system may occur
as disturbances transitional between anomia and Wernicke's aphasia.

Using this formulation, we may return to Domarus' example of
schizophrenic paralogic:

*Certain Indians are swift. Stags are swift. Therefore, certain In-
dians are stags.*

Here there is also an inability to manipulate (merge) two contrasting elements into a common third element. This takes the following form:

$$A \simeq \text{attribute x}$$
$$B \simeq \text{attribute x}$$
$$A = x = B, A = B$$

In the performance of our patient on the Cloze test there is an
identical pattern. Thus, in the phrase "he had _____ done before," the patient's solution is "he had *been* done before." Here,
the form is the following: $A \simeq x \simeq B$. With the response demanding
that x be suitable for both A and B, the patient sees x in terms of A,
or x in terms of B, but cannot sustain a sufficient detachment from
the dominant terms to invert the problem, so as to understand A
and B in terms of x. This is more than just a reduction in the
abstract ability; the one attribute of the object which is apprehended
by the patient is not seen in its partial character $(A \simeq x)$, rather it is
accepted as adequate to the full meaning of the object $(A = x)$. As in
the Cloze test, attribute and object ultimately fuse: $A \simeq x \simeq B$ (where
x is unknown); $A = x \simeq B$, therefore $x = A = B$.

The defect in logic is not imposed on the language mechanisms
from without, but is a manifestation of language breakdown. Thus,
to take a simple sentence of the form: subject (topic) : verb (action) :
object, e.g. *John threw the ball,* a cohesive narrative demands that one
phrase act as subject for the next: *It (the-ball-thrown-by-John) hit
the tree.* The discourse can rapidly become very complex, as in:
sentence A → sentence B; A + B → C and so on. The logical demands are the same as described above, e.g. sentence $A + B = x$; x
$= C$. The same situation holds within sentences as between them.
Thus, in the sentence *John threw the ball in the water, threw* may be
conceived as copula for John and ball, and *in* may be conceived as
copula for the-ball-thrown-by-John and water. These copulae have
the value of x, so that in paralogic we might expect: John $= x \simeq$ ball,
and ball $\simeq x =$ water, to become: *John was the ball from the water.*
It should be noted, *apropos* paragrammatism, that it is difficult in
this example to determine the paraphasic element, i.e. *was* or *ball.*

With paraphasic noun substitutions, this might become: *John threw the (his) arm from the water.* Here again the paraphasic element is ambiguous, for the target sentence could be "John removed his arm from the water." The sentence form, and the paraphasia therefore depend on which components (A:x:B) happen to fuse. In the category of aphasia discussed in this section, the verbal paraphasia is often a reflection of the incomplete assimilation of more than two terms in a sentence. It is evident that one cannot always distinguish the verbal from the grammatical substitution. The failure of the patient to fully apprehend the paralogical character of his utterance, and the tendency for abnormal sentence forms to serve as the bases for subsequent forms rather than be discarded, contribute to the listener's difficulty in making this distinction. Both forms of paraphasia exist together, the paragrammatism appearing to be primary and conditioned by the same disorder as the verbal paraphasia, and not a consequence of the latter. In some respects, therefore, schizophrenic speech resembles that of a deep level aphasia. Certainly, as mentioned previously, the decompensation of paralogical speech into the somewhat less common word-salad parallels the deterioration of semantic aphasia to Wernicke's aphasia and semantic jargon. This is another line of evidence to support our contention that, from whatever cause, neuropsychological regression follows a consistent pattern, the symptomatology reflecting a molar, not piecemeal decay.

Chapter 4

WERNICKE'S APHASIA

FOLLOWING MEYNERT'S demonstration of the central terminations of the auditory nerve, Wernicke (1874) argued that destruction of the sound images of words, laid down adjacent to the
acoustic projection zone in posterior T1, should result in inability to
understand or repeat spoken speech. Since patients with disorders of
speech comprehension appeared to recognize objects, and could express some needs through mimic, the concepts occasioned by these
sound images must be preserved. However, the question occurred
as to why speech could not arise independently through concepts,
rather than through the mediation of acoustic word images. In response to this, Wernicke assumed that sound images were normally
innervated coincident with expressive speech, and exercised, through
a kind of hallucinatory control, a constant corrective function on the
course of motor images. The loss of this corrective function was
responsible for paraphasia in spontaneous speech. Other basic elements of the disorder were also noted, the fluctuation in clinical
state, the lack of awareness of speech defect, the fluency, and the
absence of hemiplegia, all of which have since been accepted as part
of the clinical syndrome. Agraphia was invariably present, explained
as a consequence of loss of those sound images upon which, in
obligatory fashion, the graphic system was built. Reading was held
to be less dependent on sound images for it could be spared in
instances of exceptional native facility.

Shortly thereafter, Kussmaul (1877) isolated out of the syndrome
two components, word deafness and word blindness, though Wernicke
insisted on the common origin of these disorders. This had the
effect of an atomistic reduction of the various elements of the syndrome, and led to the brain maps of Lichtheim (1885) and others.
Over the following years, Wernicke's theories received wide attention,
his simple diagrammatic account continuing to be the predominant
force in aphasia study until the criticism of Pierre Marie in 1906.

The word of Arnold Pick (1931) once again signals the modern
era. Pick conceptualized the various receptive and expressive defects

56

of Wernicke's aphasia as interruptions in an hierarchic system, leading inward from heard speech to thought, and outward from thought to spoken speech. The basis of speech perception, Pick believed, was in those temporally organized complexes of sound which combined with the speech melody to form a total unit. In this process he distinguished the following:

1. A stage in which there is isolation of the linguistic element from the diffuse total acoustic impression. Disorder at this stage appears as a failure to respond to speech, shouts and commands, though response to gestures, as in one of Pick's own cases (Kahler and Pick, 1879), is possible. The nature of this disturbance is uncertain. It may concern a partial or complete cortical deafness, a mental reduction or a lack of attention. Related to this is the question of an isolated *sound deafness* (*quod vide*). This was denied by Pick for the reason that spoken words are among the sounds. Also, the close relationship of the speech melody and other aspects of prosody to music argues against a separation of these functions.

2. A gradual differentiation of the perceived word on the basis of recognition of it as a phonetic unit, as a component of language in general, and as a component of a specific language. Here also occurs the recognition of the musical aspect of language, particularly as concerns the speech of a certain individual, i.e. a quality of familiarity. Disorders at this stage affect the perception and the understanding of the sounds of words, *pure word deafness*.

3. At this point other mechanisms come into play to aid in understanding, and these may be differently involved in the sensory disorders. These include the following: a motor focusing on sounds heard, which is a kind of attuning of the executive speech apparatus; attention to the sentence as well as to individual words; repetition of sounds through the infantile speech reflex; speech melody; significance of the situation; emotional elements; and lip-reading.

4. Following on the perception of the word, its understanding comes about through an orderly sequence of stages. First there is an emergence of a general meaning consciousness, and the appearance of complexes of symbols. With this, a consciousness of orientation develops, an intention, and guides the process along. The next stage, that of the conception of categories of words and of the grammatical forms of words, leads finally to the recombination of words into understanding through a process of preconstruction. This is built up on the intonational pattern, which develops from the musical components heard. The syntactical model derives from this also and

plays a part in the differentiation of words for things and processes. A disorder at this deep level leads to *sensory (impressive) agrammatism* (Chap. 3).

For Pick, disturbances at various stages within this system constituted the "sensory" side of Wernicke's aphasia. With regard to the "expressive" defects, paraphasia and paragrammatism were held to be the most prominent. On a suggestion of Heilbronner, Pick postulated that a mild defect in the quantitative aspect of speech might be reflected, in severe cases, in logorrhea, and in less severe cases, abnormal talkativeness. The principal defect, however, concerned the qualitative features, among which verbal and literal paraphasia were the most important. In verbal paraphasia, the wrong word is produced out of an otherwise normal vocabulary, often related in sound or meaning to the correct word. Verbal paraphasia improves to anomia, and in mild Wernicke aphasics a conflict exists between these two phenomena. This is founded upon the instability of inhibitory forces which, in anomia, serve to prevent the appearance of inapposite words as well as to direct attention to the correct word. Word substitution can also lead to paragrammatic effects, through application to the substituted word of grammatical forms appropriate to the intended word. The substitution does not, however, ordinarily affect the sentence and intonational pattern, so that these must be formed through the action of preceding stages. Literal paraphasia can coexist with verbal paraphasia and is a disorder in the "transmission apparatus," since the correct word is evoked and the motor instrumentalities are intact. In severe cases, literal paraphasia leads to jargon aphasia. Pick also noted that paraphasia was not a product of right hemispheric function with damage to the left side, for it occurs with bilateral lesions of Wernicke's area. Especially emphasized was the lack of insight in these patients, and the course of improvement, with diminishing logorrhea coinciding with the appearance of self-correction.

Isserlin (1936) accepted Pick's formulation, and supported the existence of an "impressive" paragrammatism, the disorder appearing largely as an inability, in the face of normal understanding at a simple level, to distinguish between correct and incorrect grammatical forms. Isserlin believed that sensory aphasia derived from a disturbance of speech-sound comprehension. The understanding of sounds was held to grow out of mnesic organizations, disorder of this function giving rise to verbal and literal paraphasia, reading and writing disorders, and impairment in the comprehension of word meaning.

The work of Kleist (summary, 1962), though marred by an excessive and, to judge by the case material, unwarranted zeal toward anatomical localization, has the merit of a functional attitude to the speech receptive disorders founded on the pioneer studies of Pick. Kleist distinguished four major types of sensory disturbance, each reflecting a different stage in the passage of heard speech into thought: 1) word sound (phonemic) deafness, a perceptual disorder in the strict sense, comparable to pure word deafness, 2) word deafness, the sensory accompaniment of Wernicke's aphasia, in which the word is not comprehended as a phonemic sequence and has lost its function in determining the utterance of words; the disorder affects the time sequence of separate parts of the word, and this is reflected in literal paraphasia in spontaneous speech, naming, and to a lesser degree, in repetition, 3) sentence deafness, a higher form of the above, affecting comprehension of ordered series of words, and 4) name deafness, in which words as carriers of meaning are not understood.

Highly sympathetic to Pick's approach, Head (1926) accounted for Wernicke's aphasia as a defect in the inner speech, and in the rhythmic pattern of expression, and termed the disorder syntactical aphasia. Such patients, he insisted, revealed a range of speech disturbance, from mild semantic or verbal jargon to neologistic paraphasia. Written and verbal comprehension were impaired but less severely so than speech. Reading aloud was paraphasic but often correctly understood, writing was less impaired than speech, dictation was variable, and copying and transliteration were good. While Head's account of syntactical aphasia was aligned in a generally progressive direction, it was disadvantaged from the start by a compilation of symptoms that in some respects was uncritical, and a weak and rambling formulation. Further, the whole thrust of Pick's work, which Head so greatly admired, was directed against just such an arbitrary classification. Rather, Pick stressed the need for an independent consideration of each element in each syndrome, and of the behavior of these elements within separate linguistic classes. Thus, within the alexic component of Wernicke's aphasia, an entire range of difficulty can be seen, from complete loss, to paralexia, and in some cases to relative preservation. Similarly, paraphasia will change in the evolution of jargon, and echolalia, which also passes through a distinct sequence in recovery, is a complex phenomenon which does not clearly correspond to the symptoms which it accompanies.

Set in this light, Kurt Goldstein's classification of sensory aphasia, which has had so notable an effect on recent work, does not represent so striking an advance either, since his tri-partite division corresponds very closely to the classical entities of word-deafness, conduction and transcortical aphasia. Goldstein's differentiation of conduction (central or Wernicke's aphasia) from transcortical aphasia rests largely on the performance in repetition, but otherwise the forms are not to be fundamentally separated.

For Luria (1966), sensory aphasia is the result of an inability to discriminate phonemes in the presence of adequate hearing. Patients are able to distinguish sounds that are dissimilar, such as "r" and "m," but on paired sounds such as "b" and "p" there is great difficulty. Following on this is a disturbance in both the phonetic aspect of speech, with literal paraphasia in spontaneous speech and repetition, and in its conceptual aspect with verbal paraphasia. In addition to the defects of phonemic discrimination, disorders of the system of word meaning based on this sound structure, as well as in the memory of speech sounds, will appear. Disturbances of writing are also present, and the pathology is held to be in posterior superior temporal convolution. In his discussion, Luria particularly emphasizes the dynamic character of (auditory) perception. He argues that to hear speech is as well an act of understanding as of perception, with no definite boundary between speech perception and speech comprehension. The demonstration of these various disturbances, viz. verbal memory, conceptualization and verbal meaning, all based on defective phonemic discrimination, represents a highly original contribution. However, it is necessary to view this formulation with caution, in view of the fact that tests of phoneme discrimination, for example, paired words (peas/bees), are perhaps the least sensitive index of auditory perceptual defect.

Hecaen (1965, 1969) has distinguished two forms of auditory comprehension impairment in Wernicke's aphasia. One type approximates word-deafness with severe loss of auditory comprehension, poor repetition and verbal paraphasia in speech. A second type shows moderate auditory comprehension loss and improved repetition, but an increase in literal and neologistic paraphasia. Though it is tempting to draw a correlation with Wernicke's and transcortical sensory aphasia, it should be emphasized that the latter disorder (*quod vide*) generally has the more severe comprehension defect.

CLINICAL PICTURE

Onset is ordinarily abrupt, but may appear gradually in the improvement of neologistic jargon or in the deterioration of an anomia. Initially, there is euphoria, but paranoia often intervenes soon after, either as a manifestation of auditory perceptual loss, as in the paranoia of the deaf, or possibly as a result of some other temporal lobe mechanism. It is therefore not surprising that psychosis occasionally occurs, though unlike the case in word-deafness, it is infrequently accompanied by auditory hallucinations. Patients are generally unaware of their speech productions, whether correct or not, but are often able to distinguish, within a fairly broad range, if correct language is being spoken to them. If one speaks to such a patient either invented jargon, or jargon transcribed from a tape of his voice, there is evidence that the patient apprehends the inappropriateness of the speech. There is also a considerable tendency in this group of patients for fatigue on testing, both on general performance and within specific test categories.

Speech is fluent, often logorrheic, and characterized by verbal, and less often literal paraphasia. Augmentation and some perseveration are present to a variable degree. The amount of paraphasia ranges from 10% to perhaps 80% of words. An example of verbal paraphasia would be the following, from a patient trying to describe a picture of children stealing some cookies (Goodglass test), ". . . they have the cases, the cookies, and they were helping each other with the good." This appears also in reading aloud, as in another case who read "The spy fled to Greece," as "The spy field to grain." A more extensive form of verbal paraphasia is semantic jargon. An example is the previously quoted patient of Alajouanine who said of a fork, "Ah fork, thats the need for a schedule," or a personal case who, asked what a spoon was used for said, "How many schemes on your throat." Here the meaning of the expression can no longer be understood. Verbal paraphasia usually coexists with phonemic paraphasia, as in ". . . taken for a curson (i.e. person) who advised people to join his company which is the same thing as you tried to have as many tires in your job handling, using the telephone." When phonemic paraphasia is severe, especially in the presence of augmentation, it becomes neologistic, as in ". . . it was my job as a convince, a confoser, not confoler but almost the same as a man who was commersed." The more disturbed form of this is neologistic jargon, as in "Oh posho oh pat and he indent have the pat. Letenseped anyeted, oh how in kennel." Further, neologistic and verbal paraphasia may occur together to produce strikingly bizarre expressions. Thus an aphasic physician, asked if he was a doctor said, "Me? Yes sir, I'm a male demaploze on my own. I still

know my tubaboys what for I have that's gone hell and some of them
go." Neologistic jargon will clear into either predominantly phonemic
or verbal paraphasia, while semantic jargon ordinarily improves to
the verbal paraphasia of Wernicke's aphasia. It is of interest that
semantic jargon may fatigue on testing to neologistic or phonemic
jargon. The conclusion seems to be that neologistic jargon is a
phonemic distortion of severe verbal paraphasia, usually in the presence of augmentation.

   In the typical Wernicke's aphasic, grammar and sentence pattern
are not grossly disturbed, and prosody and intonation may be surprisingly normal. When paragrammatism and defects in stress pattern occur, they appear more closely related to the verbal rather than
the phonemic defect.

   Comprehension is always disturbed, but in varying degree. In patients with moderate difficulty on formal testing, but able to follow
a conversation fairly well, there will also be difficulty in understanding foreign accents and rapid speech, in spite of the patient's own
logorrhea. There may be better comprehension of the speech of
family or friends than of the examiner, and better understanding of
casual speech than in the test situation. Patients will often be able to
carry out some simple commands, e.g. lift your hand, close your eyes,
though object pointing may be nil. If able to point to occasional objects on command, there may be great difficulty with simple questions
which demand a response specification, as on yes or no questions
(e.g. Is it raining?), or pointing to objects described (e.g. Something
you sit on). In severe cases all speech comprehension may be lost,
and at best only such commands may be carried out as "Take off
your glasses" or "Stand up." While the reason for the preservation
of these commands is obscure, they can often be helpful when given
sotto voce in determining that the patient is not peripherally deaf.
Musical identification may or may not be affected, while sound
identification is ordinarily spared, though testing of these items is
often quite difficult. According to Goodglass, body-part names and
names of letters are the most difficult categories for comprehension
and may be more severely impaired in Wernicke aphasics.

   The various syntactical constructions used in the study of "receptive" aphasia have been studied by Parisi and Pizzamiglio (1970) and
correlated with certain aphasic subgroups. It is important to recognize, however, that many of the tests used in comprehension testing,
such as passively-voiced questions, genitive formations, before-after
type questions, and so on, can be impaired in the absence of true

aphasia. While nonaphasic brain-damaged patients may do fairly well, patients with mild dementia often fail. In such cases, the difficulty may be well out of proportion to the minimal disturbance in word-finding which is frequently present.

Repetition is impaired, usually with literal and/or neologistic paraphasia, thus representing a deterioration over the verbal paraphasia of conversational speech. At times, echolalic repetitions of single words or even short phrases are possible, aligning the disorder with transcortical aphasia. Other cases improve toward conduction aphasia where the perceptual defect is mild, and the phonemic paraphasias in repetition more marked. With regard to the repetition which is still possible, Wernicke's aphasia is similar to conduction aphasia (*quod vide*) in types of errors, facilitation of number repetition, etc. In the Wernicke aphasic with moderate verbal paraphasia, repetition may exhibit an increase in verbal substitution over the conduction aphasic, though verbal paraphasias, often within sphere (e.g. door for window) are found in the latter form as well. The occurrence of such verbal paraphasias indicates that the disordered repetition does not represent solely a defect in phonemic discrimination, as stressed by certain workers.

Word-finding is usually impaired, and is similar to conversational speech in the presence of verbal and literal paraphasia. In the typical form of Wernicke's aphasia, with predominantly verbal paraphasia and/or paragrammatism in ongoing speech, confrontation naming may be quite good in the presence of circumlocutory speech. This indicates (*vide supra*) that there is a stage between anomia and verbal paraphasia where lexical entry is retarded in spontaneous speech flow, but facilitated on naming objects. Patients with more severe verbal paraphasia in speech may show increased literal paraphasia on naming or repetition. The increasing specification of the verbal task will accentuate the phonemic paraphasia. Patients with disturbances of this kind tend not to be greatly helped by phonemic or contextual cueing. Also in this group, color naming may be superior to object naming, and errors in the former will be distinguished more for verbal than phonemic substitutions.

Writing is always impaired, equal to or worse than speech. In severe cases, patients may be capable of writing little more than their name. Dictation is possible in patients with some ability to comprehend spoken speech, but is ordinarily distinguished for misspellings even of simple words, and limited ability on longer words or phrases. Copying and transliteration are often quite good, even for unknown or nonsense words. According to Hecaen and Angelergues (1965), patients are more conscious of written than spoken errors. *Reading* is variable. In the restricted case of Wernicke's aphasia, with considerable defect of comprehension and moderate verbal paraphasia, reading may be quite good indeed, well out of proportion to the difficulty in auditory comprehension or speech. This topic is discussed at length with the alexias.

Case 2

A sixty-one-year-old right-handed woman was admitted to the hospital in February, 1971. A history of sudden onset of right hemiparesis and "global aphasia" was obtained in October, 1970. Some improvement occurred to a state of fluent jargon, at which time transfer to the Aphasia Unit was arranged. The patient was repeatedly evaluated between February and June, 1971 with essentially no change in language function during this time. Neurological examination demonstrated a right visual field defect to threat, a right-hemiparesis, and a right sensory deficit. Brain scan demonstrated a strongly positive uptake limited to the left posterior superior temporal region. The patient was highly educated, and fluent in English and Yiddish.

Conversational speech was fluent, with from 30–80 per cent neologistic jargon. The sentence pattern was vaguely preserved, and sentences were organized into definite word-like groupings. Word-stress and sentence intonation were present, the patient gestured actively during speech and appeared to be unaware that her speech was incomprehensible. Verbal and literal paraphasias were lost in the neologistic jargon. There was augmentation, clang-association and mild to moderate logorrhea, but speech only occurred on initiation by the examiner. There was some depression, which was situational rather than related to speech frustration. Articulation was excellent and her jargonized speech was clear and precise. There was no cooperation with motor series or singing. On occasion, intelligible phrases were heard though ordinarily bearing no relation to the subject at hand. For example, at the end of one burst of jargon, the patient suddenly exclaimed, "yeah, will you come to us?." The prosodic aspects of speech were preserved.

Spontaneous: "Then he graf, so I'll graf, I'm giving ink, no, gerfergen, in pane, I can't grasp, I haven't grob the grabben, I'm going to the glimmeril, let me go."

"What my fytisset for, whattim tim saying got dok arne gimmin my suit, suit to Friday . . . I ayre here what takes zwei the cuppen seffer effer sepped . . . I spoke on she asked for clubbin hond here, you what, what kind of a siz sizzen . . . and she speks all the friend and all that is in my herring."

Conversational:

Q. What is your speech problem?

A. "Because no one gotta scotta gowan thwa, thirst, gell, gerst, derund, gystrol, that's all."

Q. What does "swell-headed" mean?

A. "She is selfice on purpiten."

Comprehension was impossible to test, with failure on the simplest commands. There was no evidence of speech understanding, although at times responses were related to questions asked in conversation. On rare occasions, there was response to simple whole-body commands. Occasionally, some words of a command were repeated without response, e.g. asked to point to a spoon, she said "spoon, poon, yes" and then pointed to another object. Asked to touch her nose, she said "Stuch tux news, nose" but made no response. *Repetition* was possible for some simple three or four-letter words, but on longer words phonemic paraphasia was evident, e.g. "cable" for table, "kowt" for kite. At times, words were repeated correctly and then augmented into a stream of neologisms. Single-digit numbers and letters could be repeated, but more often than not with paraphasia. *Naming* was neologistic, e.g. "galeefs" for comb, "errendear" for yellow, "this is howert, heaven, g'dark" for red, and "my ear tuck me here" for ear. There was response to phonemic cueing, but only rarely was the cue utilized to achieve a correct response. Naming of colors and body parts was slightly superior to object naming. *Writing* and copying were nil. Initially, *reading* aloud demonstrated neologistic jargon, while reading comprehension, as tested on matching and sentence completions, was nil. Numbers and letters could neither be matched nor read aloud. Gradually, some improvement in reading occurred, such that simple words, e.g. "cat," "dog," "school," were read aloud, usually followed by a stream of jargon. Reading words aloud was superior to number reading and identical to letter reading. At this time, there was still no response to simple written commands or matching tests. She was unable to copy a simple cube, carry out simple written additions, or perform simple movements to command or imitation.

The patient was tested under continuous auditory feedback, varied over a two-second delay. Some interruption of speech-flow was produced, though the impairment was judged to be less than experienced by most normal subjects.

Comment

This patient demonstrates the preservation in neologistic jargon of sentence pattern and intonation, and the organization of the phrase into word-like groupings. The frequency of neologism varied from moment to moment, at times constituting more than 80 percent of words produced, at other times, 10-20 percent of speech. Occasionally, intelligible though irrelevant five to six-word phrases were produced. There was moderate logorrhea and impaired speech awareness, although the patient recognized jargon speech when given to her by the examiner in the form of a question or a command. The brain scan localization in left temporoparietal region is consistent with recent findings by Kertesz and Benson (1971).

Case 3

A 67-year old right-handed woman was admitted May, 1971 to the hospital with a history of sudden onset of right-hemiparesis and aphasia one month previously. On initial examination she was noted to have minimal speech but some comprehension. An EEG demonstrated left temporoparietal slowing, and brain scan was reported as showing uptake in the distribution of the left middle cerebral artery. Examination on the Aphasia Unit revealed a dense right sensorimotor hemiparesis and right visual field defect. Brain scan demonstrated superficial and deep uptake over most of the left frontal lobe, extending to the immediate post-Rolandic and anterior temporal region.

Conversational speech was fluent, consisting of streams of speech sounds. There was a loss of intonation, word-stress and sentence pattern. Utterances were not organized into word-like units, although occasional recognizable words were heard. There was a tendency for perseveration and clang association of sounds; there was active gesture during conversation, no self-correction or frustration, and awareness of the speech defect was doubtful. Articulation was good. Speech was active and confident but without logorrhea. Motor series were done poorly, e.g. on number series, she said "one, tooz, adidiling, adeeda." A melody could be successfully produced, but lyrics were jargonized.

Q. Can you tell me how you got sick?

A. "Ha dan de fafafa?"

Q. How did you get sick?

A. "Eeh, oh malaty? Eeh, favility? Abelabla tay kare. Abelabla tay

to po stay here. (stay here?) Aberdar yeste day. (yesterday?) and then abedeyes dee, aaah, yes dee, ye ship, yeste dey es dalababela. Abla desee, abla detoasy, abla ley e porephee, tee arabek. Abla get sik? (get sick?) ."
Q. What is your name?
A. "Ablayedish . . . arabek, alabistik."
Comprehension was possible for a few simple commands, e.g. "make a fist," "close your eyes," and on rare occasions, pointing to single objects presented before her. Yes-no questions, object descriptions and serial commands were not possible. When the patient was asked questions in jargon by the examiner, or asked to point to objects with jargon names, there was clear though inconstant recognition of the inappropriate nature of the request. *Naming* of objects, body parts, and colors, and *repetition* were both identical to conversational speech. For example, a comb was called "aleladeeda," a pipe "bai heedadaidah," and boy was repeated as "danallot." Repetition of numbers or letters was impossible. *Writing*, copying, reading aloud and reading for comprehension were impossible on a variety of tests. Written calculations were not possible even at the simplest level. The patient was able to copy little more than a square. On praxis testing, some imitative movements were possible, but for the most part, imitation was impaired. There was some improvement with objects though performance was still imperfect. There was no response to whole body commands.

The patient was tested with delayed feedback. No apparent interruption of speech flow or content occurred with continuous feedback at delays varying over a two-second time-frame.

Comment

In this example of phonemic jargon, there are several points to be emphasized. The predominantly anterior location of the lesion on brain scan, the preservation of singing in the presence of jargonized lyrics and the fact that comprehension was possible for simple commands and some object pointing suggest a relationship with the anterior aphasias. Moreover, the tendency towards phonemic reiteration is of great interest. Although the jargon contained a full range of English phonemes, there was a tendency for persistence of certain jargon forms. This suggests a comparison with those phonemic jargon stereotypies which may accompany Broca's aphasia. Differentiation from the latter rests largely on the variety of phonemes employed, the stereotypies containing only a limited number of speech sounds re-

iterated in constant fashion. The speech anosognosia for both jargon
streotypy and phonemic jargon is another point of similarity. Although
the anatomical correlation of phonemic jargon is uncertain, this case
indicates the possibility of an anatomical and functional continuum
with jargon stereotypy. Finally, it should be noted that, in contrast
to semantic and neologistic jargon, phonemic jargon no longer maintains a sentence pattern, word stress, or to a great extent, sentence
intonation. What phonemic groupings do occur seem almost accidental.
Moreover, while we infer a lack of awareness for the patient's utterance, it is clear that such patients are able to recognize jargon spoken
by the examiner.

DISCUSSION

Evidence has been discussed in the preceding chapter to show that
disturbance at an early stage in language formulation will lead to
comparable deficits in speech comprehension and expression, reading and writing. At an intermediate level in this process each of these
performances will be affected in a more or less equivalent manner,
whereas with involvement at surface levels, the end-stage of each
language performance may be disrupted in relative isolation. The
constellation of deficits which goes to make up the picture of Wernicke's aphasia concerns this intermediate phase.

The *comprehension* disorder appears to cover that middle ground
between contextual interpretation and response to single words or
speech sounds. This contrasts with the patient discussed in the preceding section, who had excellent comprehension of individual words
in the presence of difficulty with contextual formations. It also
contrasts with word-deafness where one often observes the ability to
follow a conversation, particularly in talking with relatives, but complete failure on single word comprehension, pointing to objects and
matching spoken to written words. These are instances of the variability of defects within a system of speech perception, the progression
being not from word to understanding but from contextual understanding to the perception of individual words. The typical
Wernicke's aphasic will often have some sparing of context and some
sparing of single word responses.

The *speech* defect also covers that middle range between the lack
of words characteristic of anomia, and the phonemic paraphasia of
the conduction aphasic, i.e. between lexical entry and phonemic encodage. It is not clear whether the verbal substitutions of Wernicke's
aphasia and the more extreme form of semantic jargon represent

truly unique disorders or only paraphasias of varying severity. The logorrhea of the Wernicke aphasic, as well perhaps as the lack of awareness with which it is usually accompanied, probably contribute to the development of verbal paraphasia. In contrast to the anomic, the Wernicke aphasic can neither delay nor circumlocute while waiting for the correct word to come up, nor is he able to suppress irrelevant discourse. Occasional verbal paraphasias may or may not be at a conscious level, for the patient will at times reject a correct utterance, or appear to accept a paraphasic one. In addition, many patients, having given a word related to the target word, will then build their discourse around the paraphasia. Or, asked to point to an object, they will at times repeat the object name paraphasically and then point to the (incorrect) object of their misnaming. This lack of awareness for paraphasias has been mentioned by Weisenburg (1935) and by Schuell (1950).

Bay (1962) holds that "sensory" aphasia is distinguished from anomia mainly by the presence of nonlinguistic factors such as euphoria and unawareness. These account for the logorrhea, and produce an increase in the paraphasia. There appears to be a difference, however, between the verbal paraphasia of the anomic and that of the Wernicke aphasic. According to Kaplan (personal communication), anomic paraphasias tend to be semantically related to the target word, while those of the Wernicke aphasic are more random. This is particularly evident on naming tasks where the target word is known. When the relation between intention and word becomes more distant, semantic jargon results. In another study, using an unselected group of aphasics, Schuell (1950) demonstrated that paraphasic and paralexic errors fell into categories similar to normal responses on word-association tests. As a partial explanation, she suggested that preparatory phases of the concept present themselves, in verbal paraphasia, as though they were the final phase. Also noted was an inability to select the appropriate word from closely related alternatives, and with this, an occlusion of some processes related to volitional choice. Certainly we may say that the appearance of verbal paraphasias with lesions sparing T1 indicates that the disorder is not sensory-dependent, as supposed by Wernicke. More importantly, the transition from verbal paraphasia and paralexia complicating (i.e. as an expression of) an anomia to the verbal paraphasia or semantic jargon of Wernicke's aphasia, seems due rather to the disinhibition of alternatives presenting at the lexical entry stage. This inability to inhibit inexact responses occurs with increasing logorrhea and diminishing self-awareness. This finding seems to indicate that discriminative ability, an ability which presupposes the control of verbal flow, is bound up with the experience of awareness.

It would seem then that within the Wernicke aphasia group, a number of interrelated syndromes can be defined. Severe disruption at a stage in lexical entry in advance of that damaged in anomia results in verbal paraphasia. When verbal paraphasia is minimal, it is accompanied by an anomia which is the predominant symptom. At the next stage there is less anomia but a looser relation between word and meaning. Here also, are mild logorrhea, euphoria and diminished awareness of the utterance. These symptoms always appear together as a unit, and correspond to cases of the semantic aphasia type. Involvement at succeeding levels appears with increasing verbal paraphasia, which is of a more random type, and accentuated euphoria, logorrhea, and speech anosognosia. This corresponds to Wernicke's aphasia. As the paraphasia becomes more pronounced, it also becomes more random, and produces the picture of semantic jargon. If defects in phonemic encodage intervene, the result is neologistic jargon. Here, either there is phonemic substitution of semantic paraphasia, or the phonemic substitution is so severe that correct semantic units can no longer be discriminated. It may be that each of these states can produce neologistic jargon, and may determine whether the jargon will evolve to Wernicke's or conduction aphasia. The participation of both semantic and phonemic paraphasia in the process is supported by evidence (Kertesz and Benson, 1969) that neologistic jargon improves to either Wernicke's or conduction aphasia. It is probable that undifferentiated jargon represents disarray of the phonemic encoding system in the face of loss of the abstract lexical frame (Fig. 3).

The appearance of logorrhea and diminished self-awareness can

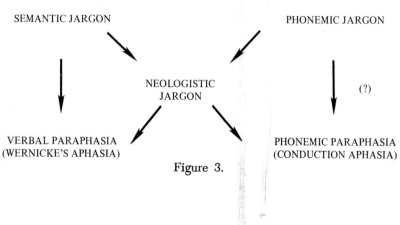

Figure 3.

be explained along the same lines. With interruption of language at a moderately advanced stage in its course, there occurs an increase in the automatization of speech and a shortening of the latency. Moreover, since the patient's speech will partake of a smaller part of the total process, i.e. the segment prior or subsequent to that interruption, there is an incomplete experience of self-awareness which it (language) generates. In addition, echolalic repetitions of single words will occur, as manifestations of the lability of the distal segment and the lack of participation of earlier contents in the final expression. This leads to a consideration of those patients with an accentuation of the echolalic component.

TRANSCORTICAL SENSORY APHASIA AND ECHOLALIA

Lichtheim (1885) postulated this disorder as the result of an interruption in a pathway from the sensory speech center to the area of concepts. Thus, speech could be perceived (as judged from excellent repetition) but could not be understood. A case was reported characterized by loss of speech and reading comprehension, preserved though paraphasic speech and writing, and good reading aloud, dictation and copying. The signal ability in this patient was that of repetition, which was excellent and of the echolalic type.

Subsequently, Bastian (1897, 1898) suggested a partial functional impairment of the sensory speech center, an idea later supported by Heilbronner, and especially Pick, for whom the disorder was but a mild or regressing Wernicke's aphasia. Pick was particularly interested in the echolalic repetition of these patients, which he held to be a disinhibited primitive acoustic-motor reflex, no longer under the control of volitional speech and cognitive processes. Following Arnaud (1887), who first distinguished automatic from mitigated echolalia, Pick demonstrated a fundamental difference between echolalia and volitional speech, and defined a series of stages in the recovery of echolalia from parrot-like repetition without understanding, to mitigated or questioning repetition with appropriate substitution of terms and partial understanding.

The major contribution to the subject, however, was by Kurt Goldstein (1915). In his monograph, as well as in later studies (1948), Goldstein emphasized the complexity of the repetition process, and the varieties of echo performance. The condition, he thought, was the reverse of that expected in sensory aphasia, for understanding is usually superior to repetition. In these patients, however, understanding is usually severely damaged, while spontaneous speech is fluent, empty and paraphasic. Series speech is good with no trouble getting started. Repetition tends to be echolalic but is not necessarily so, and there is impaired acoustic attention and speech memory. While transcortical sensory aphasia may occur in the improvement of a "severe total sensory aphasia," it is not due to a partial lesion of the sensory speech area, but more than likely, a combination of slight damage to acoustic speech perception and of its relation to the nonlanguage mental operations. In echolalia, Goldstein emphasized the importance of frontal lesions but accepted a temporal localization for transcortical sensory aphasia. After Goldstein, Henschen (1925) distinguished two forms on a pathological basis, one with diffuse brain atrophy, and another with focal cortical or subcortical temporal lesion. The locus was in Wernicke's area, as a partial lesion of posterior T1. Isserlin (1936) agreed as to the occurrence of transcortical sensory aphasia in improving Wernicke's aphasics, but stressed that this was not a milder degree of the latter. Rather, it was a complication of Wernicke's aphasia, obscured by severe word-deafness, which reappeared after comprehension improved.

More recently, Stengel (1947) has commented that the transition, demonstrated by Pick, from automatic echolalia to an almost deliberate repetition, speaks against the assumption that automatic repetition is of a fundamentally different nature. In one of his cases of transcortical sensory aphasia, postmortem revealed complete destruction of the speech area on the dominant side, leading Stengel to raise the possibility of a minor hemisphere role in the echolalia. This recalls earlier suggestions by Bastian and Liepmann and has yet to be fully studied. Stengel was the first to notice the completion phenomenon in such cases, as in responding to the question, "How did you sleep last _____" with "night," and held this to be a proof that the repetition was not wholly automatic. He pointed to the occurrence of echolalia in other organic and psychotic states, and suggested, as a common explanation, a regression to an identification at a primitive level. Other recent contributions include those of Symonds (1953), who has applied the old terminology of word-meaning deafness without word-sound deafness to a suggestive case, and Bay (1962) whose explanation of echolalia as aphasia plus "lack of ideas" (Einfallsleere) recalls similar accounts in the early literature.

Currently, there does not seem to be great interest in transcortical sensory aphasia, many workers, with good reason, being doubtful as to its very existence. Unanimity does not even exist as to the major performance in these patients, that of repetition. Although it is generally held that whatever repetition is spared is of an echolalic nature, some consider that voluntary repetition should be possible for the diagnosis to be made. Yet if the repetition were to be voluntary, an inconsistency with the Lichtheim scheme would be evident, since the concept field (Begriffsfeld), the source of volitional utterance, was held to be separated from the sensory speech center. A further problem with "volitional repetition" is that the condition is frequently mimicked by dementia. It is common to see otherwise nonaphasic dements repeating questions or commands to which they utterly fail to respond. With regard to echolalic repetition, a distinction is sometimes made between echolalia at the word and at the phrase level, the former being a common occurrence in sensory aphasics, the latter more specifically associated with transcortical aphasia, isolation syndrome cases and the echolalia of dementia. Echolalic repetition of one or a few words is a frequent accompaniment of Wernicke's aphasia, and often coexists with complete failure in voluntary repetition. The length of the string echoed, particularly in sensory aphasics, does not appear in itself to be a critical factor in differentiation. This may only reflect span limitations, or the competing paraphasia, or possibly, if accomplished through minor hemisphere, the maximum capacity for echoing in that hemisphere. Most certainly it does not, as Geschwind *et al.* (1968) suggest, represent a performance within the limitations of the ability to repeat, for even at the single word level the echolalic response and the volitional repetition are thoroughly different utterances. This echolalia for single words and short phrases is the more common appearance of transcortical sensory aphasia, and usually occurs within those Wernicke's aphasics with severe comprehension loss. Transcortical sensory aphasia can be diagnosed when the paraphasic element is reduced, and echolalia becomes the dominant symptom. Thus, transcortical sensory aphasia stands in relation both to the moderate perceptual loss and verbal paraphasia of the Wernicke's aphasic, and to the severe perceptual loss without paraphasia of the word-deaf.

As the echolalia improves there is a change to a mitigated form with semi-automatic repetition of shorter phrases, or the last word or two in a phrase, often expressed in the interrogative with appropriate grammatical alteration. Echoing of this type gives the appearance of an aid toward correct comprehension. This repetition dissolves into a simple questioning reiteration of words or phrases, which may exhibit phonemic paraphasia and thereby suggest a relation to impaired auditory comprehension. As comprehension continues to improve, the phonemic paraphasia may disappear, may remain as a sign of disordered acoustic discrimination, or may change into the phonemic paraphasia of the conduction aphasic, which is largely independent of any difficulty in comprehension. True voluntary repetition with lack of comprehension does not occur, while on the other hand, automatic echolalia does not appear with good understanding, or at least, good understanding of that item which is echoed. Similarly, the more automatic the echo, the less likely is it that the echoed content has been understood.

Regarding echolalia in general, it is, according to Pick's definition, ". . . an immediate, compulsive and irresistible imitation of everything spoken, often to the most minute articulatory and musical detail, even of utterances not understood, in foreign languages, or long chemical formulae or meaningless sequences of letters." The disorder has been described in toxic and twilight states, fatigue, psychoses and degenerative diseases. In mental deficiency, echolalia has been suggested to be the final stage of speech development. There is usually good series speech, while echopraxia and echographia (Pick, 1924; Sittig, 1928) and occasionally palilalia (Critchley, 1927) have been reported as accompaniments. The picture is simply that of brief latency, often sudden and at times explosive repetition, with no evidence that the echoed item has been understood. This may coexist with normal or paraphasic volitional repetition, as well as with intermediate states where understanding of the repeated item is uncertain.

The echolalic repetition is ordinarily accurate, nonparaphasic and without dysarthria. Even strongly automatic forms show the completion phenomenon for well-known phrases, as "Roses are ---." The "isolation" case of Geschwind *et al.* (1968) gave relatively complex completions, as in "I love coffee, I love tea, etc." to the word coffee, but this is less common. The echolalia may be for only the last word of a phrase, or more rarely, the initial words, and the echo-response may begin midway through the examiner's statement. As the echo is usually more rapid than the presented item, at times the patient will conclude his repetition on the heels of the examiner. Improvement occurs to a mitigated form in which grammatical changes occur, so as to personalize the repetition. Thus, "How are you?," becomes "How am I?", or "Close your eyes" becomes a questioning "Close my eyes?." Such repetitions may be then followed by a correct answer or response. When asked to "say, horse," or "say the word, horse," patients will usually drop the imperative. Improprietous phrases may block the echo response entirely, and induce the patient to say "No, No." This "social" aspect to echolalia has been discussed by Stengel (1947), who notes that echolalia occurs primarily in the conversational situation, and not if the examiner turns his back on the patient.

Finally, it has been mentioned that echolalia appears to be related inversely to speech understanding, except perhaps in the motor variety of transcortical aphasia (*quod vide*). This relationship is apparent also in the fact that patients may be echolalic only in imperfectly learned languages, and not in the mother tongue. Pick and Schneider (1938) have described such cases, and a good example was provided by the case of Bastian, an Italian woman conversant also in Spanish and French, who, following a cerebral hemorrhage, lost completely the first two languages and retained French only to the degree of echolalic repetition without understanding. Clearly, the language which is least understood is best echoed. This contrasts with the situation in conduction aphasia, where the later acquired language gives more difficulty in repetition.

Echolalic repetitions and echo-like responses are common features in aphasic patients, and it is only when they become the predominant symptoms is a diagnosis of "isolation syndrome" or transcortical aphasia justified. A fundamental problem, however, in all such states, is the relation of echolalia to other language processes. Certainly, in their automaticity, clarity and lack of awareness, a parallel can be drawn with the stereotypic utterances of Broca's aphasics. Moreover, echolalia is free of the paraphasic features which characterize Wernicke's aphasia, just as stereotypies do not show the agrammatism or dysarthria of Broca's aphasia. Stereotypies seem to occur without participation in the full extent of the speech-development system. If the stereotypy can be said to lack full awareness because of incomplete participation in this process, the same can be said for echolalia; i.e. the echo-response does not partake of early stages in speech formulation. The fact that echolalia is mitigated by increasing the familiarity of the test phrase tends to support this assertion. It is possible that the deep organization of speech perception is coextensive with the speech productive system at a stage in advance of the latter. In pathological states, this permits the modeling of a received signal to expressive processes without obligatory passage through earlier cognitive stages. If this modeling process is allowed to determine the subsequent course of expressive speech, only the distal (word-close) portion of the process will be traversed by the developing utterance. All of the evidence from aphasia indicates that that speech or behavior which passes through a limited range of this system, whether echo-responses, jargon, stereotypies, or disconnexion responses, without a bond to the deeper cognitive source, is not accompanied by an awareness of the content. Further, the more limited range of participation accounts for the brief latency, rapidity, and explosive quality of these performances.

This should not be interpreted in support of a strict division between conceptual and linguistic organizations. What is disturbed is that process through which heard speech becomes a part of the same deep level which gives rise to verbal expression. Finally, it is of interest that echolalia has been described with lesions affecting the substance or fringe of both posterior and anterior speech zones. The symmetry of the pathological involvement is most intriguing, and leads us, in passing, to speculate whether the frontal and temporo-parietal speech regions may be organized in parallel fashion, rather than in the traditional posterior-to-anterior direction. Much work is needed, however, before this possibility can be seriously defended.

Chapter 5

CONDUCTION APHASIA

ACCORDING TO THE FIRST description by Carl Wernicke (1874), if a lesion should occur between the center of sensory speech memory and the center for motor images of words, the following picture, termed *conduction aphasia* (Leitungsaphasie) should be observed: 1) normal comprehension, 2) paraphasia in spontaneous speech, 3) paraphasia in repetition, 4) impaired writing (spontaneous and to dictation) and reading (silent and aloud), though copying would be possible. The errors in speech were thought to be similar to those of sensory aphasics, and were explained through disruption of a common mechanism, the unconscious control of the motor speech area by the sound images. The alexia was explained by the fact that learning to read involves a total dependence of the "optical image" on the sound image, without association to other centers. Thus, reading, unlike speech, could not take place through the arousal of concepts independent of sound images. Wernicke believed that in educated individuals, reading might free itself from sound imagery and in some instances, be spared. The disorder of writing was explained by the proximity of the optic-motor (writing) to the acoustic-motor (speech) pathway. This latter pathway, presumably traversing the insula, was thought to serve for the learning of speech through childhood imitation, as well as for regulation of a later acquired system by means of which speech could be produced through concepts. In this early paper, Wernicke presented two cases of conduction aphasia, remarkable for the lack of any mention of their ability to repeat. Both patients were anomic, with alexia and agraphia, and illustrate the fact that at this stage Wernicke placed at least as much emphasis on the reading and writing difficulties as those of repetition. In a later article (1908), he referred again to conduction aphasia, noting that, after 30 years, it was still ". . . impossible to describe a uniform clinical picture on (an) empiric foundation." At this time, he emphasized the deficit in repetition as of central importance, as well as the patient's ability to criticize his own errors in speaking. He also admitted that the conducting path-

way had not been clearly correlated with insular lesions, and postulated the pathway to have the additional functions of automatic or
echolalic repetition, and repetition of unknown or meaningless
words.

Lichtheim (1885) supported Wernicke's description, adding a case
of his own with autopsy. This patient, a 46-year-old laborer, was able
to repeat single words fairly well, but showed defects in sentence
repetition similar to those of "volitional" speech. Perhaps because
of the findings in this case, Lichtheim argued that since repetition
and spontaneous speech could occur through conveyance of impulses
from the "concept" center to the motor speech center, both functions should be disturbed in similar fashion by interruption of the
older pathway. In the same year, Dejerine devoted a paper to the
problem of localization. He argued that the insula was the site of
passage of two tracts, one connecting the center of visual and auditory
memory with the motor center, subserving automatic repetition, and
another tract, connecting ideational centers with the motor speech
center for voluntary speech. A lesion of insula involving the first
tract alone would spare voluntary speech, while if both pathways
were involved, there would be defects in voluntary speech as well
as repetition. The subject was then discussed at length by Freud in
1891, who noted that in spite of all the controversy, not one acceptable
anatomical case had yet been observed, nor did he think it likely
that one would ever be observed. Freud argued that repetition and
voluntary expression were not independent functions subserved by
separate pathways, and for this reason rejected the Wernicke-
Lichtheim account.

Pick (1898; 1931) described another case with autopsy, and discussed the act of repetition in some detail. He pointed out the close
bonds between repetitive and volitional speech, and attempted to
explain the defect in conduction aphasia by an impaired attention
factor, directed chiefly to the motor act of speaking. He also pointed
out that many patients will give the appearance of better comprehension through lip-reading, thus helping to eliminate one possible
source of error in the evaluation of such cases. The notion of
Wernicke's that paraphasia resulted from damage to the sensory
speech center was refuted by the finding of paraphasia with lesions
outside this area. Pick described disorders in which the word: is
neither understood nor repeated; is not understood but automatically
repeated; is not understood but voluntarily repeated; and is understood through a correct repetition.

Goldstein (1948) devoted much attention to this syndrome. He thought that the condition had been misnamed, for the symptoms did not reflect an interruption of a conducting pathway, but an impairment of the central part of language. For this reason, he termed it "Central" aphasia, placing emphasis on the paraphasia as reflecting a disturbance of inner speech. The syndrome was thought to consist of: impairment of spontaneous speech and, to a lesser degree, comprehension; paralexia and paragraphia; literal, and less often, verbal paraphasia; disturbances in repetition; and spelling difficulties. Goldstein argued that the symptoms related to a de-differentiation within a central speech apparatus outside the primary auditory speech area, which, following Wernicke, he mistakenly localized to insula. In regard to the repetition disturbance, he commented *a propos* a case of partial word-deafness, that speech comprehension may take place through the arousal, by the sound complex, of a sphere of ideas even though the perception is insufficient to awaken the individual idea, i.e. to repeat the presented word. In this explanation, he foreshadows a more contemporary account of the repetition disorder as a function of the specificity of the task demanded, rather than the interruption of a particular function-pathway.

Following Goldstein, the importance of inner speech was stressed by Conrad (1948) and Hecaen *et al.* (1955), the latter authors considering the disturbance to be deep (prelinguistic) along the path from thought to speech, affecting that process which elaborates the temporal organization of the phrase.

Konorski *et al.* (1961) discussed the condition as audio-verbal aphasia and postulated an interruption of the arcuate fasciculus. They emphasized the repetition defect, the good comprehension, and a "fluent agrammatism" (*sic*) in speech. Repetition was particularly impaired for nonsense and unfamiliar words. Naming was variable, but could be superior to repetition. Subsequently, Geschwind (1965) more fully described the clinical picture, as consisting of fluent well-articulated speech with literal paraphasia, circumlocution, and marked naming difficulty. Comprehension is quite good, but repetition is poor, often with a dissociation in the repetition of numbers and words. Geschwind accepted Konorski's view of the importance of arcuate fasciculus, and discussed in some detail a proposed anatomy. It is of interest that, in spite of the observation of poor naming in these patients, it is the repetition that is singled out for consideration.

In addition to these interpretations, conduction aphasia has also been considered a variety of sensory aphasia (Liepmann and Pappenheim, 1914), an abortive form of word-deafness (Kleist, 1962), a combination of partial auditory aphasia with inattention to external stimuli (Stengel and Lodge Patch, 1955; this representing essentially a synthesis of the views of Liepmann and Pick), and for Luria (1966), either a failure to adequately discriminate the phonemes of presented words or a form of (kinesthetic) motor aphasia. The condition has been extensively studied from the linguistic standpoint by Dubois *et al.* (1964). These authors point out that repetition is not an autonomous linguistic process, and characterize conduction aphasia as a disturbance of encodage (expression) at the level of phonemic programming. They consider it to be an expressive aphasia which relates to motor aphasia as, in the area of gesture, ideomotor apraxia relates to limb-kinetic apraxia. In a recent study of phonemic errors in patients with Wernicke's aphasia, Boller and Vignolo (1966) found support for this view, and argued on the basis of their findings that defects of repetition and naming reflect a common underlying disorder, ". . . the disruption of the mechanism of phonemic encoding."

The pathological anatomy of conduction aphasia has always been in great dispute. In his first work, Wernicke postulated lesions in insula, but later, as mentioned, had reason to doubt this localization. Goldstein also initially emphasized insular lesions, and only later stressed some of the uncertainties. In one of the first cases in the English literature, Pershing (1900) argued that the supramarginal gyrus, not the insula, was the site of pathology, and most current opinion (Ajuriaguerra and Hecaen, 1956) would now seem in general agreement with this localization. The principal anatomical theories consistent with this localization are those of Kleist (1916; 1962; see also Liepmann and Pappenheim, 1914; Goldstein, 1948; Konorski *et al.*, 1961; and Geschwind, 1965). Kleist's most important case (Spratt) was a fifty-year-old ambidexterous man with difficulty in repetition developing out of an initial word-deafness. Comprehension was good and reading aloud was preserved. On postmortem examination, lesions were in T1 and T2 on the left side extending to supramarginal gyrus, with undercutting of left Heschl's gyrus and destruction of left auditory radiations on that side. Kleist argued that the destruction of left auditory area was so severe that comprehension must have occurred through right temporal lobe. He goes on to say that "the pathways for repetition . . . must have passed from the right temporal lobe through the damaged left temporal lobe to the frontal lobe, but were blocked by the gross left temporal softening.

This resulted in difficulty in repetition with paraphasic distortion of literal elements." The problem with this explanation is that if the patient has, in effect, an isolation of the receiving right auditory area, it should be impossible to carry on a conversation with him at all, since no speech whatever will pass over to the left side. If on the other hand, commissural pathways posterior to the connections between auditory association areas are utilized, then it would not be the disconnection *per se* that is responsible for the repetition difficulty. Another possibility of course is that the right hemisphere both comprehends and carries out repetition, the imperfections in the latter due to intrinsic right-sided limitations rather than interruption of a connection to the opposite hemisphere. Geschwind (1965) has discussed the problem of the anatomy of this disorder in detail. The lesion is held to involve the arcuate fasciculus, a multisynaptic (and monosynaptic) bidirectional pathway, presumably serving auditory-verbal responses, passing from T1 posteriorly under the supramarginal gyrus and forward in parietal operculum to inferior frontal gyrus.

Before passing on to a more current account of conduction aphasia, it is worth pointing out some of the shortcomings of the classical approach. To begin with, repetition of incomprehensible or meaningless words, which for Wernicke was mediated by a postulated acoustic-motor pathway, is the most difficult of repetition tasks for all aphasic patients, so that with this disability, which should be characteristic of conduction aphasia, we are dealing more with an index of the complexity of the task than with a primitive function. Further, automatic repetition or echolalia, which has been attributed to the function of the conduction pathway, does not occur in the normal state, all repetitions passing through the "voluntary" or conceptual system. Thus, with regard to meaningless or foreign phrases, conduction aphasia would represent only the subtlest of repetition disturbances, and with regard to echolalia, but the absence of a pathological symptom. Another problem is that of the account of paraphasia in speech and repetition as due to the loss of a regulating influence by the earlier pathway on a later acquired voluntary system. This notion was obviously somewhat *ad hoc,* necessitated by the need to explain paraphasias in "sensory" aphasia with destruction of the "sensory speech area." The theory, however, requires that the paraphasia of the conduction aphasic be accounted for along the same lines. Thus, we should not expect much difference in speech between the Wernicke's aphasic (with damage to T1) and the conduction aphasic, with interruption of arcuate fasciculus, which is an outflow tract from Wernicke's area, i.e. there should be no difference between lesion of the "center" and lesion of its projection. Yet the speech of the Wernicke's aphasic is distinguished mainly by verbal para-phasias, the conduction aphasic by literal paraphasias, a difference which the classical account does not explain.

One principal source of trouble for the classical view has been the separation of repetition into automatic and voluntary forms. The fact that there should be two systems, one for imitative learning and one for speech through concepts, seems highly unlikely. As Freud (1891) pointed out, ". . . it is impossible to understand how practise in the use of a fibre system should result in its abandonment and in the choice of another." Certainly, there is not even strong evidence that names are learned by repeating them. The repetition may be the manifestation, not the origin, of speech learning. Indeed, for the most part, children do not simply echo words they have heard; rather, words are learned in relation to concepts. The latter are not devel-oped through the action of a secondary system after imitative learn-ing, but are acquired *with* the words themselves. Further, it could be argued that the sounds of language are not truly learned at all, only their concatenations. In pre-language babbling, infants spontaneously produce the articulations of all languages. Thus, learning a language is as much a matter of losing irrelevant speech sounds through disuse. Jakobson (1968) quotes with approval Van Ginnekin's characteriza-tion of language development in a Dutch child as progressing ". . . from general human language to Dutch." Moreover, the lack of resemblance of the approximations of childhood imitation to the precision of echo speech, commented on by Isserlin (1936), and the utter difference between rapid echolalic repetition without awareness, and labored repetition of foreign words with awareness, as well as the variety of echolalic responses seen clinically, are not at all ac-counted for by Wernicke's theory, nor does his theory account for the relation of these performances to learning and word understand-ing. These clearly go beyond the capacities of a word-memory center independent of comprehension, for the young child repeats poorly what the echolalic repeats well, and in echolalic patients there is often better performance with unfamiliar languages than with the mother tongue, i.e. echolalia is inversely related to language learning. Finally, if the arcuate fasciculus transmits *all* auditory-verbal material, it must be explained why word-associations, numbers and conversational speech are less impaired, and why gram-matical words are more difficult to repeat than substantives. If some of these functions occur through other pathways, why is the defect in spontaneous speech similar to, though less severe than, that of repetition?

With regard to the anatomical basis of the syndrome, there is evidence (Geschwind, 1965) that the tract is also present in apes. We may wonder what function it serves, since most primate vocalizations are seen across species lines, suggesting innate rather than learned factors. If the limitations in the ape are "peripheral," why then is a functionless structure so prominent in their brains? Further, as this is a multisynaptic as well as monosynaptic pathway, and bidirectional, can we speak strictly of a defect in conduction? Surely, cne must suppose some processing to take place between Wernicke's and Broca's area apart from transmission. That this is the case is indicated by the localization of conduction aphasia to one point in the arcuate fasciculus, the supramarginal gyrus, whereas were this truly a conduction defect lesions anywhere in the pathway should produce a similar picture. While it is true that lesions along the Sylvian lip will produce disturbances in repetition of various types, so will such lesions interfere with conversational speech. If processing along the path of the arcuate fasciculus is admitted, the arcuate zone would boil down to the classical speech area. The disturbance in repetition would then represent only a disturbance of expressive speech tested under the conditions of repetition. It is necessary, therefore, to look for alternatives to the associationist view of the arcuate fasciculus. The most probable of these are that it acts as an "internal feedback" control on a posterior speech generating system, that it modulates activity between two systems organized in parallel, or possibly, going back to Wernicke's original idea, that it exerts a synchronizing or priming effect on the anterior articulatory apparatus. Such interpretations would satisfy the objections raised to the classical account, account for the pathway in apes, and obviate the postulation of a special function of repetition.

CLINICAL PICTURE

First of all we may say that at least as a clinical syndrome there is no doubt that conduction aphasia exists, and that, as Geschwind (1965) has pointed out, it is much more common than generally supposed. The syndrome may, uncommonly, be the presenting feature of a traumatic or vascular lesion, though more often appears as a deterioration of an anomic condition, or as a stage in the improvement of Wernicke's or transcortical sensory aphasia. Once established, it is not unusual for the conduction aphasic to remain stable over prolonged periods. The clinical picture is as follows.

   Comprehension ordinarily is mildly impaired, though in some cases, especially in those which develop out of an anomia, or with a history of left-handedness or ambidexterity, it may be exceptionally well-preserved. Patients are able to respond to complex commands and distinguish correct from incorrect grammatical forms. They are able to select the word failed on repetition from a group, either written or spoken. Difficulty in phonemic discrimination is not a common finding. The possibility of lip-reading should be checked for, though it is uncertain to what extent this facilitates repetition.

   Conversational speech is fluent, usually containing abundant literal paraphasias, particularly where the disorder is in relation to a resolving Wernicke's aphasia. Verbal paraphasias though present are less common. In cases associated with an anomia, paraphasia may be minimal or absent (e.g. cases of Hecaen *et al.,* 1955; Goldstein and Marmor, 1938). In the former group, speech is ordinarily active and more easily elicited while in the latter group there may be considerable poverty of expression. Ideally, the patient should have more speech available to him than a few words and cliché phrases, for otherwise the dissociation between spontaneous and repetitive speech, essential to the diagnosis, cannot be clearly established.

   Repetition is impaired to a degree that appears surprising in view of the conversational ability and preserved comprehension. Errors consist of literal paraphasias, and occasional verbal paraphasias within sphere. The target word or word meaning usually can be distinguished in the response. The paraphasia may be evident even at the phrase level, where it strives toward a simpler form, e.g., "What is the time" for "What time is it." Characteristically, the difficulty is greater for polysyllabic than monosyllabic words, particularly where the length has a low information content, and usually worse for phrases than single words. Dubois *et al.* (1964) have pointed out that for significative items, multisyllabic words are repeated better than monosyllables, while for nonsignificative items, the reverse is true. According to Hecaen (1967), up to three syllables, neologisms are more disturbed than words, but beyond this, both are impaired to an equal degree depending on length. Similarly, there is a greater difficulty with unfamiliar than familiar words of the same length, up to three or four syllables, and in polyglots, more difficulty with later acquired languages. The importance of the information content to repetition is reflected in the greater difficulty with grammatical words than with substantives. Some cases may show improvement for words which are embedded in phrases over those presented in isolation. This may be seen at the simplest level. For example, a patient unable to repeat the word *man,* when presented with *the man,* may produce "man" successfully, dropping the article. Complex phrases, phrases with dependent clauses, or two clauses joined by "and" are extremely difficult for these patients. Single letters may be repeated better than words and numbers better than letters. Patients are said to have greater difficulty with opposites requiring a morphological addition, such as just-unjust, than with those differing in structure, such as false-true (Dubois *et al.,* 1964). A fairer test, however, is that requiring morphological subtraction; if this is done, little difference may appear with the two opposite forms. Word associations may be done somewhat better. Repetition of tapped or spoken rhythms is poor, though apraxia may intervene. There may also be lability of attention to word presentations, suggesting a deficit in auditory attention. This, however, does not appear to be a decisive factor as disorders of repetition may, at times, be accompanied by intense concentration on the examination and repeated frustrating attempts. In spite of efforts at self-correction, there is inconstant awareness of the utterance. At times it seems that patients are less aware of correct than incorrect repetitions. If the incorrect repetition is repeated back to the patient, it will usually be judged as incorrect, but not always recognized as the response given by the patient on the repetition test. Repetitions very similar to the target word, e.g. vindow for window, are more likely to be accepted by the patient as correct than those which are quite different (see also discussion).

An important part of the testing is for digit and word-span. The patient should be able to remember a series of digits or words sufficiently long enough to rule out a short-term memory deficit as a factor limiting repetition. This is particularly important, since patients who are able to repeat single words are often included in the conduction aphasia group, because of a difficulty with phrase or sentence length material. At the other extreme, patients with poor span should not be considered conduction aphasics for their failure to repeat sentences.

Naming is invariably poor, with defects identical to those in repetition. This is true for confrontation naming as well as naming to description. Colors may be named better than objects, in contrast to amnesic aphasia, where colors are generally poor. Cueing is directly related to repetition. If the patient can repeat single words fairly well, then some degree of phonemic, and to a lesser extent contextual, cueing will be possible. If repetition is impaired for single words, there will be no response to phonemic cueing, even if the cue provides all but the final syllable of the word. *Reading* comprehension is usually preserved. Reading aloud is often poor, with literal paralexia. The ability to read aloud ordinarily corresponds to repetition and naming performance. In Kleist's case of presumed "disconnection," reading aloud was possible, and in the similar case of Liepmann and Pappenheim (1914), words could be read correctly which were repeated with paraphasia. This suggests the possibility that the conduction aphasic with the anatomical situation observed by Kleist should be able to read aloud, a capacity which would allow the two anatomical forms to be distinguished. In Case 4, however, where this mechanism may well have been present, reading aloud was markedly defective and in another personal autopsied case with good auditory and poor reading comprehension, complete destruction of left Sylvian region and Wernicke's area suggested a dissociation in the hemispheric action concerning these two functions. *Writing* is poor, spontaneous and to dictation, with paragraphia comparable to that in speech. Copying may be possible. A dissociation between spontaneous writing, and writing to dictation, such as that in speech, has not been observed. Spelling is usually quite defective. *Facial and limb apraxia* are common though not invariable accompaniments. According to Stengel (1955), pain asymbolia may also occur.

Case 4

A fifty-eight-year-old woman was admitted to the hospital in August, 1968 with a two month history of headache, memory impairment and difficulty in speaking. Examination disclosed mild right-sided weakness, an "expressive" speech defect, and inability to carry out movements with her arms on verbal direction. EEG showed left fronto-temporal slowing and a left carotid arteriogram demonstrated a tumor mass in the left posterior parietal region. At craniotomy, a large subcortical cystic mass was demonstrated, biopsied, and drained of 40 cc fluid. Frozen tissue diagnosis was astrocytoma grade III, and no attempt at further removal was made. Following surgery some improvement was noted, but her condition stabilized and little change occurred until May, 1969, when she precipitously went into coma with signs of herniation. Management was conservative; death occurred one week later. The results of repeated examinations between February and April, 1969 are described below.

Neurological Examination

Cranial nerves were normal except for difficulty in eye movements. Though E.O.M. were full and conjugate, at times there was impairment both of following a moving object, and in maintaining fixation on an object once motionless. At times she was unable to look at, touch or point to an object in either field, though at other times difficulty maintaining fixation was the only disturbance. OKN was absent with movement into the left visual field (loss of quick component to R), inconstant into the right. The visual fields were full on tangent screen testing, though initially right inattention and later, right homonymous hemianopia could be demonstrated. *Motor* testing revealed mild inconstant right hemiparesis. The patient was apraxic; *reflexes* were increased on the right side but both toes were flexor. *Sensory* testing was normal to pin, light touch and vibration, but position sense and graphesthesia were slightly reduced on right. Stereognosis was normal.

Coordination testing, gait and Romberg were normal.

Mental Status

The patient appeared bright and eager to cooperate. Her memory for current and past events was good. She gave a history of left-handedness in early life, converted to right-handedness at age 4. There was a suggestion that she may have stuttered at this time. Past age four there was evidently no speech difficulty, and she has always written with her right hand. Family history was negative for left-handedness.

Comprehension was relatively well-preserved. Verbal and written commands were done well, and she could engage in a fairly complex conversation. Spoken words were matched well with object-pictures or written words. She discriminated 24/24 paired words, responded well to yes/no questions, and distinguished grammatically and semantically correct from incorrect sentences.

Spontaneous speech was fluent with occasional literal paraphasias. There was frequent hesitation, stammering, difficulty initiating a phrase and repeated interjections such as ". . . your baby could do better than I can," and "I can't do anything, what's wrong with me." An example of her speech is given below:

Q. How have you been feeling?
A. How am I going to get my spellum . . . my spelling . . . writing . . . my bye . . . bye . . . what are you going to do with this?
Q. Have you any headaches?

A. Had one three to four week . . . days, Monday, Tuesday, Wednesday, Thursday, and Thursday it started to go away. I thought I could come back in the hospital for three or four days they would tell me what was the matter so I could get, I want to go to work again.

Q. Are you having trouble with your eyes?

A. Comes and goes. As long as I don't use them it's fine. If I use them its law . . . lawn, so I leave them alone.

Q. Can you give me the date (Feb. 6)?

A. It's the fu . . . 1–2–3–4–5, oh I don't know, there seems to me there must be something I could do but I don't know what it is.

Q. How long have you lived in California?

A. About thirty some odd years or more and practically all or par, our p . . . p . . . par. Oh, anyway what am I going to do?

Q. Where do you live now?

A. I have been spa . . . staying with a friend of mine, but I do hate to imp . . . impose on her. I want to pay my own way. Do they have some sort of chart where you can take this tee . . . tee?

Counting was performed well forward if given the first unit of the series, but she was unable to count backward.

Repetition performance was extremely variable, ranging from 0 to 80% success on monosyllabic words on different days. This variability appeared out of proportion to the fluctuation in other speech functions. Failures were characterized by hesitations, perseverations, stammering and literal paraphasias. Verbal paraphasias were uncommon. There was contamination by previously (successfully) repeated words. Polysyllabic words were generally worse than monosyllabic, as were words from a foreign language. Relatively automatic words such as Coca-cola were also performed poorly. At times, long phrases were handled much better than single words but usually with some change in the phrase. For example, *I am feeling very well* was repeated as "I am feeling very well thank you." *Can you get me a glass of water* was repeated as "Would you get me a glass of water?" However, when asked to repeat each word of these phrases individually, she failed completely. This was also true for long numbers. For example, 3,407 was repeated accurately, but she could not repeat 3, 4 and 7 separately. In general, numbers were not handled strikingly better than words. For example, "the eleven plus A" was given for 11 plus 8 and "three-fourths" for three-quarters. She was unable to reproduce tapped rhythms, and had great difficulty with sound repetition. For example, "burz" for buzz;

"shush" for sh; "k/puk" for k/p; "m/nut" for m/n. She was able to give the opposite of words such as poor and true, but had great difficulty with words requiring a morphological addition, such as sincere, visible, happy. Simple word associations were done fairly well. Repetition of nonsense and improprietous words was done poorly; nor did she seem to notice the inappropriateness of the request. At times she would repeat single words correctly, in echolalic fashion, but seemed unaware of having done so for she would then attempt to evoke the word again. It appeared that successful repetitions, of which she was aware, had a slightly longer latency (three seconds or so) and at still longer latencies (3–10 seconds) repetition was almost nil with evidence of considerable frustration. Similarly, if a series of single words was repeated well in an automatic, though not necessarily echolalic manner, a slight change in the rhythm of the presentation would bring about complete failure of repetition. Giving a word and showing the object simultaneously did not facilitate repetition. Finally, that the failure to repeat was not due to a defect in verbal memory was shown by her ability to point to an object named after a few minutes delay though still unable to repeat its name.

Naming was markedly impaired and showed rapid fatigue but was aided by contextual cueing. Tactile and auditory naming were similarly impaired. In contrast she could point to objects, match objects and select the appropriate spoken or written name from a group. Color naming and object-picture naming were impaired to an equal degree.

Reading aloud was almost impossible because of marked literal paralexia. Written commands were followed poorly, but matching of written to spoken words and words to pictures was done well. On one occasion, she was seen reading the *Saturday Review* in the waiting room. *Spelling* aloud was very poor, but she recognized a short word spelled to her. *Writing* was markedly impaired, perhaps done better with the left hand than the right. Occasionally she would voluntarily switch to her left hand in exasperation. There was only slight improvement on writing to dictation. Copying was better but nonetheless quite disturbed, with no difference noted between words, numbers, or familiar anagrams such as USA. Transliteration was possible. There was no improvement with eyes closed.

Calculations were performed poorly. Simple computations could be done on paper though not mentally.

Constructional ability was markedly impaired for simple cube reproduction, overlapping figures, drawings, matchstick construction and mapdrawing. She was, however, able to find her way about the city by streetcar quite well. Facial identification was normal. There was no right-left discrimination. Finger identification was relatively normal. Stereopsis and visual memory were normal.

Musical recognition was normal. She could not be encouraged to sing, nor did she read musical notation in the past.

Praxis showed considerable impairment. Spontaneous handling of objects and use of hands was normal. She was unable to yawn, whistle, chatter, blow a kiss, nor could she wave goodbye, pretend to light a match, knock on the door, or thread a needle to command. There was substitution of body part for object, such as putting her hand in her mouth on being told to brush her teeth. There was only slight improvement with mimicry and object use. There was disorganization of complex actions such as lighting and smoking a cigarette or calling someone on the telephone, with or without objects suggested an ideational component. There was no dressing apraxia. Routine audiometry was normal and sound localization was normal. The patient was able to indicate accurately the number of tones (from 1–10) presented to either ear.

Wada Test

Following angiography, an intracarotid injection of 200 mg Sodium Amytal® in 10% solution was performed. The left and right side were done at a three-day interval. On *left* injection, there was momentary dazing and confusion which lasted about 30 seconds, followed by uncontrollable crying which cleared in about two minutes. A slight right hemiparesis was noted. Thereafter, she was able to point to objects named and perform appropriate facial movements to command. Repetition, which was about 50% accurate for monosyllabic words prior to test, was not appreciably changed; motor series were performed well and conversational speech was not altered by the injection. After *right* injection there was sudden loss of consciousness, deviation of the eyes to the right and dense left hemiparesis for four minutes with clearing by six minutes post-injection. Gradually, speech returned with marked literal paraphasia approaching jargon. She was able to point to objects on command. Repetition was nil, with severe perseveration and literal paraphasia. There was no mood change.

In summary, a fifty-eight-year-old right-handed woman with a possible history of left-handedness in early life, who developed symptoms of a left parieto-occipital tumor ten months prior to her death. There was inconstant right hemiparesis, bilateral limb and facial apraxia, constructional deficits with labile fixation and inability to locate objects presented in either visual field. Speech examination revealed good comprehension, reduced but fluent speech with marked difficulties in word-finding and repetition, characterized by literal paraphasia, stammering or complete failure. Silent reading was apparently preserved, but reading aloud, response to written commands, writing and copying were severely impaired.

Neuropathological examination (by Dr. N. Malamud, Letterman General Hospital) revealed a surgical defect 3 × 5 cm (Fig. 4a), oval-

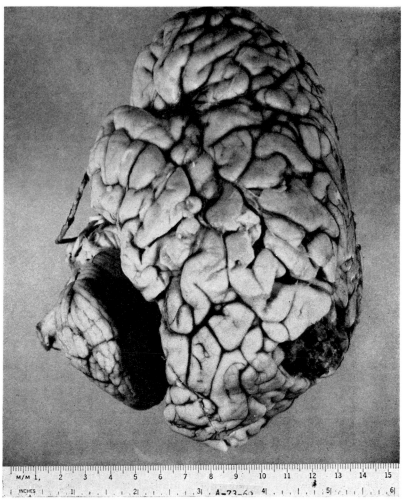

Figure 4a.

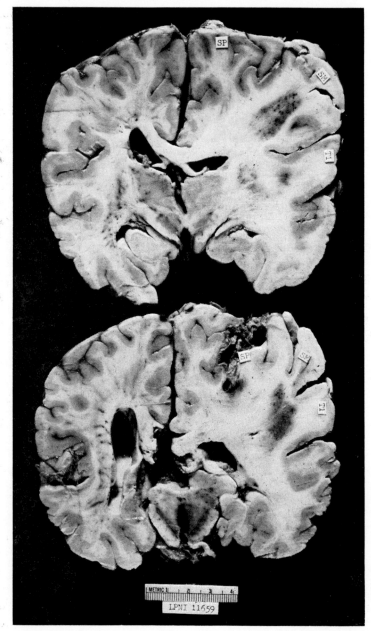

Figure 4b.

shaped, extending from the posterior aspect of the superior parietal gyrus as it joins the superior occipital gyrus, lateralward, and extending into the occipital cortex and the upper half of the angular gyrus. The lesion was well delimited and healed. In coronal sections (Fig. 4b), there was considerable edema of the white matter of the left parietal lobe, causing deviation of the midline and a mild subcallosal herniation, and edema and terminal hemorrhage in the white matter of T1 and the supramarginal gyrus. Microscopic diagnosis was meningioma.

Case 5

A seventy-one-year-old right-handed man, was admitted to a nearby hospital in December, 1969 with a presumed stroke, after a sudden collapse followed by confusion, agitation and transient right-hemiparesis. Speech was described as mumbling and logorrheic. He was transferred to the Aphasia Unit, Boston Veterans Administration Hospital six weeks later. Neurological examination was normal except for minimal weakness in the right arm and mild reflex asymmetry. Sensory examination, cranial nerves and visual fields were normal. The general mental state was one of agitation and depression, with constant reference to dying. The brain scan showed uptake in left posterior Sylvian region.

Speech was fluent, logorrheic and grossly paraphasic with many neologisms. He seemed intermittently aware of errors in speech and expressed great frustration in repeated attempts toward a correct statement, though he was not able to self-correct his errors. Asked to explain his difficulty in speaking, he said: "Well, its very hard to because I don't know what it would my pi why what's wrong with it, but I can't food, its food and rood, to read the way I used to do all right off but I can't now you see its arise taw eat and everything read and write and read and vite and everything I did my own self no help. . . ." Motor series were performed with many neologisms and literal paraphasias. In fact, automatisms appeared to increase the paraphasia. For example, for *roses are red, violets are blue,* he said: "waves is pees, varets a roo."

Comprehension was fairly good if he could be silenced during testing. He was able to point to single items and body parts well, handled simple yes/no questions, and simple functional descriptions accurately, and was often correct on questions of even greater grammatical complexity, such as "Do you have lunch before breakfast?" He could indicate which sentence of a simple group spoken to him was grammatically correct. However, above a simple level of testing, comprehension was certainly impaired, with difficulty in prepositions, genitive and passive-active sentences. On one occasion, he was given, with eyes closed, a series of 13 sounds such as knocking on a door, dialing a telephone, and was asked to name the sound, point to its source, or duplicate it. On this test, he recognized 5 of 13 sounds, only 2 of which, whistling and coughing, he identified by name. There was also difficulty recognizing familiar melodies hummed or whistled to him.

Naming was extremely poor for objects, body parts and colors, with marked literal paraphasia, neologism and augmentation. For example, for cheek he said "expee," for cup "pepva," for pipe "pope." There was no modality preference. Slight improvement on cueing was observed, and he could usually select the correct name from a group. At times he would name quite correctly. They were usually rapid and immediate responses, and most of the time he did not seem to be aware of having given the correct word. For example, asked to show his wrist, he replied, "wrist, wrist, I can't say it, I can't pronounce it (touching his wrist) ." He was then asked to name (wrist) , and said: "exfier, what do you think, gee whiz it's terrible." He was unable to name objects from description. *Spelling* was markedly deficient and he could not point to objects orally spelled. *Reading* aloud was paraphasic, e.g. "mout" for house, "sime" for climb. He was unable to follow written commands or point to written objects named. Matching objects to simple written names was about 50 percent accurate, and matching written to printed names still better. He could match written to spoken words fairly well if the words were simple and dissimilar. He could point accurately to letters and numbers named.

Writing was very poor (spontaneous and to dictation) , with only his signature possible. Copying was nil.

Repetition was similar to naming, with marked literal paraphasia and augmentation. Giving the word and showing the object at the same time did not facilitate repetition. For example, cow was "how," horse "hoise," spoon "spoze," pen "expen." As in naming he not infrequently gave the correct response but then continued to supply paraphasic variations without seeming to have awareness of a successful performance. For example, for hammer, he said: "hammer farmer pammer . . . I don't know, I don't know." Most of the time the correct repetitions were among the first few responses given, usually the initial repetition. However, accurate repetitions occurred in the middle of a flow of responses, these also having a somewhat labile and explosive character suggestively different from his other responses. At times, he would pause after such a response, uncertain as to whether it was correct or not, or registering surprise at having achieved an accurate repetition.

At such times, if asked whether the word was correct or not, he would generally say, "Yes, I think so" or "I think it was, I'm not sure." Also, he would occasionally show unexpected echolalic responses to commands during testing. For example, when asked to show how he would saw wood, he said: "saw wood what a saw would I would. . . ." Repetition of letters and numbers was paraphasic, e.g. "v" for g, "fee" for three. He showed a similar echolalia without awareness for these, as for words. For example, asked to repeat "s," he said: "s,s,w,f, I don't know, I can't hear it." At times a sentence could be repeated fairly well while the individual words were impossible. For example, for *The boy and the dog*, he said, "The boy and the bug," but was unable to repeat any of these words singly. At times also, overlearned phrases, such as "How are you" could be accurately repeated. Repetition of tapped and oral rhythms was poor.

Praxis was quite impaired in either arm, with slight improvement on imitation, considerable improvement on object use. Facial apraxia was also present. Whole body commands were done somewhat better than limb commands, and he was able to perform better on the latter (e.g. saluting) when it was a part of a whole body sequence (e.g. coming to attention) rather than if given alone.

Constructional ability was considerably diminished. He was able to draw a square, a circle, and a triangle to command, but had difficulty copying these figures. There was no right-left disorientation or finger agnosia. Map locations and facial recognition were normal.

Comment

This patient presents a clear picture of repetition disorder with a "sensory" aphasia, in which both comprehension and expression are less impaired than repetition and naming. It is of interest that, with improvement, this patient progressed through an initial stage of moderately impaired comprehension with echolalia of single words (rarely 2 to 3 words) accompanied by increasing neologistic paraphasia in speech, to improved comprehension, mitigation of the echolalia, transition of neologistic to phonemic paraphasia, and aggravated repetition difficulty. This was not a transcortical aphasia for comprehension was too good and echolalia too infrequent and limited. But the transition through improving comprehension, diminishing echolalia and increasing repetition defect, is one that is often seen in transcortical patients. Once reaching the conduction aphasia stage, there was no further improvement over a six-month period of observation. Another feature worth emphasizing is that the patient's speech became markedly paraphasic and jargonized under the imposition of a specific task. This was seen not only in repetition, but in object naming, evocation of a specific word to description or on sentence completion, over-learned rhymes, and writing and spelling. The patient, therefore, demonstrates a transitional stage between neologistic jargon and the true or anomic, form of conduction aphasia (Case 4).

These cases illustrate the range of repetition disturbance with different aphasic syndromes. In Case 4, a posterior anomic aphasia, there was reduced, mildly paraphasic self-critical speech, with excellent comprehension. Repetition was characterized by infrequent, though definite, correct echolalic responses of single words, more frequent though still uncommon correct repetitions with uncertainty, paraphasic repetitions, and finally, complete failures which merged into the anomic disorder. In Case 5, a "sensory" type of aphasia, there was logorrheic, highly paraphasic speech, impaired self-awareness with only moderate comprehension. Correct echolalic responses of single words were given, at times 2 or 3 words were not uncommon, though most repetitions were marked by literal paraphasia. Complete failures were unusual; there was almost always some attempt toward the correct word.

Discussion

It is important to understand that in a patient with fluent paraphasic speech, with mainly literal paraphasia, good articulation and good comprehension, repetition and naming will invariably be worse than spontaneous speech. In fact, given such a patient, the diagnosis can be predicted without testing repetition. The repetition defect is not *added on* to this picture, as inferred by the tract theory, but is an inherent part of the total syndrome. Essential, therefore, to an interpretation of conduction aphasia is an account of the act of repetition, for this is the pivotal defect in the syndrome, and the most difficult of explanation. The conduction aphasic does not merely fail to repeat; he may of course fail completely, but he may also repeat accurately, he may repeat erroneously with various kinds of errors, and he may or may not be aware of his correct or incorrect repetitions. This variability is seen in the two cases presented where at least four different repetition performances were observed, these varying according to the time elapsed after word-presentation. The most immediate and echolalic repetitions, though infrequent, were accurate and appeared to be outside the patient's awareness. Words repeated after a slight delay, but still in a relatively automatic way, though successful, might be followed by "No, that's not right," or "That isn't it," the patient then going on to attempt to evoke the correct word. A slightly longer delay, of perhaps 2 seconds or so, gave even more trouble in repetition with increasing paraphasia and self-correction, and if the patient delayed (or was asked to delay) for a still longer time, e.g. 3 to 10 seconds, repetition could be reduced to zero, at which point the disorder seemed clearly to be a part of the word-finding difficulty.

At times, as in Case 4, correct repetitions without full awareness occurred during a logorrheic burst, along with paraphasic attempts. Although here we are not dealing strictly with the latency after presentation, there is a factor of brief latency with respect to the verbal flow that appears significant. In either case, however, as the automaticity of the response decreased, repetition passed from a nonparaphasic echolalic stage, through literal paraphasia, to a stage in which scarcely more than the first sound or syllable of the word could be produced. Further, awareness of speech output seemed to parallel this change in repetition, passing from nonawareness, to uncertainty, to awareness of paraphasic errors with self-correction, and finally, to awareness of failure in word-evocation with a great deal of frustration. Stengel (1955) has also described in one of his patients: 1) correct repetitions without awareness, 2) correct repetitions with surprise or uncertainty over their occurrence, 3) paraphasic repetitions and 4) complete failure. These four varieties of repetition are seen, to a greater or lesser degree, in most conduction aphasics. In Case 5, for example, echolalic, echo-like, and paraphasic repetitions were seen, the anomic form adumbrated by the logorrhea. These different repetitions are important clues to processes taking place at evolving stages in speech production, and for this reason, each form will be discussed separately.

With regard to the echolalic responses, these, if looked for, are seen in a good number of patients, and though ordinarily only at the single word level, are nevertheless a link to the transcortical aphasias. Although these might be explained by the action of the opposite hemisphere, this is unsatisfactory for a few reasons. Firstly, one might ask why they should occur at all, what with the limited speech function of the minor side, or why they should be limited to single words. There is the problem of their occurrence in the flow of speech, and, if left frontal region is the "final common pathway" for speech production, it remains to be explained how the opposite hemisphere can assume control. If on the other hand, the left frontal region is involved, why should there be lack of awareness? Further, both transcortical and "isolation-syndrome" echolalia could also be explained in this manner, and then we have not really settled the repetition problem, only shifted it to the other hemisphere. Another and more compelling alternative is the possibility that echolalic responses, whatever their hemisphere of origin, reflect a stage in the development of speech within that hemisphere, i.e. as a point of transition on the dominant side to a higher level, or on minor side as the furthest attainable stage. At any event, the echolalic responses are clearly more common in the "sensory" form of conduction aphasia than the anomic form. Further, as in Case 5, there may be occasional bursts of echolalia for commands as well. It is easy to see how this patient might have shifted, with a little more speech imperception and a little more echolalia, to the category of transcortical sensory aphasia. On the other hand, a mitigation of the echolalia and an improvement in comprehension would bring him closer to the type of conduction defect seen in Case 4. This transition we have seen occasionally in our aphasic population. In the improvement of transcortical aphasia there is passage from a state of poor comprehension with echolalia to one of improved comprehension with infrequent echolalia and marked paraphasia in repetition (i.e. conduction aphasia).* The second form of repetition disorder, echo-responses with uncertainty or surprise, indicates that the echoing is related to a process that is continuous with normal speech. This also argues against an origin in the opposite hemisphere. The problem of echolalia in general, and a tentative explanation, are discussed more fully with the transcortical aphasias.

With regard to the next form of repetition disturbance, paraphasia with self-correction, the following points can be made. Firstly, the paraphasia in repetition does not differ markedly from that in naming, or in spontaneous speech. The occurrence of literal paraphasia in repetition is not the outstanding feature for it occurs in all forms of verbal expression, except in echolalia. Therefore we may ask, what is the significance of self-correction of paraphasic responses, and why is repetition quantitatively more severely paraphasic than conversational speech. Certainly we can say that while in Wernicke's aphasia there is no attempt to self-correct at all, the conduction aphasic will try to produce the demanded word, and may, like the anomic, be frustrated by his unsuccessful attempts. Probably this reflects an interference in some system responsible for internal control. That is, the attempts at self-correction do not indicate that the mechanisms

---

*This, incidentally, is to my mind a decisive argument against the tract theory of conduction aphasia, as we can hardly expect the repetition pathway to be undergoing deterioration as the patient continues to improve.

for self-correction are intact, but rather that the conduction aphasic has awareness of speech productions *without* good ability to correct them, whereas the Wernicke's aphasic, unaware of his errors, does not utilize these mechanisms, whether intact or not. In the latter, the comprehension disturbance interferes with "external" monitoring, while the internal system may be relatively unimpaired. In the conduction aphasic, there is "external" monitoring and an impaired internal mechanism. Probably, literal paraphasia is the manifestation of involvement of this system; thus, most Wernicke's aphasics show verbal, not literal, paraphasia. Concerning the difference in severity between repetition and spontaneous speech, it does not appear necessary to invoke a separate pathway to account for this. If one presents the conduction aphasic a word for repetition (e.g. key), and at the same time allows him to see and touch the object, i.e. key, there will ordinarily be no change in his performance. Or if one asks the conduction aphasic to give the name of a specific item which is not present, being careful to avoid obvious cueing, such as "An object to open a lock," he will show defects identical to those in repetition and naming. This is usually taken to indicate an accompanying anomia, and the patient is described as having two separate defects, one of naming and one of repetition, the paraphasia contaminating both performances. This derives from the fact that anomics ordinarily repeat well. Yet, repetition is never impaired in the face of normal naming. In part, the problem concerns the specificity of response demanded. Thus, in visual or tactile naming, the patient is required to give a specific word (i.e. name) for a discrete object. This demands a high degree of specificity of both perception and expression. In repetition, the situation is the same, it only appears more striking for one expects an easier match between given and spoken word. Yet an equally demanding particularization of perception and expression is required. In this respect, there is a relation between naming and repeating. Further, the greater difficulty in repetition than spontaneous speech has to do with the greater specificity of the former. As Stengel (1934) has pointed out, repetitive speech may be interpreted in some instances as the criterion of word implementation, for the demand is for a highly specific response. This is comparable to the disparity in the anomic between objects named to command and randomly. With regard to this problem of specificity, it is worth noting that patients with disorders of comprehension also show a tendency to understand well in conversation, but deteriorate when tested with specific words or phrases.

As the auditory perception of the conduction aphasic improves, the condition becomes, as mentioned, more noticeably a part of an amnesic aphasia. There is a shift in repetition performance from echolalia toward the paraphasic and evocatory forms. Dubois *et al.* (1964) point out that the absence of literal paraphasia in anomia is determined by the ineffective search for a word in memory, whereas in conduction aphasia, the word is known but its verbal execution impossible, this appearing as an absence of literal paraphasia in the anomic and the presence òf phonemic approximations in conduction aphasics. It is along these lines, in terms of a relationship with anomia, that one should study conduction aphasia. Certainly, the final type of repetition disorder seen, complete failure, is essentially the same as one finds, after a longer latency, in anomics. That there is not an underlying deficiency in verbal memory can be ascertained by having the patient indicate objects corresponding to the demanded name, or select the name from a spoken group, many minutes after the failure in repetition has taken place.

Regarding the *anomic* aspect of conduction aphasia, the problem is mainly one of output specification since comprehension is relatively normal. Conversational speech is less impaired for it is under few constraints, whereas naming, and especially repetition, demand a highly specific response. This is why repetition is not facilitated by giving the object for touch and vision simultaneously with the demanded name, for this only accentuates the specific nature of the task. Further, it is possible to see within anomic patients a transition to conduction aphasia. This is seen in the ability of the anomic to cue. The anomic form of conduction aphasia may be thought of as a failure of the patient to name with the most obvious of cues, the demanded word. Indeed, in conduction aphasics who recover to an anomic stage, one can often show a transition to a state where monosyllabic words can be repeated just before the time the patient begins to respond to phonemic cues. Conversely, the anomic, whose ability to cue phonemically deteriorates, will still be able to name, i.e. repeat, when cued with the whole word. This problem is also discussed with the anomic aphasias.

Thus, it will be clear why neologistic jargon improves to conduction aphasia, but the latter improves to anomia. It will also be clear why true Wernicke's aphasia with verbal paraphasia does not evolve to conduction aphasia, for the phonemic substitutions of the latter represent a level in advance of verbal encoding. The direction of these transitions is constant and predictable, and again and again indicates that the major language categories tested—speech, comprehension, naming and repetition—all change together as a unit. The anomia which evolves out of conduction aphasia is not there all the time obscured by the phonemic paraphasia. The impaired "word-finding" element in conduction aphasia has gained the level of phonemic encoding and will now have its effect in this category. Similarly, when the comprehension and speech of the jargon aphasic improves, a concealed conduction aphasia is not suddenly exposed. This improved level of comprehension and speech *constitutes* conduction aphasia.

Chapter 6

BROCA'S APHASIA

ALTHOUGH REFERENCES TO speech loss from cerebral lesions can be found as far back as the *Hippocratic Corpus* of 400 BC, the modern era is usually taken to begin with Franz Joseph Gall.* In spite of the disreputable light into which his work was subsequently thrown, there is no question but that it played an important part in drawing attention away from holistic approaches current at the time, and in opening the possibility of a cerebral localization of speech. The most influential disciple of Gall was Bouillaud, whose great contribution to the developing study of aphasia was the forceful championship, after Gall, of the frontal representation of speech. This idea was originally advanced in 1825, at which time he also distinguished between disturbances of the sign function of speech and its articulatory apparatus (i.e. internal and external speech), and noted the dissociation between gestural and vocal language. On the basis of a few cases, Bouillaud proposed that the "legislative organ of speech" resided in the anterior lobes of the brain, an hypothesis later to be confirmed by Paul Broca.

In his first paper (1861a), Broca presented the clinicopathologic findings of a fifty-one year old man (Leborgne), epileptic since youth, who presented with loss of speech of indeterminate duration. Comprehension was excellent, but all that remained to him in speech was the utterance "tan," which he used to respond to all questions. Postmortem examination revealed a large Sylvian lesion, the center and most involved point of which Broca reasoned to be the third, possibly also the second, frontal convolution. In this paper, Broca also commented that language concerned the establishment of a constant relation between an idea and a sign. The loss of speech he termed "aphemia," which he took to consist of a loss of the faculty of articulating words, in the presence of good understanding of spoken

---

*For further historical information the reader is referred to the fascinating account by Head (1926), to Benton and Joynt (1960) and to Riese (1947). The *Bulletin de l'acad. Imp.*, vol. 30, 1864–65 contains a spirited discussion, by all the principles, of the entire range of this early work.

and written language. He pointed out that utterances consisted of only a few syllables, at times only a monosyllable; he described the occurrence of stereotypies and oathes, and speculated that the condition was a kind of ataxia of movements serving for the articulation of words. Accordingly, word memory was not affected, only the movements necessary for the production of words. The impairment of the speech movements with preservation of the primitive oral motility was explained as a return to an earlier childhood stage in speech development. This paper provided the fullest account of Broca's views on the clinical picture and pathogenesis of "aphemia," and was received with considerable interest.

A few months later (1861b), a second case appeared that was to lend considerable support to Broca's position. This patient (Lelong), an eighty-four year old man with sudden onset of speech loss, one and a half years previously, had, in spite of good understanding, only a few words at his disposal. In response to questions, he replied "oui" or "non" appropriately, said "tois" (for trois) for all questions requiring numerical answers, when asked his name, said only "Lelo," and at all other times responded with "toujours." On the basis of the post-mortem findings, which revealed a more delimited lesion than in the first case confined largely to F3, Broca argued that normal speech required an intact third frontal convolution. In his third paper (1863), he commented on a series of eight autopsied cases with lesions in F3, noting the fact that all were on the left side. In his paper of 1865, he pointed out the high incidence of right hemiparesis in aphasia, and the occurrence of cases of right frontal lesion without aphasia and confirmed the left hemispheric preference and the possible role of handedness. In this paper, Broca also mentioned the hitherto unknown work of Dax (1836), in which the subject of possible left-hemispheric dominance was discussed. This paper by Dax, in view of its never having been presented or published, and the cursory and uncritical fashion in which it was composed, deserves little more than passing mention. Reviews can be found in Benton and Joynt (1960) and Critchley (1964).

Another important figure of this period was Trousseau, who is remembered today largely for a series of articles in which he criticized Broca's use of the word "aphemia." He argued that this term connoted "infamy," and suggested in its place "aphasia." Subsequently, it became customary to use "aphasia" for instances of loss of speech *and* writing, and aphemia for aphasic loss of speech alone. In London, Hughlings Jackson was well aware of the startling discoveries on the continent. Though generally sympathetic to this work, Jackson (1866) gently criticized Broca's view that the word-memory is separable from the articulatory process, arguing that those signs through which thoughts become known consist only in our power to reproduce them, word-memory being just another term for this capacity to produce words. Jackson also stressed, following Baillarger, the dissociation between voluntary and involuntary speech in aphasia, suggesting that the more habitual utterances were in special relation to minor hemisphere. In a later paper (1878), he went on to advance his important dictum, that aphasia consists of loss of the ability to *propositionize*, defining a proposition as a relation of words such as to make one new meaning. He also proposed a classification of aphasic utterances, listing:

A. Recurring Utterances
  1. Jargon (single words, e.g. "Yabby" or phrases, e.g. "Me, me committimy, pittimy, lor deah").
  2. Words (without propositional meaning, e.g. "man," "one").
  3. Phrase (without meaning, e.g. "Come on," "Oh my God").
  4. Yes and no (with or without propositional meaning).
B. Occasional Utterances
  1. Nonspeech (e.g. "Oh," "Ah," "Oh dear").
  2. Inferior speech ("That's a lie," "Yes, but you know").
  3. Real speech (occasional sentences).

Concurrent with Jackson's writings, Wernicke (1874) published a monograph which supported Broca's localization and description, but which advanced the view that the "motor speech area" was not the only speech zone. Wernicke's postulation of a posterior speech center, connected to the motor area by conduction pathways, tended to redirect thinking away from the functional approach of Broca and Jackson, toward a more anatomically oriented position. This tendency was encouraged by the writings of Bastian (1898), Lichtheim (1885), Broadbent (1878) and others, their common contribution being little more than the division of Broca's aphasia into pure motor, pure agraphic and mixed forms. This led finally to the aggressive paper of Pierre Marie (1906), in which all of these theories were criticized, however justly, but from a point of view equally severe. Head's review of this period under a chapter entitled "Chaos" is apt and exhaustive, and it is not until the papers of Pick and Isserlin that a proper reformulation of the problem appears.

According to Pick (1931), motor aphasia represents a disturbance at the most word-close stage in the process of speech development, a process which he conceptualized as an hierarchic unfolding of laminae on the path from thought to speech. Though in agreement with Broca's localization, he defined the function of this area in a somewhat different manner, viz: ". . . the physical processes corresponding to the simultaneous consciousness of meaningful thought, formulated as inner speech, are converted via Broca's center (through kinesthetic mediation) into motor sequences, which are modulated in accordance with the intonational pattern. . . ." According to Pick, there is a gradation from the mild case, with stuttering or hesitation of speech, to admixtures of defective grammatization, particularly with incorrect use of the preposition, to a stage of "motor agrammatism" in which only uninflected nouns and verbs are retained, with dropping of the small grammatical words. In more severe cases, one sees the end stage of agrammatism, viz.: the one-word sentence; and finally, only a few syllables (e.g. yes, no, the patient's name) or sounds (vowels, consonants) are possible with defects of phonation and breathing. Pick also described what he termed "linguistic puerilism" in some of these patients, a return to an infantile form of pronunciation. He noted that in milder cases, the character of the language spoken may become modified (e.g. French becomes Germanized), and that a second tongue, affected more severely than the mother tongue, may develop the accent of the former, i.e. a German's perfect English now reveals a German accent. He considered that disturbances of reading and writing were somewhat variable, and related this to the equally variable involvement of inner speech. This, along with a general functional reduction and poor speech retention, figured in the mild comprehension defect present in most patients. Pick was outspoken in his praise of Jackson, forcefully stressing the primacy of the sentence (i.e. the preposition) in the utterance. He differed from Jackson, however, in his reluctance to attribute automatic speech to the right hemisphere, noting the gradation in voluntary control that occurs and the stages of improvement of the automatism, and preferring in general to assign to automaticity a place in his unitary model of speech development, either through joint hemispheric action, or within the major hemisphere.

An excellent account of motor aphasia was given by Isserlin (1936). Following Pick, he stressed the gradation in the disorder from mild hesitation and stammering in speech, through agrammatism, to a severe stage of near muteness. In his valuable discussion of agrammatism, he noted the predominance of nouns and verbs (especially, infinitive forms), the lack of prefixes and suffixes, pronoun confusions, and the resemblance to an early stage of childhood speech, and he remarked on the occasional dissociation of spoken agrammatism and correct writing. With regard to the more severely affected patient, Kleist's demarcation of "sound muteness" and "word muteness" was strongly criticized. Isolated sounds, he pointed out, are an abstraction, and cannot be treated as units; the sounds "a" and "b" are not present in "ab," nor is the latter simply an inverted "ba." Thus, even in the simplest speech formations, linguistic factors must be recognized. Isserlin discussed the varieties of paraphasic error in Broca's aphasia, distinguishing, after Pick, Bouman and Grunbaum, and others, omissions, transpositions and distortions, as well as the great frequency of exchange between related phonemes (e.g. "b" and "p"). Isserlin noted further that polysyllabic words were more easily expressed than monosyllables, if the constituents of the former were possessed of significance. He accepted earlier statements about the accompanying defect in reading and speech comprehension, noting that for the latter, it concerned not only longer or more complex material, but also lower frequency individual words, again a most modern conception. The localization of Broca and other workers was not questioned.

Though the contribution of the German school was of major importance, particularly in the study of agrammatism and the renaissance of a functional approach, the principal interest of these workers, from the time of Carl Wernicke, was in the posterior forms of aphasia. More recent investigations of the problem, following the line of Broca and Marie, has been carried out largely in France, where the work of Alajouanine (1956; 1968) and Sabouraud *et al.* (1963) may be considered representative.

Alajouanine has been particularly concerned with the evolutive aspects of Broca's aphasia, and the dynamic interrelationships between the various symptomatic forms. Following the approach and classification of Hughlings Jackson, he emphasized the automatic nature of stereotypies, and the lack of awareness which accompanies them, in contrast to the full awareness of language deficit, and distinguished four stages over which the stereotypy resolves. Firstly, there is a stage of modification in which, through intonational adjustments, the stereotypy comes to express a wide variety of emotional states. Then, a stage of checking the stereotypy, which signals the patient's first awareness of his utterance, followed by a fluctuant period in which other expressions, stereotyped or not, come to accompany the original, now impersistent, stereotypy. Finally, there is abolition of the stereotypy, with the gradual return of speech having characteristics which are the exact opposite, viz.: slowness, laboriousness, aspontaneity and critical self-awareness. From this stage, there is resolution through either a phase of slow but grammatically correct speech, or a stage of agrammatism. Alajouanine stressed the reduced awareness of agrammatic formations in contrast to the normal grammar of spontaneous utterances, salutations, exclamations and so on, and noted a difficulty in word-finding and an articulatory defect, suggestive of a disturbance of scansion or stuttering.

Sabouraud and co-workers have characterized the fundamental defect in Broca's aphasia as an inability, at different levels, to pass from one complete utterance to another, resulting in a loss of contrasting features in the expression. The authors noted that those oppositions which provide for lexical definition are ordinarily conserved, while contextual contrast is lost. This leads to stereotypy in the severe form, and in the milder case, agrammatism. Within the phonological system, phonemic contrast is impaired in the presence of a preserved catalogue of phonemes. This results in anticipation, perseveration, fragmentation of the utterance, and recourse to more primitive phonemic linkages. With respect to agrammatism, the authors suggested its essential features to be a difficulty in moving from one designation to another and the loss of contextual relations. Agrammatism is a form of compensation in which the preserved lexical items are utilized to the maximum (as in a telegram), relying on the listener to supply the missing matrix. The authors were among the first to point out in these patients the interesting phenomenon of greater impairment for literal than verbal reading. Such patients can neither read by literal analysis, nor phonetically, but rather see words as ideograms (see Chap. 29).

Finally to be mentioned is the work of Luria (1966), in which two forms of frontal aphasia are described. The first of these, afferent (kinesthetic) motor aphasia occurs with left inferior post-central lesions, in relation to oral apraxia. It is characterized by the absence of dysarthria, and (apraxic) substitutions of correct individual articulations. In severe cases, there is confusion of very different phonemes, such as "k" and "t," while in less severe instances, the substitution occurs only between similar sounds such as "l" and "n," "b" and "m." There is greater difficulty for the individual utterance than, at times, for the phrase. The speech melody is retained, grammatical defects are more often in the form of paragrammatism, and writing is similar to speech with an increase in errors if articulation is prevented, as by holding the tongue between the teeth. Repetition may be altered, and when affected, the disorder may resemble the conduction aphasia of other authors. In the second form, efferent (kinetic) motor aphasia, the localization is in left premotor area. The picture is one of diminished fluency, good naming and pronunciation of individual words, but failure to inhibit individual articulatory movements, and to shift from one articulation to another. Thus, a patient trying to say the word window, might say "win . . . wim . . . win . . ." and only with assistance achieve the whole word. Repetition, writing and the speech melody are impaired. Agrammatism, when it occurs, is attributed to a disintegration of kinetic melodies, as well as the scheme of the expression itself, particularly affecting all predicative words. In this regard, a disturbance of inner speech is postulated.

Luria argues that these two independent disorders constitute what is traditionally called Broca's aphasia, viewing the kinesthetic element as providing for the differential composition of a complex movement, and the kinetic element as providing for the smoothness of movements in series. However valuable such a differentiation, it must be admitted that neither the occurrence of these forms in isolation, nor the separate localization has been adequately documented. Further, if the kinesthetic form corresponds to conduction aphasia, the more posterior variety must be assimilated to this model. Finally, the primary defect in kinesthetic motor aphasia, literal paraphasia, is a ubiquitous and complex disorder which requires explanation in terms more sufficient than those of an apraxic-motor theory.

Although there has been much quibbling over the exact borders of Broca's area, there is general agreement on the central importance of F3, particularly pars triangularis and opercularis. Goldstein (1948) cited evidence (especially, Niessl v. Meyendorf, 1911), for a more extended speech zone, involving the precentral operculum where, he thought, lay foci for the musculature of mouth, tongue and larynx. According to Goldstein, large lesions in this wider speech area produce motor aphasia, while small lesions in F3 may produce no, or only transient, aphasia if callosal fibers are spared. Deep lesions in F3 produce severe motor aphasia through callosal involvement. Goldstein followed Bastian (1898) in accounting for related syndromes through dedifferentiation within a single region. Thus, severe damage produced no speech activity, less severe damage permitted direct, reactive speech only, and mild damage prevented only voluntary speech (i.e. transcortical motor aphasia).

AGRAMMATISM

One of the essential features of Broca's aphasia is a reduction in grammatical use and flexibility. In mild cases, this may appear only as an occasional dropping of inflection, pronoun confusion and a preference for certain forms of the verb, while in the most severe cases, only single words, with or without volitional control, are possible. In the typical instance, however, the picture is that of loss or impoverishment of those small functional units which serve to indicate relationships between lexical words. Thus, a patient of Goodglass (1962), in describing a picture of a child stealing a cookie, said "Ah . . . little boy . . . cookies, pass . . . a . . . little boy . . . Tip, up . . . fall. Wipe dishes . . . ah, dishes, wipe . . . Water spill off." A patient of Alajouanine's greeted him with, "Today, Doctor. Good evening. Talk literature."

This picture, especially prominent in highly inflected languages like German, was first fully described by Pick (1913), and later studied by Isserlin (1936) and Bonhoeffer (1923). More recently, Goodglass (1967; 1968) has provided important correlative studies of aphasic grammar, and of agrammatism. According to Goodglass, agrammatic speech is characterized by a simplification of the sentence pattern with a tendency for holophrastic sentences of the subject-verb-object type, and an inability to initiate speech with unstressed words. There is omission and/or substitution of articles, prepositions and personal pronouns, gender reversal, as in "The wife, he says . . . ," confusion and/or dropping of subordinate clauses, and loss of the speech melody. Speech is emitted in short bursts, rarely followed or preceded by more than a single unstressed morpheme. There is omission of the final "s" in the possessive and noun-plural form, especially the extra-syllabic "es," as in horses, though these changes are not specific to agrammatism. The final "s" of third person singular verbs may be omitted, reflecting a preference, in English speakers, for the present progressive (Goodglass) and in French and German speakers, for the infinitive form. Ordinarily, the disorder is apparent not only in spontaneous and conversational speech, but in reading aloud, repetition and writing. In reading aloud (see Low, 1931), there is a greater difficulty for letters and asemantic phonetic groups than for words, so that the patient will pronounce only the major nouns and verbs in the sentence. Further, since these appear to elicit speech largely by virtue of their ideogrammatic character, the word is simplified as it is read. Repetition may be very limited, but it is often possible to establish the preservation of grammatical function if only by the fact that each syllable of the test phrase is replaced, in repetition, by a grunt. Writing and speech may be unequally impaired. Writing may be severely agrammatic in the presence of speech that is nearly absent or nearly normal. Conversely, agraphia may persist as speech improves to agrammatism. Those cases with grammatical writing but agrammatic speech, or anarthric but grammatically correct speech, should be distinguished from the wider category of agrammatism. This probably represents more strictly an "economy" of speech or writing (Bay, 1962). Alajouanine (1968) has noted that agrammatism spares automatic or stereotypic expressions, and that once agrammatism is established there is generally no further resolution toward normal speech.

According to Goldstein (1948), agrammatism is related to pathology in Broca's area. The concept of von Meyendorf, that agrammatism is the result of right hemispheric activity with destruction of the corresponding region on the left side, has been discounted by Weisenburg (1935), who points to the greater severity of the disorder with bilateral lesions.

For Pick, agrammatism was an attempt by the patient to get the best possible result with the least expenditure of work, with the fullest application of his linguistic reserves. Goldstein argued that an impairment in the abstract attitude would affect the function words preferentially, for they were more abstract by virtue of a lack of a referent. Other accounts stress the fact that grammatical words achieve their meaning through their relation to lexical words, and therefore, would be especially vulnerable in speech made up of one-word utterances. According to Goodglass, agrammatism is not a linguistic phenomenon, but largely a result of the increased threshold for initiating and maintaining speech flow. For this reason, the patient must rely on words of great informativeness, phonological prominence and/or affective quality. Particularly important is the factor of word stress, which is reflected in the frequent omission of the initial unstressed word in a phrase. Thus, Goodglass has shown that the initial stressed negative interrogative "can't," in spite of its greater grammatical complexity, is easier for the patient to pronounce than the simple interrogative, "can," this related to the differing stress patterns of phrases beginning with these words.

Clinical Description

Broca's aphasia occurs most often with pathology in the distribution of middle cerebral artery, and is accompanied in perhaps 80 per cent of patients by a right hemiparesis. When acute in onset, the patient may be initially mute or nearly so and often appears globally aphasic. Conversely, most global aphasics recover toward a Broca's-like picture. This may reflect an initial obscuration of speech comprehension by the severe expressive deficit, or perhaps a diaschisis-like effect within the wider speech system. Generally, the patient is self-critical, often self-corrective, and usually moderately depressed, though stereotypies may be accompanied by euphoria. It is uncertain whether the depression is a reaction to the disorder or an inherent feature. Gesture is often quite active, the patient at times resorting to complex pantomime to aid in expression. There is usually good visual memory. Digit span is often, though not always, impaired, and is frequently associated with defects on sequential tasks such as hand sequences or the reproduction of tapped rhythms. The Lichtheim test, tapping the number of syllables (or letters) in a word, has been used as an index of inner speech, but the patients' performance will parallel that on other sequencing tests. Other aspects of memory or intellectual testing must often be approached through multiple choice tests; nonverbal IQ is usually mild to moderately reduced, as a general effect of brain injury.

Spontaneous speech is nonfluent, slow and laborious, usually with only a single sound or word uttered per expiration. In severe cases, no more than a toneless "uh, uh" may be possible. What words are uttered are usually aspontaneous, dysarthric and prolonged in emission. There is a gradation from 1) the patient with single sounds (e.g. aye, aye) or words (yes, no, fine, one), with or without inflectional or propositional meaning, to 2) those with an assortment of sounds or the full range of English phonemes approximating the desired words (e.g. "mum fi" for "I am fine"), accompanied or not by stereotypic words or phrases, to 3) the patient with agrammatism and some literal paraphasia. Some speech is usually possible, if only name or address, motor series, rhymes and prayers. Utterances are usually amelodic, and a patient able to produce sentences may be unable to inflect an interrogative, or even repeat two notes of a different height. This may contrast with his ability to carry the melody of a song once initiated. At times, lyrics are possible in the face of markedly limited speech. As the patient improves, there may be reluctance to speak or stammering due to an awareness of the difficulty. There may be passage into or through a stage of agrammatism; at times spontaneous speech alone is agrammatic, with good reading and repetition.

Defects in articulation and literal paraphasia are a part of the clinical picture at all stages. As Cohen *et al.* (1963) have pointed out, there is particular difficulty with liquidals, these tending to be replaced by /d/, and trouble with the palatal sibilants /ž/ and /š/ and with the velar /g/ although substitution may affect all phonemes. In French, the nasal quality of /n/ is often lost. Among the vowels, only /u/ requires some effort, whereas s-consonant groupings (sl, st, sm, sk) are troublesome. Words are also distorted through "anticipatory determination," in which the vowel influences a preceding consonant. For example, the initial consonant of a CVC tends to become /k/ when the vowel is /o/. Metathesis is frequent, e.g. risi for siri, often striving toward a phonemically simpler form. Perseveration and augmentation occur, and especially common is the tendency to end a word with an open vowel. Complex consonants may have deleted elements, e.g. srue for screw, and consonantal anticipation, e.g. babbet for abbot, is often seen. Common changes are the substitution of /θ/ for /s/, /š/ for /č/, /d/ for /t/ etc., with literal paraphasias tending to follow distinctive feature distance.

Usually, though not invariably, some trace of agrammatism is present even though there may be fairly good use of grammatical forms in ongoing speech. In addition, difficulties in finer grammatization occur, though these are not specific to Broca's aphasia. Phrase completion can be used to demonstrate difficulty within a wide range of forms, e.g. plural ("one horse, two _____"), possessives ("That is John's bike. The bike is _____"), tenses ("Today I walk, yesterday I _____"), pronouns, dependent clauses, etc. The use of plurals and possessives can also be tested through sequences (after Goodglass) of the type: My sister lost her gloves. Q1 "Whose gloves were they?," Q2 "What did she lose?." The patient should be tested with different inflectional endings, of tense (e.g. passed, waited); third person singular verbs (e.g. swims, blushes) and so on. There may be difficulty in sentence completion, e.g. "You shave with a (razor)," with a tendency to elaborate on the word provided, e.g. "a shaver." This may reflect a mild word-finding problem present in most patients. When impaired, naming is invariably helped by phonetic cueing. Giving the patient one or two words out of which to construct a sentence may result in bizarre forms, and there may be inability to rearrange a given sentence into passive or active form, e.g. "Tom hit John" to "John was hit by Tom."

Comprehension may be quite good but still imperfect. Patients will err on complex yes/no questions, particularly those involving adverbs such as before and after, e.g. "Do you have lunch before breakfast?," and they will have difficulties with passive-active transformations, e.g. "With the pen touch the spoon," to "Touch the spoon with the pen." It must be noted, however, that nonaphasic mild dements also have difficulty on these tests, though right hemispheric patients may perform quite well. A frequent though not invariable accompaniment is a reduction in pointing span. This is often found with impaired reproduction of tapped rhythms and imitation of hand sequences, though in a given patient there is no constant agreement among these tests.

Repetition will usually be better than spontaneous speech, with clearer articulation, less agrammatism, and success with longer strings. When this discrepancy is great, transcortical motor aphasia must be considered. This is partly a reflection of an akinetic component in speech, which is mitigated by the diminished speech demand of repetition. In testing repetition, responses should be rated for deletion of grammatical words, even if repetition consists of unintelligible sounds. Stress patterns should be varied, as in the Goodglass phrase: "If he moves, shoot" versus "Shoot, if he moves," and the patient should be made to reproduce a wide variety of grammatical forms.

Naming is similar to repetition. If the latter is superior to spontaneous speech, then so also is confrontation naming. In the patient with a transcortical element, word lists and naming to description should be inferior to object naming. Usually the target word is discernible within the paraphasic response. Patients respond well to phonetic and contextual cueing.

Writing is invariably impaired, though at times differing in severity from speech. Usually it is more seriously affected than speech with only the patient's name and perhaps, a few simple words possible. At times, words may be written under duress which cannot be written to command. There is often hesitancy initiating speech, at times improving to dictation. Substitution of letters within words and of dictated letters is common, and numbers are usually written better than letters. Copying and transliteration of unfamiliar words are often possible in the face of severe agraphia. Testing is usually carried out with the left hand, and thus mirror reversals are to be expected. Ordinarily there is no improvement to typing or to word construction by anagram letters. Spelling and reading, naming and constructional ability have been discussed elsewhere.

Case 6

A seventeen-year-old right-handed boy was admitted to the hospital in May, 1971, with progressive right hemiparesis and aphasia. Evaluation disclosed a left frontal subdural mass. At surgery, a large abscess was found over the entire left frontal lobe, extending to the immediate retro-Rolandic area. Following evacuation of the abscess, language examination disclosed the following.

Conversational speech was nonfluent and limited almost exclusively to the word "mommy," repeated in a pathetic and resigned manner. Initially, the stereotypy was labile and rapid, with doubtful awareness by the patient, but by one week after surgery, a change could be demonstrated in the utilization of the stereotypy. The patient was now able to select the stereotypy from a group of words presented him, could inflect on command the first or second syllable of the word, prolong voluntarily either syllable of the word such as "maaa, me" or "ma, meee" and could produce either syllable, "me, me, me" or "ma, ma, ma" separately to command. The stereotypy could also be reversed, as in "meema." During this time, he was unable to produce any other speech sounds spontaneously, on naming or on repetition tasks. Motor series were not possible nor could the patient carry a melody. The following day, the patient could count "one, two, three, tor . . .," give Monday as "muhdee," and could produce some nouns through a combination of naming and sentence completion. His first name, Jose, was repeated as "Ho kay." This improvement coincided with almost complete suppression of the stereotypy. Three days later, testing disclosed the return of confrontation naming, with improved repetition, the latter showing some phonemic substitution and a slight agrammatic quality. Conversational speech tended to be somewhat more agrammatic than repetition or reading aloud.

Comprehension was excellent for pointing to single objects, and objects in series of two, with failure on serial pointing to three or more objects. Pointing to body parts and colors and performance on questions in the active or passive voice was good. There was confusion of subject and object on passively-voiced commands. The patient was able to read and respond to simple written commands and was able to match words to objects. Writing was possible for his name and a few simple words, though misspellings and incompletions were the rule. He was able to write numbers from 1-10, and the first 5 letters of the alphabet. As writing returned, written agrammatism was not a notable finding. Simple written additions could be carried out, constructional ability was preserved, right-left orientation and finger identification were intact. There was mild apraxia in the buccofacial muscles and in the nonhemiparetic right arm.

Comment

This case is included only as an illustration of the course of recovery in a patient with a rapidly resolving Broca's aphasia. The progression from labile streotypy through volitional control of the stereotypy and ability to manipulate elements within the stereotypy while still being unable to utter any other speech sounds is characteristic of the initial stages of recovery. Eventually, suppression of the stereotypy is achieved, followed by return of speech with single-word utterances. These tend to be dysarthric and paraphasic in contrast to the stereotypy which is clearly and correctly articulated. This stage leads through agrammatism to full recovery.

TRANSCORTICAL MOTOR APHASIA

The history of transcortical motor aphasia, as with the sensory form, begins with the description by Lichtheim in 1885. On the strength of a personal case without pathology, Lichtheim postulated the interruption of a pathway from concept to motor center, leaving the acoustic-motor pathway intact. This would produce loss of volitional speech and writing, with preservation of reading and speech comprehension, and good repetition, reading aloud and writing to dictation. The principal finding, however, is superior repetition, reduced spontaneous speech and good speech understanding. Lichtheim's view was rejected by Bastian who argued that mild disturbance of the motor speech center could produce a state of heightened threshold for spontaneous speech, but sufficient reactivity for repetition. The problem was discussed critically by Freud (1891), who concurred with Bastian, and was among the first to point out that, according to this theory, repetition should be superior to spontaneous speech in the recovery of motor aphasia. This conclusion has since been widely accepted, both in the earlier literature by Pick, Foerster, Dejerine *et al.*, and more recently, by Goldstein (1948) and Gloning *et al.* (1963).

Kurt Goldstein (1915, 1948) made fundamental contributions to this subject, and distinguished two forms of transcortical motor defect. The first, due to partial damage of the motor speech area, results from a (usually transient) heightening of the speech threshold. It is characterized by modestly superior repetition, impaired series speech and agrammatism, with good writing, reading aloud and object naming. The second and more typical form is a result of diminished speech initiative, with lack of speech in response to questions or emotional stimuli. Repetition is good even for long phrases, and does not have an echolalic quality. Object naming and writing are better than spontaneous speech. Series speech is good if the initial item is provided. The localization is frontal, just rostral to, and perhaps mildly involving Broca's area.

Goldstein also commented on the relation of transcortical motor aphasia to anomia. This was pointed out many years earlier by Wernicke, who considered the latter only a variety of the transcortical defect. More recent studies (e.g. Gloning *et al.*, 1963) stress that anomia occurs as a residual of recovered motor aphasia, and indicate the need for a closer look at this relationship. The similarity between anomia and transcortical motor aphasia was also discussed briefly by Nielsen (1940), who emphasized that the transcortical aphasic ". . . does not have a clear idea of the word he wishes and repeats any word one offers him . . . has equal difficulty with all parts of speech . . . (and) talks very little if at all, while in amnesic aphasia the patient talks well." The only legitimate difference here is the relative fluency of the one and the limited speech of the other, the factor of fluency in the anomic reflecting the availability of small grammatical words. This is consistent with the idea that frontal anomia occurs in a manner which is the reverse of posterior anomia, i.e. from grammatical to content words. Most cases of transcortical motor aphasia, in fact, do have some conversational speech available, and are at times severely agrammatic. Substantives are fairly secure, and patients cue rapidly both phonemically and contextually. Repetition may be grammatically correct, i.e. not exhibit the agrammatism of many motor aphasics, and patients can repeat long phrases in a volitional manner with understanding. The volitional character of repetition can be seen in the superiority of better learned languages in the polyglot, which is in contrast to the direction of echolalia, as well as the heightened difficulty for unfamiliar or nonsense words. There may or may not be facilitation on number repetition, though often, at a time when the patient is nearly speechless, one sees single digit repetition as the first stage of returning speech. In certain cases of an evanescent nature, it is possible to observe a transition from near-speechlessness, through agrammatism to normal speech, repetition remaining excellent throughout. In such instances, the "frontal anomic" quality of speech is particularly evident though direct naming may be quite good. Such cases suggest that the transcortical disturbance may be at the very center of Broca's aphasia, the difference relating only to severity and the imposition of dysarthria and/or vocal apraxia.

PURE MOTOR APHASIA

In this disorder, also called subcortical motor aphasia, anarthria (Marie), and by some aphemia, speech is said to be impaired in a manner similar to Broca's aphasia but, in contrast to the latter, inner speech and, therefore, writing is preserved. The earliest case appears to be that of Boinet (1871), followed by Charcot (1883) and Dejerine (1885). Dejerine (1914) later reported the case of a cultivated young woman, able to say only "Oh non," but appropriately. Repetition, singing and reading aloud were impossible though reading comprehension was intact. Writing, both spontaneous and to dictation, was facile and correct; copying, transliteration and the composition of words with anagram letters were quite good, and comprehension was preserved in four languages. At postmortem, a large cortical inferior frontal and opercular lesion was found. According to Dejerine, this case demonstrated that "aphemia" could be produced by cortical as well as subcortical lesions. Other early cases, as well as a good discussion of the disorder, can be found in Weisenburg and McBride (1935).

Perhaps the best case on record is that of Souques (1928), a thirty-year-old man, seen two years after the onset of right hemiparesis and speech loss. Comprehension of written and spoken language was intact, but expressive speech was greatly reduced, only a few syllables without meaning being possible: *que, e, aou.* There was no improvement on reading aloud, repetition or singing. Writing with the left hand (spontaneous, dictated and to copying) was excellent. He was able to indicate the number of letters and syllables in a word he could not pronounce (Lichtheim maneuver). Respiration was normal but he could not cough on request. With therapy he progressed from an anarthric to a dysarthric state. Postmortem revealed a large anterior lesion in the left hemisphere, completely involving the frontal lobe and the anterior half of the corpus callosum. The temporal, parietal and occipital lobes were spared, and the right hemisphere was normal, except for a small lesion in the inferior parietal region. Shortly after, another case was reported by Nielsen (1936), who considered the disorder "distinguishable from Broca's aphasia in that in the latter the patient can always say something but cannot write, while in subcortical motor aphasia, the patient can say nothing at all but can write."

The problem was next taken up by Alajouanine, Ombredane and Durand (1939) from a somewhat different point of view. These authors attempted to demonstrate a continuity between the defect in Broca's aphasia and the anarthria of Marie, and stressed the hierarchic nature of the disintegration in phonemic realization within a range of motor aphasic forms. Three aspects of the disorder were noted: a paralytic problem, demonstrated on spirometry, with weakness of respiration and articulation; a dystonic problem, marked by hypertonic and synkinetic innervations; and an apraxic disorder, particularly apparent on imitating facial attitudes of the examiner, in which substitution of movement occurs, and other instances of facial apraxia are evident. These three aspects refer to different levels of organization, apraxia being the highest, paresis the lowest, and possibly relate to cortical-subcortical-striatal pathological localization. With respect to speech, there is slowness and effort at onset, instability and substitution of phonemes according to their articulatory demand, and commonly a lack of control over the positions of the articulatory organs requisite for proper phoneme production. Thus, because of the difficulty in checking certain movements, replacements will occur (e.g. dentals for fricatives), while weakness in vocal cord vibration will have a similar effect (voiceless for voiced). There is also a tendency to abandon movements once started, difficulty in passing from one movement to another, and impairment in the smoothness of relaxations. Phenomena of assimilation (e.g. intoxication: "kakro" for casserole"; anticipation: "mammer" for "hammer"), metathesis and elision also occur. After a comparison of this picture with that of childhood speech, the authors conclude that this "syndrome of phonetic disintegration" is a unique disorder, contained within the category of the anarthria of Marie. That it is not an evocatory defect, involving, "phonological leit-motives," is apparent in the manifestations of paralytic, dyskinetic and apraxic phenomena, as well as the fact that in one of their cases, writing, which would be expected to be impaired in the case of a disorder of evocation, was entirely normal, and in three other cases, the disorder in writing did not at all correspond to the phonetic disturbances of speech. This major work has contributed greatly to the understanding of anarthria (i.e. pure motor aphasia) in terms of the relation to lower-level motor dysfunctions, and in separating the disorder from Broca's aphasia, in much the same manner that pure alexia, and pure word-deafness, have been distinguished from neighboring aphasic syndromes.

More recently, the condition was discussed by Goldstein (1948), and accepted as a distinct entity (peripheral motor aphasia). It differed from Broca's aphasia (central motor aphasia) in that, while speech is diminished, the intention to speak is great, and the defective speech is not aided by repetition or motor series. Goldstein emphasized the occurrence of agrammatism in both conditions (see also Ombredane, 1926), but did not place great stress on the preservation of writing. Following von Mayendorf, he localized the disorder to the operculum of pre-central convolution (thus, not subcortical), considering this the most specific facial-motor area of the wider speech zone, which included F3 and which, when damaged, resulted in Broca's aphasia. The disorder was also considered by Liepmann an apraxia for speech, though in later writings he abandoned this view. More recently, Denny-Brown (1963) and Luria (1966) have proposed that, at least in part, apraxic disorders play a role in Broca's aphasia. Morsier (1949) has reported impairments in swallowing and tongue movements in these patients, though here the differentiation from a pseudobulbar state is important. Ajuriaguerra and Hecaen (1964) have reviewed the clinical picture, and comment that speech is slow, scanning and spasmodic in the severe state, and simply deformed in the milder case. This is in contrast to the past emphasis on total, or near-total loss of speech. Hecaen and Angelergues (1965) have noted severe facial weakness in the pure motor aphasic, in contrast to Broca's aphasics where facial weakness is generally quite mild. Bay (1962) has spoken of this condition as cortical dysarthria.

If one attends to this literature closely, it is apparent that there are at least two disorders under consideration. First, a form of muteness or near muteness with preserved writing, which may, in the absence of bilateral findings, be difficult to distinguish from a pseudobulbar state involving the speech musculature selectively. This form, corresponding to the anarthria of Marie, improves to labored and dysarthric, but *nonaphasic* speech. A second form, that of "pure motor aphasia," may also begin with near muteness, and show dysarthria in improvement, but recovering speech is clearly agrammatic with paraphasic errors. Confusion occurs in that both of these forms occur with or without writing impairment. Also, agrammatism may be simulated in a patient for whom speech is labored as an attempt to convey the greatest amount of information with a minimal effort (i.e. speech economy). It is necessary, therefore, to demonstrate agrammatism through other means, as in reading aloud, repetition, etc. The following case is an example of this disorder.

Case 7

A fifty-eight-year-old right-handed man, employed as an inhalation therapist, was admitted August, 1970 to the Aphasia Unit with a history of two strokes, one in May, 1959 and another in July, 1970, both presumed to be embolic in origin. The initial episode, occurring with an acute myocardial infarction, consisted of a sudden left hemiparesis clearing over a week or two, and dysarthria lasting only a few days. The left facial weakness was noted to be severe, but this too disappeared rapidly. On WAIS (Form II), given two weeks after admission, there was a verbal IQ of 113, performance IQ 63; this was repeated (Form I) two weeks later, with verbal IQ 119, performance IQ 90. There was not specific mention of aphasia, but the history and high verbal IQ at the time would make this unlikely. Except for two left focal seizures in 1959, the patient did well after discharge and returned full-time to work.

The second episode, occurring with atrial fibrillation, also developed abruptly with right facial weakness and speech loss. There was mild facial inexpressiveness but moderately good bilateral movement spontaneously and to command. The palate elevated symmetrically and gag was active. Mild deviation of the tongue to the right and slowness of movement were noted. There was minimal weakness of the left arm, a presumed residual of the previous hemiparesis. No other motor, sensory, reflex or coordinative defects were noted. Babinski's were absent. Gait was normal. There was no dysphagia or bladder dysfunction. Brief hyperventilation produced an abnormally long delay before resumption of breathing, suggestive of pseudobulbar impairment. No pathological laughing or crying was seen. Brain scan revealed left inferior frontal lesion.

Speech was reduced to single phonemes, often repeated (ta, ta . . . ba, ba) in stuttering fashion. Simple words were occasionally possible, usually preceded by repetition of the initial sound, as in "k, k, kupa, k . . ." for *cup*. Articulations were crisp and explosive, with brief latency and a tendency toward augmentation and persistence. There were attempts at self-correction. The patient was unable to give single sounds corresponding to each of the letters or syllables in a word, possibly due to the palilalic tendency. There was slight improvement with numbers, but other series were impossible. Occasionally, strings of numbers were pronounced quite well and without dysarthria, but in a loud and explosive manner. There were no stereotypies, and there was acute awareness of the speech difficulty.

Comprehension was good with failure only on very complex tests; *repetition, reading aloud* and *naming* were identical to spontaneous speech. *Reading* comprehension was excellent, spelling comprehension fairly good. In contrast to speech, *writing* was excellent, both spontaneously and to dictation. Penmanship was very good both in print and cursive, copying and transliteration were preserved. There was an agrammatic tendency noted in spontaneous writing, with occasional spelling errors, and in longer samples a mild syntactical defect. Writing to dictation was not agrammatic. Asked to describe his speech difficulty, he wrote:

> My speech problem, anxiously, I use haste, I'll do bit more slowly, I'll do everything bit more slowly. I'm conversant with Webster dictionary Collier (Americanna) antonyms, synonyms, and I'll do everything to annunciate/pronunciate the word more carefully. And I was to retire 1956, myocardial infarct, physical advercity. After all the salesman stock in trade in expertise in experience thru the hospitals/doctors in pulmonary function/inhalation therapist.
>
> Respectfully submitted,

Calculations were good; constructional performance was mildly impaired; right-left orientation was fragile; finger gnosis was intact. Limb praxis was good, but there was severe *facial apraxia* with only slight improvement on imitation. On WAIS testing, verbal IQ was 116, performance IQ 99. Lesions were presumably bilateral and frontal.

The speech characteristics of this patient (also Case 10) differed from those of the typical Broca's aphasic by their fulminance, rapidity, ease and clarity. Utterances suggested an apraxic, rather than dysarthric or aphasic difficulty. This was consistent with the presence of severe facial apraxia, such that the patient was unable to achieve even the correct positioning of the tongue or mouth for individual speech sounds, either on command or imitation. Moreover, a persistence of movements once initiated was observed, with failure to pass smoothly from one phoneme to another. Facial weakness was mild, and clinical evidence for a generalized pseudo-bulbar state was not impressive. Nevertheless, it seems possible that a pseudo-bulbar condition was present, restricted largely to the vocal musculature, and apparent mainly as bucco-facial and speech apraxia. This disorder we believe to be a true apraxia for speech, and distinguishable from Broca's aphasia in which the (inconstant) apraxic element is not primary. The relative preservation of writing, with agrammatism, suggests a diagnosis of pure motor aphasia, while the mild pseudo-bulbar features suggest an anarthria.

DISCUSSION

Previous attempts to account for this disorder have in one way or another been hampered by the early interpretation of Broca's aphasia as a defect or loss of articulatory patterns of motor-speech images. As a consequence, Broca's area was thought to serve for the realization of utterances prefabricated in a more posterior zone through the faculty of inner speech. In two-stage models of this kind, whether as disparate as those of Bastian (1898), Marie (1906) or Bay (1962), there is in all a distinction between an intellectualistic stage of speech formulation and a motor stage of expression, the distinction lying, so far as Broca's aphasia is concerned, in whether motor-word or articulatory images are held to be involved. The functional approach, initiated by Pick (1913), and subsequently extended by Isserlin (1936), Schilder (1951), Conrad (1947) and others, envisages Broca's area as but a distal way-station in an unfolding process of speech formation, a process which consists of a series of transformations successively applied to the developing sentence pattern. Moreover, the primary speech area, that region along the supra-Sylvian lip between and including Wernicke's and Broca's area, is held to underlie this process. The different forms of aphasia are, in fact, manifestations of its orderly hierarchic breakdown. Accordingly, Broca's aphasia would result from interference at a distal point in the speech continuum, and should reflect both that level in the hierarchy attained and the activity still possible at subsequent stages.

If one accepts this view, a precise delineation of the syndrome becomes to some extent arbitrary. Certainly, one of the central defects in Broca's aphasia is agrammatism. Patients neither recover nor deteriorate through agrammatism to a Wernicke's or fluent anomic state, probably as much for pathoanatomic as functional reasons, nor do posterior patients in resolution pass to agrammatism. Prior however to agrammatism, and leading to agrammatism in recovery, is a stage in which all intentional speech is severely limited. This is, in fact, the most common presentation of Broca's aphasics, and represents an extension of the agrammatic defect to a failure in the production of content words. The typical Broca's aphasia is a combination of agrammatism, with loss of small grammatical words, and anomia with loss of substantives. One can see a certain reciprocity with the anomia of posterior lesions which begins with a failure at the level of abstract, then concrete nouns and, with increasing severity, encroaches upon grammatical words as well. In Broca's aphasia, the sequence is simply reversed. This may be seen especially in transcortical motor aphasia, where a recovery occurs from near-speechlessness, through agrammatism to normal speech. One possible explanation for this lies in anomic change over the speech area. Since grammatical words and inflections are terminal additions to the sentence pattern, they are more affected by an anterior anomia, while a posterior anomia would affect those elements, i.e. nouns and verbs which are the first to appear in the sentence structure. Just as the posterior anomic will recognize the intended noun in a group, and is sensitive to the anomic speech of others, so agrammatic patients can distinguish agrammatic from correct writing, and will reject perceived agrammatic speech. Those posterior anomics who do not accept the intended word, and who fail to respond to cueing, have their counterpart in the agrammatic who does not improve on repetition, given the grammatical model. In sum, word-finding passes through a series of pathological stages from: 1) a defect of nouns, then verbs, and in severe cases grammatical words; through 2) verbal substitution; to 3) an intermediate stage where both content and grammatical words are impaired with phonemic paraphasia; to 4) an increasing difficulty with the finer units of speech, affecting ultimately grammatical words and inflections. A severe disturbance at this terminal stage will limit content words as well.

The literal paraphasia of Broca's aphasics is similar to that of more posterior forms. Phonemic substitution in general tends to follow distinctive feature distance. Cohen *et al.* (1963) have discussed the effects of anticipatory determination. Here the strongest element of a term is the final syllable, particularly the initial vowel of this syllable. Thus, /k/ and /g/ give way to /t/ and /d/ when followed by /i/, and occasionally other vowels, as in kedi for kegi. In addition, there is intoxication from preceding items, deletion or augmentation of syllables, elision and epenthesis of vowels, and metathesis. These difficulties are not occasioned by loss of certain phonemes, for in most patients showing this disturbance all phonemes of the language can be produced. The trouble seems to lie in the serial programming of phonemes, determined by some abstract representation of the emerging word. The occurrence of such contextual effects as anticipation and metathesis indicates that the word exists in some form prior to its phonemic realization, and is not achieved simply *in seriatim*. A differentiation of phonemic paraphasia from dysarthria is not always easy. It is usually held that sounds which are not transcribable are likely to be dysarthric, for the latter does not clearly lend itself to feature analysis. Though phonemic paraphasia and cortical dysarthria occur independently, most Broca's aphasics show elements of both.

Thus, without wishing to attach a greater fixity to these forms than is their due, we can define the following arbitrary patterns of loss in the Broca's spectrum.

1. *A severe loss of intentional speech.* This corresponds to a severe frontal anomia, affecting substantive as well as grammatical words and inflections. If repetition is preserved, the restricted condition is transcortical motor aphasia. With Broca's aphasia, stereotypies may constitute the only possible speech. This latter state will pass into a stage of one-word utterances, often beginning with a modification of the stereotypy, and will improve to stage 2.

2. *A disorder of the terminal grammatization (agrammatism).* Through this disorder small functional words and inflections are combined, with the aid of prosodic values, into the emerging sentence pattern. Articulation may be excellent. Sentences which are produced are the products of intact preceding stages.

3. *An impairment in the initiation, selection and serialization of correct phonemes by the more or less completely grammatized sentence pattern.* This stage, intermediate between grammatization and articulation is often accompanied by disorders in both of these (i.e. agrammatism and dysarthria).

4. *An articulatory phase in which the sentence pattern and phonemic choice may be substantially correct, but passage into articulation is impaired.* Disorders which can occur at this stage are speech apraxia, pure motor aphasia and anarthria or the syndrome of phonetic disintegration. The relationship between these conditions is uncertain.

It is to be emphasized that overlap is common between each of these forms, the pure variety being a rare if not imaginary occurrence. The overlap is, in fact, a reflection of the instability and arbitrariness of any symptom grouping. A second point implicit in this classification is that in recovery the sequence of changes will correspond, within limits, to the normal sequence of stages on the productive side of speech. This is an important principal of great generality, but particularly so in Broca's aphasia because of the seeming independence of the various symptomatic forms. Yet the matter must be interpreted with care. Recovery from the one-word stage to agrammatism implies that the speech level of the more severe condition precedes the agrammatic state.

A narrowing of the possibilities of expression leads to the concrete synthetic productions, or expletives close to the emotional life. This helps us to understand the nature of the stereotypy. This is speech realization at an incomplete level of development. It has the flavor of echolalia, as an auto-repetitive response to stimulation where true echoing is not possible. Yet it may come to define a particular affectual or cognitive state, and is not completely isolated from the personality. To attribute the stereotypy to the activity of right hemisphere, whether justified or not, does not relieve us the obligation of relating the stereotypy to language function in that (the minor) hemisphere. In the major hemisphere, the stereotypy appears to reflect a pathological limitation of speech capacity, whereas on the minor side, it may well be the highest vocal achievement. Further, the differentiation of a content in speech goes hand in hand with awareness of the content. The lack of awareness, so characteristic of the residual automatisms of Broca's aphasia, is a reflection of incomplete participation by the utterance in the full process of speech development. The stereotypy does not undergo that complete development of which the experience of self-awareness is the highest accomplishment.

Regarding the state of inner speech in Broca's aphasics, several attempts have been made to determine the extent of impairment. Perhaps the earliest was the so-called Proust-Lichtheim maneuver, in which patients were required to tap the number of syllables in words which they were unable to pronounce. This test has certain disadvantages, however, for both praxis and rhythmic limb movement must be intact, and even if the test is performed successfully, it is not clear whether inner speech or the preverbitum is being tested. Luria (1966) has shown that immobilization of the mouth and tongue in motor aphasics defacilitates writing, suggesting that inner vocalization plays some role, and other authors have used a similar argument to account for alexia in Broca's aphasics. Alajouanine (1956) has discussed anosognosia for speech, as in stereotypies, and takes the view that awareness of a disability may be inversely proportional to its automaticity. This is an important principle which applies not only to stereotypies, but other speech automatisms and echo phenomena. With regard to the thought life of the Broca's aphasic, Critchley

(1955) has remarked that it is ". . . probably not a type of reverie in which verbal symbols participate . . . (the patient) is probably a passive vehicle for a series of images, mainly of a visual character." From these and other studies we may infer that voluntary speech and speech awareness are inseparable phenomena, and that an important feature of volitional speech is its active productive quality. Ach has written that awareness during a voluntary action has the personality, the ego, in the more prominent position. It is not at all unlikely that processes of verbal development are the mediators of this ego state. The sense of volition and the awareness of a voluntary act, speech or motor, appear to require a microgenesis across the full range of these processes.

Chapter 7

WORD DEAFNESS

PURE WORD DEAFNESS was originally described by Kussmaul in 1877, after noting cases with lack of comprehension of spoken words in the presence of good speech and hearing. The defect was thought to involve that process whereby perceived speech sounds (i.e. vowels and consonants) were combined into acoustic word-images. Subsequently, Lichtheim (1885) described a case of word deafness in a fifty-five-year-old man with presumed vascular disease. This patient had defective understanding of spoken speech, but no difficulty in speaking, reading or writing. Recognition of music was also impaired, but nonverbal sounds could be identified. In the absence of post-mortem examination, Lichtheim postulated a subcortical lesion interrupting fibers from both auditory nerves to the left auditory word center. The first case with postmortem, recorded by Pick (1892), was a twenty-four-year-old man unable to understand or repeat spoken speech or recognize familiar tunes, and indifferent to sounds around him. He responded to calls, clapping or the ringing of bells, and on one occasion said, "I hear quite well, but I don't understand; I can hear a fly flying past me." Speech was fluent and correct, reading aloud was normal, writing was slow but accurate, though writing to dictation was impaired. Necropsy revealed softening of superior temporal lobe bilaterally, involving the posterior half of T1 and supra-marginal gyrus on the left side, and T1 and T2, Insula and inferior frontal region on the right. Bastian (1897) considered this case, as well as that of Lichtheim, examples of complete cortical deafness, and proposed, in Lichtheim's case, a lesion involving the left auditory radiations, and the commissural fibers from right to left auditory word centers.

Perhaps the best studied case with unilateral lesion is that of Schuster and Taterka (1926), a sixty-eight-year-old woman with fluent, mildly paraphasic speech, intact reading and writing, good hearing and impaired comprehension of speech, music and noises. Post-mortem revealed a lesion subcortical to left Heschl's gyrus, and

127

partially affecting posterior T1 and T2. The right hemisphere was normal.

Goldstein (1948) was somewhat ambiguous in his treatment of word deafness (peripheral sensory aphasia). On the one hand, he accepted the anatomical descriptions of Lichtheim and Bastian, and on the other, emphatically rejected the idea that destruction of pathways could produce aphasia. Goldstein conceived the area for speech perception, Wernicke's area, as a more highly differentiated and extended zone within a locus of general audition (Heschl's gyrus).

The relation of word deafness to amusia was studied by Henschen, who gathered sixty-five cases of word deafness from the literature. In only a third of these was amusia an accompaniment, leading him to postulate separate centers for word, sound and music perception. Morel (1935), in agreement with Henschen, argued that speech and music perception were not independent functions, and related each of these capacities to separate lesions, those anterior to Heschl's gyrus giving musical agnosia, those posterior to Heschl's gyrus giving word deafness. Klein and Harper (1956) suggested the common denominator of word deafness and musical agnosia to be a diminished memory span for sequential data.

In regard to the pathological anatomy, Henschen insisted that word-sound deafness was related to lesions in posterior T1, either from subcortical or bilateral cortical lesion. Nielsen's (1946) conclusion that ". . . the lesion or lesions causing pure verbal agnosia (i.e. word deafness) must interrupt fibers from both primary auditory areas to Wernicke's center on the major side" has met with general acceptance. More recently, Geschwind (1965) has discussed this problem, pointing out that the bilateral cases are ordinarily cortical, involving right auditory association area as well as a zone just anterior to Heschl's gyrus on the left side. In the unilateral cases, the lesions are usually subcortical, interrupting the commissural connections from right to left auditory area, as well as the auditory radiations on the dominant side. In both instances, however, the result is an isolation of Heschl's area on one or both sides, either from auditory input or from Wernicke's area in dominant hemisphere.

The condition usually has its onset as a more or less typical sensory (Wernicke's) aphasia, with paraphasia in spontaneous speech and, in most cases, disorders of reading and writing. As the disturbance resolves, the difficulty in speech comprehension becomes more striking as the paraphasia disappears. At this time, the patient will be aware of his deficit. He will be unable to understand spoken speech, as judged by his response to commands, auditory matching tests and writing to dictation and repetition, though according to Henschen (1925), echo speech may be possible. It is unusual for patients to be deaf to all speech sounds, and with persistence, it is often possible to induce the patient to repeat a few words. Isserlin (1936) noted that patients may recognize a word as having previously been given, while not understanding its meaning. According to Goldstein (1948), partial defects are possible, with recognition of vowels and consonants but not words, or the reverse, recognition of words but not consonants and vowels. A lack of attention to both speech and nonspeech sounds, and difficulty in sound localization may, combined with word imperception, give the appearance of deafness. Polyglots may show word deafness for a secondary language and inattention for the mother tongue. Speech may be perceived as too intense, or too weak, too near or too distant; word length is unstable and the patient may not be able to indicate word junctures or the number of syllables in a word. Some patients can grasp the number of syllables in the word though not distinguishing the vowels and consonants. Jakobsen (1968) remarks on the similarity of this phenomenon to that of ordinary word amnesia, where only the number of syllables in the forgotten word may be remembered. Words are often described as running together. A patient of Hemphill and Stengel (1940) said, "Voice comes but no words. I can hear, sound comes, but words don't separate." And the patient of Klein and Harper (1956), in describing the sound of his own speech while talking said, "I can't hear the words right, not the actual words. I can hear the voice." Commonly, patients describe a humming noise and compare it to an indistinct conversation in a foreign tongue. Pick (1931) held that patients more often report hearing recurrent sound complexes, such as "drub-arub" or "totero-tot".

In addition to the word deafness, other difficulties have been described, such as impairment in the reproduction of tapped rhythms (Luria, 1966), pain asymbolia (Hemphill and Stengel, 1940) and contralateral hemiacousia (Meyer, 1908). According to Hecaen (1965), calculation disturbance is common, but tests of intelligence, such as progressive matrices, are normal. An increase in the latency of response has been noted by some authors such that patients seem to hear words many seconds after presentation. This may underlie the mentioned defect in auditory attention. Also, some patients may have as an accompaniment so-called "transcortical alexia," ability to read aloud without comprehension. This has been explained on the basis of loss of internal monitoring of words read aloud secondary to the word deafness, though word-deaf patients who are unable to understand their own speech may not show this abnormality. Finally, it is of importance that most patients will, as a part of the Wernicke's picture, show initial logorrhea and euphoria, as well as psychotic episodes with auditory hallucinations and "depersonalization of language." This in fact may be in part responsible for the oft-mentioned paranoia of the Wernicke's aphasic. In three cases at the Aphasia Unit in which this diagnosis has been entertained, all have had auditory hallucinations at one time or another in their course and two have been acutely psychotic. These hallucinations may consist of noises, single words, or in some patients, sentences, as in the case of Ziegler (1952) who heard such phrases as "Carl, we're going this way" and "It will be all right."

It should be emphasized that the clinical picture is extremely variable. On the one hand, there are patients who are unable to differentiate language from other sounds or distinguish a male from female voice. Then there are patients who recognize some words, can follow a conversation with friends and relatives to an extent but show difficulty at the single word level, especially in discriminating between similar words and phonemes. Such patients are often helped by giving the demanded word in a sentence, or giving a functional description of the object named. At the other extreme, are patients who show little impairment for simple words, but have a questioning echolalia for more complex words or sentences, which seems to act as an aid toward understanding. A progression can be noted in some of these cases from more severe stages to those of minimal impairment, and these are quite instructive toward a functional understanding of the basic disorder. An attempt in this direction was made by Klein and Harper (1956) in a patient who passed from a state in which he could only differentiate language from noise, to individual voices, to a specific language, to a distinction between ideomatic usage of the language, and eventually to familiarity with the succession of word sounds though still unable to recognize particular words.

Some patients, as Geschwind has pointed out, will occasionally show excellent performance to whole body verbal commands. This may at times be quite striking and in dramatic contrast to failure on all other comprehension tests. One possible explanation holds that whole body commands have less grammatical and formal complexity, and are endowed with a certain automatic character. The context of the command is also important. Thus, one patient, unable to salute to command when asked to do so as a part of an unrelated series of praxis tests, was able to salute after coming to attention. Another possibility to be considered is that whole body commands do not extract the "object-concept" in the same way as most limb commands. For example, one patient was unable to respond to "how do you hold a shovel?" or "how do you hold a bat?", but when asked to "show how you would shovel snow" or "stand like a baseball batter" performed correctly and rapidly. This is not simply a matter of redundancy, for commands such as "throw a punch" when in the position of a boxer may be misunderstood while "punch" will be correctly carried out. A similar tendency may be found on limb commands, but not to the same extent. Parenthetically, some patients with the above dissociation will show the reverse findings on written commands, viz.: good limb and facial response and poor whole body movements. Here the word or object concept seems to facilitate understanding. In either case, since most written or spoken whole body commands are intransitive, comparison with appropriate limb and facial movements is essential. To complicate matters, there may also be a factor of comprehension by minor hemisphere. According to Geschwind (personal communication), the patient of Smith's (1966) with dominant hemispherectomy could carry out some whole body commands in spite of failure on tests of limb and facial praxis. It is unlikely that this represents a hemispheric specialization; rather, the residuum of impaired left-sided speech comprehension now appears as the maximum capacity of an otherwise speechless right hemisphere.

With regard to testing, every effort toward an exhaustive study of these exceptional cases should be made. In addition to tests of speech comprehension, sound and music recognition (*quod vide*) and hearing, the clinical evaluation should include a standard aphasia examination, with particular attention to conversation for there is uncertainty whether word-deafness can exist in the absence of paraphasia and/or some disturbance in narrative speech.

Clinical Testing

The following outline is intended to provide a minimal battery for testing of disorders of speech or sound perception:
  A. *Tone Discrimination* (adapted from Seashore tests)
    1. *Pitch.* Two pure tones, 0.6 sec. duration, 500 cps., should be given over a frequency range. The patient is to judge whether

the tones are the same or different. Response should be non-verbal, as by pointing to one of two sets of boxes (e.g. ☐ ☐, ■ ☐).

2. *Loudness*—two pure tones, 440 cps., differing over a range of intensities. Judgment as above.
3. *Duration*—two pure tones, 440 cps., differing in duration only. Judgment as above.
4. *Timbre*—two pairs of tones, differing only in harmonic structure. Judgment as above.
5. *Tone sequence*—two patterns, differing in one note only, ranging from 5 to 7 notes. Judgment as above.
6. *Melody*—for recognition of short samples of a familiar melody. Brief samples, same duration, comparable redundancy, single notes on piano. For matching to picture (e.g. "Happy Birthday" to picture of birthday cake).
7. *Instruments*—same sequence of notes played on different instruments. This should include the human voice (singing, humming). Matching to picture of instrument.

B. *Meaningful Sounds*

The following categories of sounds might be employed:

Animal sounds (e.g. horse, rooster).

Human sounds (e.g. baby crying, sneezing).

Object-derived sounds (e.g. clock, train).

Onomatopoetic sounds (e.g. bow-wow, moo).

Approximately 40 sounds should be presented; each over a 3–4 sec. duration, at comparable intensity and redundancy. In all cases, subjects should match sounds to one of four pictures. Included in these four choices should be an exact match, an acoustic or similarity match, a category or semantic match, and a phonically related match. For example:

Stimulus sound . . . . Sawing
Choices (pictures) . . . . Sawing (exact)
. . . . .Train (acoustic)
. . . . .Hammering (category)
. . . . .Sewing (phonic)

This set of alternatives represents an advance over other tests (Faglioni *et al.*, 1969) in which the fourth choice is to an irrelevant item. This procedure should be followed wherever possible in other test categories.

Included in this test should be a series of similar and dissimilar meaningful sounds for matching to a single object. Thus, the patient should select one of four sounds presented as the best match to a picture. This will place less emphasis on semantic, and more on acoustic discrimination. For example:

Stimulus picture .... Man whistling
Choices (sounds) .... Man whistling (exact)
.... Birds chirping (acoustic)
.... Factory whistle (category)
.... Cock crowing (category)

C. *Non-Verbal Components of Speech*

1. *Male versus female voice.* This should require a match to one of four pictures. Nonsense words might be used to eliminate possible linguistic clues.

2. *Young versus old voice.* Matching as above. Nonsense words used.

3. *Interrogative/exclamatory/declarative.* The same nonsense words, or repeated sounds (e.g. da, da, *da?*) might be given in each of these forms, with matching to punctuation (e.g. ! ? . +), or same-different response.

4. *Foreign language.* Samples of equal length and content should be given in a number of languages, with matching possibly to the written name of the language, the flag, etc., or a same-different response.

5. *English spoken with several non-native accents.* Samples in this test, as well as #4, could be given in nonsense words and/or in caricature. Matching as with test #4, or perhaps to the languages of that test.

6. *Word stress.* A simple sequence of 5 to 6 words should be given, and the patient asked to indicate which word is stressed. Identical sounds and nonsense words should be used, with matching to the correct number in a written sequence (1–6).

This test evaluates nonverbal factors in speech, and utilizes for the most part nonverbal responses. In some items, conceptual mediation is unavoidable, nor is this wholly undesirable, for it makes possible comparison of acoustic discrimination performance, as on same-different responses, with conceptual discrimination, as on matching to one of four choices.

D. *A Minimal Speech Sound Discrimination Test*

1. *Vowel discrimination.* Two meaningless C.V.C. sets should be given sequentially, differing as to vowel only (C.V.C.) for same-different response. Pairs should differ by one or more

distinctive features (e.g. /nak/ and /næk/, /nak/ and /nik/) over a range of different vowel sounds.

2. *Consonantal discrimination.* Patients should be presented with two meaningless C.V.C. sets differing as to leading or following consonant only (C̲.V.C., C.V.C̲.). Sets should differ by one or more distinctive f̄eatures (e.g. /nas/ and /das/, /nas/ and /bas/) across a range of features for different consonantal classes.

3. *Monosyllabic words.* Two C.V.C. sets, differing over a range of features, should be given but at the word level (e.g. /piz/ and /biz/).

DISCUSSION

Word deafness presents a problem quite different than sound-agnosia (*quod vide*). Whereas in the latter, tonal diversity is the prime factor facilitating perception, in word deafness this diversity has a detrimental effect. Both similar and dissimilar tones undergo sensory processing into a structural form preparatory to perception, but the perception itself breaks down in relation to the specificity of the tonal elements to be reproduced. The heterogeneous sounds of human language are processed "acoustically" with no difficulty, but rather it is the articulation of the "sound-complex" into perception which is impaired. This impairment seems to reflect both those distinctions necessary for the separation of neighboring sounds, and the particularity of each sound itself. There is a similarity here with the Broca's aphasic, for whom the terminal units of speech, phonemes, present the greatest difficulty. Such patients have trouble with the articulation of separate phonemes which differ by a single feature, and with isolated speech sounds in relation to their degree of individuation. This is characteristic of the perceptual defect as well, and is a further indication that analogous processes serve in the expression of words in speech and in perception.

As emphasized by many writers, contexts and phrases are often better comprehended than single words. In a sense, the physical stimuli which constitute the phrase have an existence prior to the full perceptual realization of each constituent, and are therefore apprehended, though perhaps intuitively, before the component parts. Thus, a word-deaf patient told to "point to a chair," may point to a bed or to the wall, or at the least will often initiate some response. In such instances the latent context is in some way understood but the specifics of the command are not fully comprehended. This contrasts with the speech-comprehension defect of Wernicke aphasics where single words, especially concrete nouns, are often understood much better than phrases. In Wernicke's aphasia, the disorder seems to be at a deeper level in speech perception so as to spare some surface units. In word-deafness the opposite is true. One can see, in fact, a passage from one form to the other. Thus, the patient with word-deafness may have mild verbal paraphasia which, when it becomes more severe, passes into Wernicke's aphasia. At this point there is a change in speech perception as described above, and defects in reading comprehension appear. This transition occurs in molar form, components of each condition appearing and disappearing simultaneously. The progression from sensory agrammatism, through Wernicke's aphasia to word-deafness, is comparable to the transition from anomia through conduction aphasia to Broca's aphasia.

It should be emphasized that the sparing of sound recognition in word-deafness is not based solely on disruption of the semantic values of language. It is not the semantic aspect of speech that accounts for its selective impairment, but the more highly differentiated nature of speech sounds as opposed to other acoustic signals. Thus, in a word-deaf patient, while noises, sounds and music may be relatively spared in proportion to the speech sound deficit, there will also be exceptionally severe impairment for speech sounds of a foreign language. For the listener these are not linguistic, though they may be recognized as being a part of another language. The ability to reproduce foreign speech sounds *qua* sounds is greatly reduced, and this is in relation to their acoustic, not semantic, properties.

Chapter 8

RELATED DISORDERS

SOUND AGNOSIA

THERE IS SOME evidence, contrary to the view of Pick, that a restricted agnosia for sounds exists. Henschen (1919) speculated on the possibility of isolated sound-deafness without cortical deafness and without word-deafness, but was unable to find any such case in the literature. For Kleist (1934), three categories were possible: inability to perceive isolated sounds, noises, vowels or consonants (perceptive Gerauschtaubheit); inability to grasp sounds in sequence (Gerauschfolgetaubheit); and inability to understanding the meaning of sounds heard, such as connecting the sound of barking with a dog (Gerauschsinntaubheit). In partial cases of the first type, words may be better understood than sounds, whereas in the third type, sound-meaning deafness, words are more difficult than sounds with particular difficulty for foreign or unfamiliar words. The second form, sound-sequence deafness, is not accepted by most workers (see Isserlin, 1936).

Although it is questionable whether such a strict classification is possible, or even desirable, there does appear to be a division between the perception of words and the perception of noises. In many cases of word deafness or Wernicke's aphasia, there is relative preservation of sound perception, this usually explained on the basis of persistence of the more primitive function. There is also a single well-documented case (Spreen *et al.*, 1965) in which sounds were partially affected without a disturbance in speech understanding. This was a sixty-five-year-old, right-handed man with left hemiparesis, who was not aphasic and had good understanding of spoken speech. There were, however, many errors on sound recognition tests. Sounds were misnamed and mismatched to objects and pictures, though on 3 or 4 trials sounds heard could be picked from a series of 4 choices played to him. Also there was poor performance on pitch discrimination tests and inability to identify the sound of an organ, a piano or a marching band suggesting a receptive amusia as well. Postmortem revealed softening in right temporo-parietal lobe. In this case it should be emphasized that sound recognition was not abolished but only moderately impaired, performances running 50–70% correct responses. The case of Wortis and Pfeffer (1948) with transient partial inability to identify familiar sounds in the absence of aphasia, also had a presumed minor temporo-parietal lesion. Nielsen's case (1939) of "acoustic agnosia" also had cortical blindness with loss of revisualization, and was unable to identify objects by vision, touch, taste and smell as well as by audition. A recent case which may fall into this category was reported by Jerger *et al.* (1969). This patient, with bilateral temporal lesions, was initially deaf, but improved to the point where he could repeat some words and write normally to dictation, at a stage when sound identification was impaired. Speech comprehension was apparently reduced on audiometric testing, though in view of the normal writing to dictation, this is hard to evaluate. Musical recognition was not clearly recorded, and the misidentifications of sounds were not satisfactorily distinguished from word-finding errors, a deficiency compensated somewhat by the extensive psycho-acoustic measurements.

Patients with auditory agnosia may well be mistaken for partial peripheral deafness, though in cases with careful audiometric examination, such as that of Spreen *et al.* (1965), this possibility can be ruled out. Inattention to sounds and impairment of auditory localization have been described. Impairment of musical recognition is a common, probably constant accompaniment. According to Kleist (1934), an isolated deafness for sounds without musical impairment has not been recorded, though in individual cases the agnosia for sounds was more prominent than the word or music agnosia. Henschen (1919) knew of no cases of auditory agnosia independent of an associated amusia.

The problem of auditory agnosia was critically discussed in recent papers by Faglioni *et al.* (1969) and Vignolo (1969). In this study, it was found that patients with lesions in the right hemisphere had difficulty in discriminating between similar acoustic presentations when semantic, i.e. verbal, designations were not a part of the interpretation or response. Thus, they were unable to satisfactorily distinguish between meaningless noises in the face of normal ability to distinguish sounds quite dissimilar in nature, such as the barking of a dog or neighing of a horse, and matching these sounds to pictures or names. On the other hand, patients with left hemispheric lesions showed good discrimination of meaningless similar acoustic presentations but impairment on tests of the semantic type. The authors concluded that this demonstrated a different specialization of the hemispheres, the right for perceptual and the left for cognitive discriminations. There is, besides this important study, other recent work in support of this idea. Over the past few years, investigations by several authors (Kimura, 1964; Broadbent *et al.*, 1964; Sparks and Geschwind, 1968) have suggested that speech and nonspeech auditory patterns are to some extent processed in different parts of the brain. These studies, utilizing dichotic listening techniques, have shown a normal preference for digits, syllables and words to right ear, and melodies and tonal qualities to left ear, and this has been confirmed in patients with unilateral left or right temporal lesion (Shankweiler, 1964; Milner, 1962). Other studies, and a guide to testing, are discussed in the section on word-deafness.

RECEPTIVE AMUSIA

Inability to recognize familiar melodies (receptive amusia) has been the subject of a few excellent studies (e.g. Wallaschek, 1891; Feuchtwanger, 1930; Ustvedt, 1937) but as yet no clear idea of the nature of this disorder has been obtained. It occurs to some extent in all cases of sound agnosia, and according to Henschen in one third of patients with word deafness. There are no clear-cut instances in which receptive amusia has occurred as an isolated problem. Most patients will complain that they no longer enjoy music, or that they cannot differentiate music from noise. Patients may fail to recognize melodies, show uncertainty in recognition, or recognize a familiar piece but without the sense of familiarity. The rhythmic element may be more resistant than the melodic. There is a dissolution from complex to primitive music. In some cases, the impairment of musical recognition is accompanied by a heightened affective reaction. Patients can often sing melodies which they cannot recognize, indicating that the problem is not exclusively in the sphere of melodic memory. The case of Spreen *et al.* (1965) could not distinguish between a piano, an organ and a marching band. Barrett's case (1910) of word deafness could not distinguish between a human voice singing, and an imitation of the cry of a cat. A case of Wertheim's (1963) could recognize a sung melody better than if played on an instrument. This unusual situation is explained by Wertheim as reflecting the fact that recognition is differently impaired for vocalization and instrumentation, the former being ontogenetically older and, therefore, more resistant to pathology. Patients may recognize rhythms but not individual tones, or the reverse, better tone recognition than for rhythms.

The anatomy of the disorder is equally in doubt. According to Henschen (1926), receptive amusia is related especially to left anterior temporal area, though right temporal lesions can also produce the picture. Wertheim (1969) cautiously accepts this localization. For Feuchtwanger, the localization is Wernicke's area bilaterally, for Ustvedt left T1, and for Pick (1931), anterior to Wernicke's zone particularly in left hemisphere.

In addition to the clinical and anatomical difficulties, the interpretation of amusia is further complicated by the nature of the musical function itself. Pick, for example, emphasized the dependence of speech on musical elements, and argued that "speaking and singing make use largely of the same peripheral executive and perceptual organs, so that the essential difference between them appears to lie only in modifications of the same function." Isserlin (1936) believed that a word must be understood not only as to its meaning, but that it must be given a pure tone sound as a part of the total intonational pattern. The subject has not been studied closely enough to ascertain whether, in receptive amusia, the musical aspects of speech are affected. Thus, would homonymous words differing as to inflection be differentiated; could patients distinguish the declarative, emphatic and interrogative forms of the same sentence, etc. At least in motor amusia there is some evidence that the prosodic features of speech can be involved in the absence of aphasia (Wertheim, 1969). This relationship of the musical function to speech is clearly very subtle, and as Ustvedt pointed out, at a level independent of the "symbolizing function" of speech.

Discussion

It is tempting to relate the preceding disorders to experimental work suggesting that verbal and nonverbal acoustic signals are processed on opposite sides of the brain, i.e. that the right hemisphere (temporal lobe) is specialized for "perceptual" or nonverbal, the left for "cognitive" or verbal functions. However, it is likely that there is not only a functional asymmetry of hemispheric organization, but that this asymmetry underlies a two-stage sequence in the normal processing of any given acoustic signal, whether verbal or nonverbal. In the first or sensory stage, the signal is received and decoded, undergoing in this decodage a construction into spatial form. That this process should have a special relation to minor hemisphere is not surprising in view of the priority of that hemisphere to spatial-constructive operations. In this, the sensory phase, mild disabilities may be overcome by augmenting the available acoustic information, for the signal goes through a synthetic process that is aided by tonal diversity. In contrast, with a defect of the second or perceptual stage mechanism, which is of an analytic type, individuation of the perception will be facilitated by simplifying the information pertaining to any specific content. Thus, verbal material escapes the sensory stage impairment, and nonverbal material escapes the perceptual stage defect.

Auditory sound agnosia (sound deafness) would represent an impairment in the sensory phase of auditory perception. This has to do with processes worked on the stimulus immediately after reception in the cortex, and prior to first awareness. Sound agnosia may relate especially to minor hemisphere lesions, for the minor side has a favored role in this stage of the acoustic process. If the lesion is complete and bilateral, there is cortical deafness, affecting all sounds. If partial, as in sound deafness, in order of severity one would expect: impairment of similar meaningless sounds, dissimilar meaningless sounds (e.g. noises), similar meaningful (nonverbal) sounds (e.g. tones), dissimilar meaningful (nonverbal) sounds (e.g. familiar melodies), similar meaningful (verbal) sounds (e.g. phonemic pairs), dissimilar meaningful (verbal) sounds (e.g. speech sounds). The impairment would be graded according to the information content of the message and the specificity of each informational "bit" to be processed. Therefore, in sound agnosia, the better performance on speech sounds than nonspeech sounds is accounted for by the greater diversity of the former, and the closer relation, in the strictly acoustic sense, of nonspeech sounds to noise. That is, the more highly differentiated nature of the speech sound provides a greater abundance of clues to the partially sound-deaf patient than do the more homogeneous nonspeech sounds. This is not to be compared to the case of the peripherally deaf patient. For him, the amplitude is insufficient for the isolated sound to emerge. In the cortically deaf patient, the problem is rather in the reduced ability of sounds (speech and nonspeech) to undergo synthetic transformation into a unique spatial form, a disorder which will be accentuated as the sounds achieve greater uniformity. Thus, the patient of Spreen *et al.,* (1965) identified rattling keys as a "chain jingling or a bell ringing," demonstrating his inability to distinguish between closely related noises. Such patients should recognize onomatopoetic sounds such as "bow-wow," while failing with the actual animal noises themselves. The more dissimilar the sounds, the easier it will be to distinguish them. But each unique sound must still be identified within its class. Such patients understand speech well, though careful testing might disclose some difficulty in comprehending isolated phonemic pairs (e.g. peas, bees). In patients of this type, one would expect fairly good ability to transcribe words from a foreign language or nongarbled nonsense words. For the patient these are noises, at least they are not semantic as in the tests of Vignolo, but with respect to his disorder, they should behave closer to the speech sounds.

In contrast to the patient with sound agnosia, patients with word deafness (*quod vide*) have an impairment at a secondary stage in perceptual development. The order of disturbance is the *reverse* of that seen in sound agnosia. The difficulty here is in the differentiation of normally "sensed" signals into perceptual awareness, a process that is facilitated by minimizing the degree of perceptual differentiation required. Thus, the most internally variable and discrete elements of acoustic perception—words, are the most difficult to generate. In this way, the final development of an acoustic perception is comparable to the development of a thought into spoken speech.

With regard to the relation of amusia to sound and word deafness, the central position of music in a sound-speech dichotomy has to be considered. In severe cases on the (cortical) *sensory* side, there is loss of sound, music and words in this order. The most differentiated sound is best recognized, for the impairment is not one of amplitude, as in the peripheral cases, but of specificity of input. On the perceptual side, there is loss of words, music and sound in this order, for here it is the least differentiated sound that is most readily perceived. Here the impairment is not one of specificity of input, which would be helped by signal variability, but specificity of "output," i.e. perceptual expression, which is negatively affected by this variability. Thus, one finds an association of word deafness with amusia, and sound deafness with amusia, while sound and word deafness are seen together only in complete cortical deafness. The pivotal position of music may account for its seeming independence from the other two forms.

PALILALIA

Though it is not, strictly speaking, an aphasic disturbance, palilalia is often confused with, and accompanies, other language disorders, particularly echolalia, and for this reason a brief review is given.

According to Critchley (1927), palilalia was first described by Souques in 1908, though there was earlier mention in the literature of "auto-echolalia," presumably the same disorder. It has been described in Parkinsonian states, particularly in post-encephalitic Parkinson's disease, degenerative diseases and diffuse vascular encephalopathies. The localization is generally held to be subcortical, involving particularly the basal ganglia, but reference to frontal lobe pathology has been made from time to time without clear justification.

The clinical picture is one of reiteration in ongoing speech, accompanied by reduced speech volume, acceleration of speech in longer passages, and a tendency for the discourse to drift off into an unintelligible mumble toward the end of the passage. Geschwind (1964) notes that in general paresis, palilalia is confined to syllables; ordinarily, however, repetition of syllables is the least common symptom. More often there is repetition of single words or phrases, usually the latter part of the phrase or the second of two successive phrases. At times, the repetition is incorporated into a following statement, tending to obscure its reiterative characer, as in "I used to work, for a time I used to work as a painter." The repetition is most severe for free, open-ended speech, with possible accentuation when the material discussed is of recent vintage. Palilalia is minimal on clinical tests of repetition (numbers, words and phrases) and there is also a minimal amount of palilalia on reading aloud. Motor series, rhymes and other speech automatisms such as prayers and songs are performed without marked palilalia. The patient seems to repeat himself only when the information to be conveyed is of an indefinite nature, as in creative spontaneous speech. In this respect it suggests the so-called "lack of ideas" (Einfallsleere) mentioned previously. Palilalia is usually associated with perseverative features in other aspects of language and behavior. Writing is often impaired through perseveration, grasp reflexes are present, and generalized or axial rigidity with both aspontaneity and festinating gait are commonly seen. Indeed, micrographia and festination also show the acceleration with diminishing amplitude seen in palilalic speech. Patients with palilalia are often aware of their defect and can, with encouragement, be made to speak without self-repetition. However, there is usually reversion to palilalia in a relatively short period of time. The question of whether or not this disorder is related to echolalia, in the nature of an auto-echolalia, has often been raised. However, in a personal case, given a binaural background of white noise, no improvement occurred. In fact, an amplified feedback of the patient's own speech proved more efficacious. The course and progress of the disorder are uncertain. In a few personal cases with palilalia as a feature of progressive supranuclear palsy, the disorder appears to have begun with phrase repetition, progressed to repetition of single words, and in severe cases, single word and syllabic repetitions. Syllabic palilalia may resemble stammering, the differentiation depending on the accentuation of the former in spontaneous speech, stammering remaining constant for all speech modes, the sense of effort in the latter and its lack of acceleration and mumbling. This may at times be difficult, for stammering is an occasional occurrence in aphasic states. Such cases may be associated with cortical pathology, and need not have a history of childhood stammering.

Finally, it should be mentioned that palilalic-like symptoms may possibly occur in association with parasagittal meningiomas in the region of the secondary motor area. Cases have been described in which there was sustained repetition of single words or sounds secondary to seizure events. Stimulation of this region produces blocking of utterances and persistent reiteration. Thus, Brickner (1940), stimulating in the region of Brodman area 6 at its juncture with the posterior superior portion of area 32, caused the patient to utter "err" repeatedly. On asking the patient to say the alphabet, repetition of the last spoken letter occurred for the duration of the stimulus, following which the patient resumed giving the alphabet. Some distortion of letters repeated was noted with a slower rate of production and full awareness of the repetition. Other examples are given by Alajouanine *et al.* (1959) and Chusid *et al.* (1954). It should be remarked, however, that this form of stereotyped auto-echolalia is rather different than true palilalia, and appears related more to those speech automatisms seen in temporal-lobe seizure states than to palilalia or aphasia proper.

PAROXYSMAL SPEECH DISORDERS

Transient aphasia, either of "expressive" or mixed type, has been reported in epileptic patients. This may occur in isolation, or as the seizure aura, or even during the post-ictal period, and is ordinarily recalled later by the patient. There is a strong correlation with a seizure focus in major hemisphere (Serafetinides and Falconer, 1963). Most patients will report, or are described as having, garbled or jargoned speech, though careful testing during the spell has rarely been performed. It would be of interest in such patients to determine whether seizure recall is correlated with the aphasic form, and to what extent the recall of the speech difficulty accompanies the recall of other seizure phenomena.

The more common seizure event, however, is speech arrest. This has been reported by Penfield and Roberts (1959) from direct stimulation at only three sites in the dominant hemisphere, the posterior temporo-parietal region, including posterior T1, 2 and 3, supramarginal and angular gyri; Broca's area; and the supplementary motor area on the medial aspect of the hemisphere rostral to precentral leg area. As described above, stimulation in this latter site may produce a perseveration of the immediately preceding utterance.

In addition to aphasic, distorted and arrested speech, one may also see speech automatisms occurring in epileptic states. These may originate in either hemisphere, perhaps more often on the right side, and may also occur before, during or following the seizures. Serafetinides and Falconer (1963) describe five forms, of which only two or three appear due to language disturbance. One form, which they describe as a warning utterance, and which may consist of such sentences as "I feel funny" or "I feel sick" just preceding the seizure, appears to be no more than a normal response to an imminent seizure. A second type, which they term the perplexity utterance, occurs following the seizure as an attempt at reorientation, and again does not appear to be abnormal. A third type, the "emotional utterance," is described as an apparent conversation with imaginary or hallucinated people. Thus, a patient might say "I don't care what you do to me" during the seizure but this is not directed at anyone in particular. This form may relate to linguistically correct sleep speech utterances such as those described by Arkin and Brown (1971). A fourth type, the "irrelevant utterance," occurs during a conversation but appears as a sudden remark out of context. Again, this may relate to distraction, or weakened attention. Their final type, the "recurrent utterance," appears to be the only form that suggests an aphasic-like state. This consists of reiterated sentences such as "that is right, that is right," which remind us of the stereotypies seen in motor aphasics. It is of interest that none of these utterances are recalled by the patient following the seizure, and all are described as being linguistically correct.

APHASIA AND THE THALAMUS

Interest in the possible role of the thalamus in language disorders has developed out of two principal lines of inquiry. In those studies in which *nu. ventralis lateralis (V.L.)* has been the primary surgical target, dysphasia has been reported as an occasional complication, in some series more commonly following surgery on the speech-dominant side. However, this is by no means a common occurrence. In Cooper's series, 2 per cent of 1500 cases were found to have (transient) dysphasia, in the study of Allen *et al.* (1966), 7 per cent of 115 cases, and in the study of Herrmann *et al.* (1966), 8 per cent of 118 patients. In most cases, aphasia is present only within the first week or two following surgery and rarely beyond three or four weeks. It is probable that many of these patients are, in fact, either mild cases of anomia, or instances of "nonaphasic misnaming" (Weinstein, 1964), both common postsurgical disorders are seen in a wide variety of nonlocalizing states. Certainly, the relatively low incidence of "dysphasia" following thalamotomy suggests the presence of other factors than the pure thalamic lesion.

Some possible explanations for persistent aphasia apart from the thalamic lesion are cortical damage from a left frontal or parietal burr hole; introduction of the probe; subsequent hemorrhage into the cryogenic lesion; and general effects of ventriculography and/or postoperative cerebral edema. In some cases, the thalamic lesion may act nonspecifically to increase the total mass of (pre-existing) cerebral pathology. Finally, it is possible that thalamotomy may occasion a defacilitation of the dominant cortical speech zone, rather than induce a deficit in a subcortical speech function. My personal suspicion, from evaluating several thalamotomy cases, both preoperatively and postoperatively with an extensive battery of language tests, is that, given an intellectually normal subject (e.g. a dystonic) and an uncomplicated surgery, thalamotomy in the speech-dominant hemisphere does not produce a distinct impairment in language, praxis or constructional ability. There may well be subtle deterioration in mentation not readily demonstrated by clinical testing. This is suggested by the fact that patients with mild preoperative linguistic or cognitive deficits tend to show postoperative regression in a functional pattern similar to that seen in aphasia, viz: minimal dementia to anomia or to nonaphasic misnaming. Patients may also show deterioration within that system which is already slightly impaired, i.e. regression limited to the area of preoperative difficulty. This indicates that the adverse thalamotomy effects may be due to *quantal* deterioration within the language system, rather than the loss of specific components within a subcortical language mechanism. In this respect then, there is little to distinguish thalamotomy complications from those of other diffuse states such as trauma, increased intracranial pressure and stupor.

A second line of study has implicated the posterior thalamus in aphasia. The anatomical relationship of *nu. pulvinaris* to those regions of cortex generally identified with language function, the posterior peri-Sylvian and parietal cortices, tends to support this possibility. Penfield and Roberts (1959) attributed to the pulvinar, by way of its partici-pation in cortico-thalamo-cortical loops, a signal importance in lan-guage function. However, their evidence is scanty and their case of aphasia with a "small hemorrhage" in the pulvinar leaves much to be desired. More recently, Ojemann *et al.* (1968) have decribed dysnomia with electrical stimulation in the pulvinar in the dominant hemisphere. In a recent study (Brown, 1971; Brown *et al.*, 1972) patients under-going stereotaxic ablation of the pulvinar (cryopulvinectomy; see Cooper *et al.*, 1971) were evaluated before and after surgery. Either transient or no effects upon language were observed following pulvinar lesion in the speech-dominant hemisphere. A conclusive case is the following:

A thirty-nine-year-old left-handed electrician with severe torticollis, unresponsive to a variety of medications. Complete examination (June 9, 1971) disclosed normal speech, comprehension, repetition and nam-ing. Writing was intact, reading excellent (Goodglass test). Spelling and calculations within normal limits. Copying, drawing, right-left orientation and finger identification, map drawing, praxis and visual imagery were intact. Preoperative I.Q. was 112.

Following *left* cryopulvinectomy* (June 10, 1971) no change in per-formance on any of the above tests was observed. Postoperative I.Q. was 116. On June 21, the patient underwent *right* cryopulvinectomy. Continuous monitoring of speech, comprehension, repetition, naming, spelling, reading, calculation and praxis during lesion production demonstrated no abnormality. In both instances, large 16–18 mm) lesions were produced through separate freezing of the medial and lateral half of each pulvinar. Thorough evaluation after bilateral pulvinar lesions (June 25–28, 1971) demonstrated no change in con-versational speech, or on a range of naming and repetition tests. Com-prehension was intact for serial pointing (to 5 objects), commands, and yes/no questions, with no difficulty on complex grammatical forms. Spelling, reading (Goodglass test) and praxis were intact. Visual imagery, map and free drawing, right-left orientation, finger identifica-tion, and digit span were unchanged, with the exception of a slight tendency toward miniaturization on drawing. Writing was also reduced

---

* Surgery performed by Drs. I. Cooper and J. Waltz.

in size, with some spelling errors and a tendency to run words to-gether. However, he could correctly write a passage descriptive of his work, such as "I am a construction electrician. This work is mainly the installation of machinery." Proverbs were done fairly well, e.g. for "A bird in the hand . . .," he said: "Anything you already have is worth twice as much as what you think you can get." Although extensive memory testing was not done preoperatively, no major impairments in recent or remote memory were apparent. On a verbal learning test of ten items, postoperative performance was impaired (5, 7, 6, 6, 5) on five trials for immediate recall. IQ following bilateral pulvinar surgery was 108. It is to be emphasized that these tests were carried out from the fourth to the seventh postoperative days. Long-term effects have not yet been studied.

It would appear that lesions of the pulvinar do not necessarily result in a major impairment of language. Moreover praxis, calculation, con-structional ability and visual imagery were also unchanged. Mild deficits in memory may occur in some patients, though this is certainly not a prominent feature. Occasionally, alteration of mood has occurred. In two left-damaged patients, increased depression and aggressiveness followed left pulvinectomy, whereas two patients with pre-existing "pathological crying" showed a great reduction in this following right cryopulvinectomy. Other cases have shown greater relaxation and placidity and in some instances mild asponteneity. These changes may be related to connections of the pulvinar with amygdala and *nu. dorsomedialis,* i.e. limbic system mechanisms, a possibility currently being studied in our department.

Regarding aphasia from natural lesions in thalamus, Cheek and Ta-veras (1966) noted the occurrence of dysphasia in 20 percent of their patients with thalamic tumor, but twice as many patients had confusion, memory loss or drowsiness, all of which may produce dysnomic states. Similarly, in the patients of Smyth and Stern (1938), speech disturb-ance occurred against a background of obtundation or dementia. A similar difficulty surrounds those reported cases of dysphasia with vascular lesion in thalamus. Certainly, such accounts of thalamic dysphasia do not refute Nielsen's (1946) conclusion that thalamic lesions affect language functions *pari passu* with general deterioration.

II. APRAXIA

Chapter 9

INTRODUCTION AND CLINICAL DESCRIPTION

HUGHLINGS JACKSON'S (1866) description of the inability of some aphasics to perform certain voluntary actions such as coughing or protruding the tongue, in the absence of weakness of the involved muscles, was the first clear account of an apraxic disorder in the literature, though most writers attribute to Steinthal (1871) the distinction of having first used the term *apraxia.** Finkelnburg (1876) suggested the term "asymbolism" for an inability to employ conventional signs (linguistic as well as perceptual), a designation soon extended to disorders of object recognition generally. It was argued that asymbolia for objects (i.e. nonrecognition of objects) gave rise to their incorrect use. Shortly after, asymboly was separated into a visual (i.e. visual agnosia) and a motor form, the latter, motor asymbolia due to loss of images of movement and localized to the precentral area. As soon as the motor form achieved an independence from the visual, it became possible for de Buck (1899) to postulate a dissociation between the concepts of an action, and the kinetic images of the action, a formulation which led directly to Liepmann's important case study.

This patient (Liepmann, 1900), a forty-eight-year-old right-handed government official (Regierungsrat), aphasic and emotionally labile, was considered on admission to be in a state of complete imbecility. He was unable to correctly select objects or carry out hand movements to command. Yet he could carry out whole body commands, such as "stand up," "go to the window," and so on, which, Liepmann thought, argued against a loss of verbal comprehension. Closer study revealed that if the patient's right arm was restrained, and the left tested alone, he was able to carry out movements quite well. In addition, he could copy a few words and do simple drawings with the left hand, a task impossible on the right. Though spontaneous movements were possible with either hand, the right hand interfered with

---

*Though Morlaas (1928) attributed to Gogol (1873) the first use of the term apraxia, as the erroneous use of objects resulting from their incorrect recognition, according to Nielsen (1946), the term was borrowed from Steinthal.

151

performances by the left, and tasks requiring bimanual coordination were impossible. Facial apraxia was also present, with no improvement on imitation, but eye movements were preserved. At postmortem, there was, in the left hemisphere, softening in frontal subcortex extending to the Rolandic operculum, a subcortical lesion in supramarginal gyrus, superior parietal lobule, and partially in angular gyrus. In the right hemisphere, there was a recent parietal infarct, and most importantly, the corpus callosum was totally destroyed with the exception of splenium. The significance of this case lies in the fact that for the first time an apraxic disorder could be shown to be principally one of motor execution and not dependent on faulty comprehension of the task or agnosic disturbances in the perception of the object or object-situation. This was particularly clear in that only one limb was involved. Although Liepmann later admitted in this case a slight left-sided dyspraxia, the relative normalcy of the left side with such a large callosal lesion is hard to explain when taken together with his subsequent publication.

This second case (Liepmann and Maas, 1907), a seventy-year-old factory worker (Ochs) was examined one month after the onset of right hemiplegia, moderate expressive aphasia and agraphia, and apraxia on the left side. Comprehension was said to be normal. The apraxia concerned mainly the more highly differentiated movements, sparing such everyday automatisms as eating and drinking. There was no improvement with objects, though he could distinguish correct from incorrect movements. Complex movements such as lighting a match were disorganized in spite of object use. The left-sided agraphia was complete and considered by Liepmann to be part of the apraxic disorder, writing being the most highly differentiated of skilled movements, and therefore, the most susceptible to pathology. The autopsy findings in this case revealed a normal right hemisphere, and in left hemisphere a lesion of the first frontal convolution, part of para-central lobule and destruction of the anterior two-thirds of corpus callosum. A lesion in the pons was held to explain the right hemiparesis. The left apraxia and agraphia were accounted for by disruption, by the callosal lesion, of the pathway from guiding left motor centers to the following right frontal motor area.

The importance of these cases, apart from their relevance to callosal physiology, lies mainly in their historical role in the development of the theory of apraxia. Because the apraxia was limited largely to one extremity, as in the first case, or present in spite of good understanding of the task, as in the second, it became possible to eliminate disorders of comprehension as causative in the impaired motor performance. Based on these cases and others, Liepmann proposed a theory of apraxia, described and discussed in systematic fashion in his paper of 1920. This discussion, which is of central importance to all later investigations of apraxia, is worth reviewing in some detail. In this paper, Liepmann divided the apraxias into three major forms according to where, in the physiological organization of movement, the pathology occurred:

1. The disruption of kinetic engrams acquired for simple over-learned movements. These engrams consist of traces of the motor innervation linked to traces of centripetal stimuli (i.e. kinesthetic sensations). This innervational-kinesthetic engram is conceived as a physiological rather than a psychological entity, having no specific locus in space or time, but only in the pattern of linkages as they are affected, moment to moment, by other conditions at the time of the movement. Such engrams serve for waving the hand, clenching the fist and for

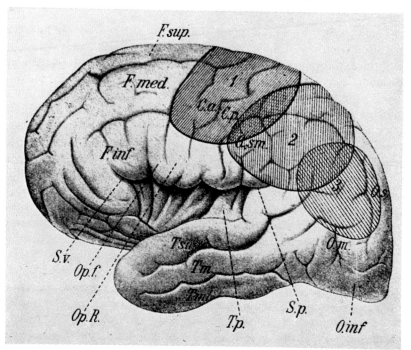

Figure 5.   1) Limb-kinetic apraxia, 2) Ideo-motor apraxia, 3) Ideational apraxia (Liepmann, 1920).

the vocalic elements of speech. A disorder here results in limb-kinetic apraxia.

2. More complex movements require an ideational outline, an idea, of the body parts to be used, the speed, rhythm and sequence of the movements. This space-time plan is embedded in sighted persons in the optical frame, and gives rise with pathology to ideational apraxia.

3. A cooperation between the above levels is required. This may be in the form of a connecting pathway, though a progression through stages of a developing process cannot be discounted. Interruption here produces ideomotor apraxia.

With respect to the pathology of these forms, Liepmann demonstrated that, in general, lesions of dominant posterior parietal area produced ideational apraxia, lesions placed somewhat more anteriorly produced ideo-motor apraxia, and precentral lesions produced limb-kinetic apraxia. His diagram (Fig. 5) suggests a kind of channel, passing from caudal to rostral, and superior to the speech zone, through which the physiological development of action takes place.

Later on in his paper, a differentiation is made among the apraxias resulting from involvement of corpus callosum. Liepmann's paradigm for this syndrome was, as indicated, the case (Ochs) written in collaboration with Maas. Yet as we have pointed out, his initial case (Regierungsrat) would appear to directly contradict the callosal explanation. In attempting to get around this objection, Liepmann later admitted a mild degree of left-sided dyspraxia in this patient, and suggested that a callosal lesion, when combined wih a left-parietal lesion, might have an additive effect on apraxia of the right arm. In any event, he listed a number of possible forms of apraxia depending on where, in the callosal system, a lesion might occur (Fig. 6).

Types (1) and (2) are characteristic of the so-called "sympathetic apraxia," occurring in patients with Broca's aphasia and right hemiparesis as an associated apraxia of the left arm. Presumably, it is due to involvement by the left frontal lesion of callosal fibers (or their origins) to right frontal cortex, separating the right frontal limb area (i.e. for left arm) from left speech area. The lesion may be subcortical on the left, catching commissural fibers to right side, or may spread more widely into corpus callosum, as in the syndrome of the anterior cerebral artery. Type (4), left-sided apraxia from solitary lesion in the corpus callosum, spares the right arm which is guided by a normal left senso-motorium. Type (5), left-sided apraxia from subcortical

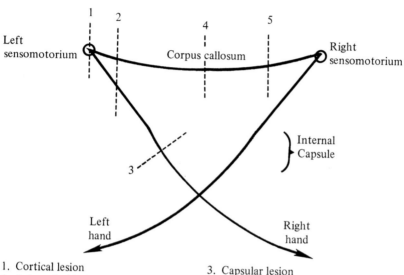

Figure 6.   Callosal Apraxias, after Liepmann (Brown, 1969). 1, 2) "sympathetic dyspraxia", 3) capsular lesion, hemiparesis without apraxia, 4) callosal lesion, with left apraxia, 5) right-subcortical lesion, with left apraxia.

lesion on right side, catching commissural fibers from left hemisphere, remains, since Liepmann's day, only a theoretical possibility. These callosal syndromes will be discussed in detail further on.

This major work by Liepmann had a profound effect on all workers in the field. Some measure of the respect given to him can be seen in the critical review by Lange (1936) where, in spite of a fair evaluation of all opposing data, Liepmann's position on almost all aspects of apraxia is sustained. However, there were different approaches, and among these the views of Sittig (1931) and von Monakow (1905) were the most authoritative.

Sittig tried to adopt as physiological a view as possible and conceived the apraxias (ideo-motor and limb-kinetic) as different degrees of hemiparesis, disposing of ideational apraxia by grouping it with the agnosias. Sittig's approach was thoroughly Jacksonian, for he characterized apractic disorders in terms of higher-lower relations, and focal versus diffuse representation of functions. Though the formulation is not as clear as might be wished, and the arguments in its favor unconvincing, it must be said in fairness that no careful attempt has since been made to evaluate this hypothesis. Certainly, even Liepmann conceded that, at least in limb-kinetic apraxia, cortical frontal lesions too mild to cause hemiparesis would produce an apraxia of the contralateral limb.

Von Monakow's (see also Brun, 1921) position is usually taken to be quite different from Liepmann's, but actually his classification, and to some extent his pathological localization, do not differ substantially. Where he does depart from Liepmann's views, is in his stress of the ontogenetic aspect of movement, its complexity, and its subconsciously-acquired character. Further he argued, as did Schlesinger, and Gruenbaum (Lange, 1936), that since movements are learned in concrete response to object situations, it is inaccurate to assign these movements to transmission effects of preinnervatory optico-kinesthetic concepts; i.e. that in ontogenesis and in phylogenesis there are no experiences corresponding to the establishment of concepts which, in adult life, will give rise to movements, that we do not act on the basis of concepts but rather form concepts on the basis of our actions. With regard to localization, von Monakow argued that the more automatic a movement, the more diffuse its representation, and therefore, the abolition of automatic motor activity will require a diffuse lesion. The effect of a local lesion is to obstruct the ecphorization of an act under a given set of conditions, while the ecphorization of the act as a whole, as under the conditions of automaticity or object use, is unaffected.

Morlaas (1928) described two major forms of apraxia, those showing disturbances in evocation of the movement, and those in its execution. In this latter group, he distinguished perseveratory, inhibitory and spatio-dyskinetic phenomena. The two groups can occur in mixed form, and vary according to intensity. Morlaas stressed that in apraxia a defect of the symbolic aspects of a system of gestures was involved, and not a simple motor performance.

Since this early work, there has been little constructive theory in apraxia. Most authors have tended to follow Liepmann's lead, concerned more with one or another subdivision of apraxia, rather than with the foundation upon which the subdivision is based. However, it is our view that the apraxias, like the aphasias, can be conceived as interruptions at sequential levels in the realization of a voluntary action. In this light, the classification of apraxic disorders to a certain extent conforms to that of the aphasias. In the following chapters a classification of this type is attempted, though hopefully future work will permit a typology on a more analytical basis. Since the differentiation of the apraxias has depended heavily upon adventitious features such as performance to command, imitation and object use, it seems best to discuss apraxia testing in general, rather than recount a special methodology in each section. For this reason a brief guide to testing is incorporated.

The diagnosis of apraxia can be determined in a patient with disorder of voluntary movement in which the presence of misunderstanding, dementia, sensory or motor paresis, and/or ataxia, is not a contributing factor. The action must be possible under other conditions than verbal command, and responses should entail incorrect, not uninitiated, movements. As most patients will be aphasic, comprehension disorders represent the most common source of confusion. With severe comprehension disorders, one may elicit movements by showing the patient pictures of actions to be performed, objects to be used, presenting a functionally-related object (e.g. nail, for hammering), or by imitation. Mild disorders of comprehension can be discounted if the patient can repeat the command on request, select the correct command, action or action-picture from a group, describe the action which cannot be carried out, and/or indicate the object to be manipulated. Further, the patient's response should approximate the desired one, except in special instances, and the appropriate body part used, especially in shifting from facial to limb commands, or from one side to the other. The ability to perform whole body movements does not in itself signify comprehension, for there is some evidence that these may be carried out by the right hemisphere.

The outline which follows is only a skeleton of the complete examination, and should serve as no more than a starting point for more intensive studies. In the formulation of these tests, I have been fortunate to receive the advice of Dr. Edith Kaplan, a pioneer in the development of apraxia testing.

A. *Nonrepresentational movements*
  1) place hand under chin
  2) place hand in front of nose
  3) touch index finger to ear
  4) put hand behind head
  5) touch thumb to forehead
B. *Facial praxis*
  1) blow out match
  2) sip on straw
  3) protrude tongue
  4) cough

     5) sniff flower
     6) close your eyes
     7) lick upper lip
     8) puff out cheeks
     9) whistle
   10) wrinkle your nose

C. *Intransitive movements (on the body)*
     1) salute
     2) scratch head
     3) throw kiss
     4) indicate full stomach
     5) make sign of cross

D. *Intransitive movements (away from the body)*
     1) wave goodbye
     2) beckon
     3) hitchhike
     4) make fist
     5) snap fingers

E. *Transitive movements (on the body)*
     1) brush teeth
     2) shave
     3) comb hair
     4) drink with spoon
     5) file fingernails

F. *Transitive movements (away from body)*
     1) saw
     2) hammer
     3) flip coin
     4) use screwdriver
     5) use scissors

G. *Leg praxis*
     1) stamp out cigarette
     2) press on gas pedal
     3) tap foot
     4) kick a ball
     5) slide foot in slipper

H. *Whole body movements*
     1) stand, sit, turn around, walk backwards
     2) stand like a boxer, golfer, batter, diver, etc.
     3) shovel dirt
     4) jump, squat, bow, shrug

  5) dancing
 I. *Bilateral (similar movements each hand)*
  1) play piano
  2) clap
  3) circle hands in air
  4) pray
  5) jump rope
 J. *Bilateral (different movements each hand)*
  1) use hand drill, eggbeater
  2) wring towel
  3) screw in bolt
  4) file fingernails
  5) thread needle
 K. *Ideational tests* (few objects, cooperative movements also J above)
  1) cutting paper
  2) opening lock with key
  3) dialing on telephone
  4) tie shoelaces
  5) button shirt
  6) tie necktie
 L. *Ideational tests* (multiple objects, sequencing)
  1) take cigarette and match from pack, light and smoke
  2) pour coffee into cup, add sugar, stir and drink
  3) fold letter, seal in envelope, stamp
  4) put tobacco in pipe, pack, light and smoke
 M. *Ideational series* (single objects, sequencing)
  1) hammer in a series of 5 nails
  2) cut paper into 8 parts (or fold in half)
  3) file fingernails in series
 N. *Miscellaneous, sequencing tasks*
  1) reproducing tapped rhythms
  2) reproducing sequence of hand positions (after Luria, 1966)

Items K–M are done only with objects. All other tests should be done to command, imitation and where applicable, with objects. Both right and left hand should be tested separately, as well as sequentially, noting improvement on one side following correct performance on the other. Proximal-distal differences, latency of movement and any tendency to substitute a part of the body for the object (e.g. rubbing the fist on the cheek on shaving) should be noted. Imitation should be tested, with and without the real object in the examiner's hand. With respect to object use, the patient should be examined for facilitation by: 1) wrong objects, both structurally (stick for hammer) and conceptually (screwdriver for hammer) related; 2) functionally related objects (e.g. nail for hammer); 3) objects related through similarity of movement (key for screwdriver); and 4) an object in one hand, on an action in the other. One can give the object at the start of a movement, then withdraw it and note any decay in performance. Cueing may be done by beginning the action, and allowing the patient to complete it, or by giving commands contextually which cannot be carried out alone, such as saluting from a position of attention, punching from the position of a boxer, etc. Care should be taken to explore the effect of the command itself, for the phrasing of the command will influence ability to carry out the action. Thus, telling a patient to "Use a hammer" or "How would you hold a baseball bat?" is often less effective than telling the patient to "Hammer" or "Stand like a baseball batter." One patient consistently failed to demonstrate how to "Hold a shovel," but immediately responded when told to "Shovel snow." Other tests that can be carried out in selected patients involve the learning of movements, as in tracing a maze, as well as transfer of motions passively acquired from one hand to the other. The patient should be observed in his daily routine for difficulty in spontaneous complex movements such as during eating, shaving, toilet and brushing his teeth.

Finally, it is important to recognize the demands placed upon patients by actions in pantomine, whether to command or imitation. Impairment on these tasks to some extent may be said to differ from the normal condition only in degree. Most normal subjects are unable, without the real objects, to tie their shoelaces or necktie, or pick up a pen and pass it between their fingers to a writing position. Though highly overlearned, just as brushing the teeth or hammering a nail, these actions, nevertheless, cannot be reconstructed either in pantomine or in the imagination. One should, therefore, be cautious about concluding that a patient has an intact idea of the motion, interrupted in its passage to motor form, for some ideas at least can be realized only through the completed movement.

Chapter 10

IDEATIONAL APRAXIA

THE FIRST DESCRIPTION of ideational apraxia was by Pick (1905), who recorded the case of a forty-three-year-old right-handed man, globally aphasic with echolalia, but able to understand simple orders. There was some paresis of the right hand and a preference for the left. Many actions were carried out well with no, or few, mistakes, but on using objects there were many errors. Single objects were misused, as for example, employing a razor as a comb, but the difficulty was particularly marked when the task required a sequence of actions with two or more objects. Thus, given a candle to light, he held the match with both hands, and did nothing more. On repeating the command, he inverted the match and tried to grind it into the candle. Upon lighting the match for him, he lit the candle and then put it into his mouth. Pick recognized the role that visual agnosia could play in this disorder, and insisted that objects could be named correctly in spite of their misuse. In addition, errors could result from disturbance of a) the temporal sequence of individual movements, as in the anticipation of a movement which should be carried out later. This is the so-called Kurzschluss-Reaction (short-circuit reaction), b) premature terminations of a movement sequence, c) condensation of two movements into one, d) derailments through faulty association and e) perseveration. Pick concluded that the disorder in this case resulted from a loss of attention directed to the inner voluntary action. This was conceived as a persistence, or a recognition, of the purpose of the action which held the subordinate activities together. Loss of this factor resulted in the disintegration of the movement plan into a series of individual actions only secondarily related. Pick believed that ideational apraxia was intermediate in nature between agnosia and ideo-motor apraxia, leading to Grunbaum's use of the term "apractagnosia." Pick also gave the name "pseudoapraxia" to an inertia or fixing of ideation, or perseveration, and "parapraxia" to the situation in which an unintentional movement occurs in the place of the intended correct movement.

About this time, Marcuse (1904) described a condition which he termed "amnesic apraxia," a disorder which, following the studies of Kurt Goldstein on amnesic aphasia, came to be applied to patients with inability to evoke appropriate movement concepts at the right moment. The principal finding is a total inability to evoke the desired movement in the presence of an understanding, by the patient, how to proceed. However, the patient does make correct movements, does well on imitation and distinguishes correct from incorrect movements performed in front of him. Comparable to amnesic (anomic) aphasia, this apraxic syndrome is apparently quite rare and little studied, though it has been revived to some extent in a recent paper by Zangwill (1960).

Pick's description was accepted by Liepmann with the qualification that ideational apraxia was only a more severe form of ideo-motor apraxia. Later, however, Liepmann (1920) accepted it as a distinct form, characterized by preserved simple movements, and some complex movements, with impairment on tasks requiring an action sequence utilizing more than one object. Though often associated with perceptual difficulties, ideational apraxia does not depend on these, but rather relates to an inadequacy of the ideational plan of action. Failure to arouse the correct movement pattern results in the amnesic form, while insufficiency of the plan once evoked leads to ideational apraxia. The pathology was assigned to left occipito-parietal region, though diffuse conditions were frequently associated.

The work of Monakow (1905) should also be mentioned, if only for the reason that it tends to support the views of other workers. Three posterior forms were distinguished: a) parapraxia, which is associated with optic agnosia, b) amnestic apraxia, similar to that discussed and c) an ideogenic form, corresponding to ideational apraxia proper.

This early work was elegantly summarized by Lange (1936), who was in agreement with Pick and Liepmann that ideational apraxia should be applied only to those cases in which actions with objects, particularly serial actions with multiple objects, were disturbed. He pointed out that the condition was always bilateral, though at times more severe in a limb already affected with ideo-motor apraxia, and emphasized the role of occipito-parietal lesions (as well as lesions of posterior T2) in producing the syndrome.

Paul Schilder (1935) regarded ideational apraxia as closely related to "object-apraxia," hesitating to admit a primary disorder of the "utilization of movement-sequences." According to Schilder, voluntary action first develops out of a broad schema, constructed of visual-spatial and kinesthetic images. This schema contains the body image, and the object which is the aim of the action, and evolves toward a completely unfolded form. Ideational apraxia, he believed, was a form in which there were inhibitory effects from an object apraxia (i.e. agnosic apraxia) upon the movement sequence.

Morlaas (1928) reviewed the subject, added some personal cases, and concluded that the disorder was in the psychic, not the gestural, sphere. He pointed out that while the defect appears in complex serial acts, the underlying disorder does not lie in the ability to produce these acts, but rather in an incapacity to correctly use the test objects. Since patients can name and manipulate objects which are used inappropriately, there must be adequate recognition but an "agnosia of utilization."

Recent contributions include those of Zangwill (1960), Hecaen (1968) and De Renzi *et al.* (1968). Zangwill has discussed this topic with customary insight. He noted that cases of ideational apraxia without either an ideo-motor or visual perceptual component were not to be found in the literature, and that, if one excluded this latter group—the optic-apraxias—all ideational apraxics would be severe instances of ideo-motor apraxia; that is, impaired praxis to command, to imitation, and finally, even to object use. Recalling earlier work, he suggested a relation to amnesic aphasia, in the failure to evoke the right movement at the precise moment in the action sequence.

For Hecaen, ideational apraxia is an impairment of the logical and harmonious sequence of the several elementary movements that make up a complex act, though each movement by itself is executed correctly. There is agreement with Zangwill that ideational apraxia is a more severe stage of ideomotor apraxia, the objects no longer having a facilitatory effect on the disordered movements.

De Renzi and co-workers have studied the relation of object use to apraxia in a group of brain-damaged patients, in an attempt to determine whether, as emphasized by many workers, there is a quantitative relationship between the ideo-motor and the ideational forms. In their study, patients were given a series of intransitive gestures, as well as a series of movements with objects, and the results of the tests were compared. Their finding was that the two forms were relatively independent, with ideational apraxia showing a closer statistical relation to aphasia than to any of the other parameters examined. For this reason, they conceived ideational apraxia as a disturbance in concept formation, linked with the aphasias. Although this study is open to criticism on many grounds, it provides the first statistical treatment of the problem, and is a hopeful sign of renewed experimental interest in a very neglected area.

Case 8

A sixty-year-old right-handed man, transferred to the Aphasia Unit in January, 1970 with a history, in September, 1969, of a four-day period of confusion, inappropriate speech and weakness of the right hand. This problem stabilized and transfer to the Aphasia Unit was arranged. The patient's background was inexceptional, except for a brother with left-handedness.

Neurological testing revealed: right homonymous hemianopsia with visual acuity 20/40 or better in left hemi-field; EOM full and conjugate; inability to consistently follow moving objects in either direction and difficulty in diverting gaze to objects presented in the good field, to the left of fixation. There was impairment of visual pointing, and he was unable to count more than one object in the left field. Fixation was labile and uncertain. Completion of semicircles into the impaired field was noted. Other cranial nerve functions were normal. Motor testing disclosed minimal weakness of the right arm (pronator sign) with some increase in tone on that side. Otherwise no weakness or incoordination to formal testing was found. Reflexes were normal and equal, Babinski's absent bilaterally. Sensation normal to all primary modalities, though impaired tactile localization in all limbs, with foreshortening, and a tendency to extinguish on the right to simultaneous stimulation were noted. Brain scan revealed left occipito-parietal lesion; EEG showed biparietal slowing, more marked on the left side.

The patient was oriented to age and location of hospital, but could not give the hospital name, his own birthdate or the current date. He was unable to perform on serial 7's, did poorly on recent memory, word list and proverb testing. Digit span was 6. In spite of his poor performance on these tests, he was alert and attentive to questions, responded promptly to all commands, conversed easily, and was active and social on the ward.

Speech was fluent, though empty, aspontaneous and circumlocutory with occasional perseverations. There was no paraphasia or echolalia, and except for its anomic quality, speech was nonaphasic. Singing and series speech were normal. *Comprehension* was fairly good at a simple level, for pointing and yes/no questions. Many questions which were not responded to appropriately were repeated, in nonecholalic fashion, back to the examiner. In part, testing was limited by a visual and somatic disorientation, and by the perseverative tendency. The disorder did not appear to be one of perception, as in a sensory aphasic, but one of organizing a response to a situation adequately perceived.

Repetition was intact for words, letters, sounds, numbers and long phrases, and simple tapped rhythms could be reproduced.

Naming was accurate visually and tactually to 80 per cent, for objects and body parts, in a word-frequency dependent manner. Auditory naming was similarly impaired. Misnaming was partly a result of perseveration and confabulation, and also dependent in the visual sphere on fixation on the test object. Once an object name was confabulated, he could not select the right object from a group. Colors were named better than objects, but still impaired. He was unable to select a color named from a group of colored skeins in front of him, presumably a reflection of simultanagnosia. He could name line drawings of objects and actions fairly well, but on magazine pictures failed badly, usually noting only one or two elements of a larger scene.

Writing was impaired in either hand, though his name and some words such as horse or dog were possible. There was greater difficulty writing individual letters or numbers than words. Copying was no better, nor did writing improve with his eyes closed. Reading was possible for small words such as cat, chair, and sky, and occasionally for longer words also. He was unable to read individual letters or numbers, match them or point to them on command. Though able to hold up fingers to command, or to a series of drawn lines, he could not match fingers to written numbers. *Spelling* and comprehension of spelled words was quite good. *Calculations* were limited but possible mentally. *Constructional* ability was severely impaired for drawing, copying and Koh's blocks. Fingers were misidentified, mismatched and mislocalized, and right-left orientation was fragile. There were similar though less severe confusions on other body areas. Identification of well-known faces was impaired, though he accepted the correct name. He could find, but not trace, embedded figures; no dressing apraxia; visual imagery was impaired.

Facial praxis was fairly good, mistakes consisting largely of perseverations of previous movements. Intransitive movements to verbal command, with either hand, were fairly good, though occasional errors occurred, improved by imitation. Transitive commands, without objects, to verbal command were fair, accurate to 75 per cent in such tests as sawing wood, hammering a nail, combing hair and so on. Poor performances were improved with imitation. No difference was noted for movements toward or away from the body, or directed to the head or other body parts. Poor performances were not facilitated by object-use, and in fact, movements with single objects were usually worse than without objects. For example, when told to demonstrate how to brush his teeth, he did so promptly, but when given a toothbrush and asked to demonstrate its use, he first brushed his nails, then his pants, and only with much prompting did he finally use the toothbrush correctly. Manipulation of objects was usually correct, in the presence of improper use. More complex movements were severely disorganized.

For example, the patient is given a pitcher of water and a glass, and instructed to pour water into the glass and take a drink. He picks up the pitcher with his left hand, tilts it toward him spilling water on the floor. On filling the glass in his right hand (assisted), he puts the glass down and drinks out of the pitcher.

The patient is asked to call the operator on the telephone. He picks up the receiver and holds it properly to his ear; then with his right hand presses down on the tone button, saying, "I don't know how to do it." Encouraged, he continues to push on the button, then runs his fingers over the dial, stumbles into the second hole, and dials #2 repeatedly.

Some complex movements such as sealing a letter, were performed slowly but accurately. Other actions, done without knowledge that he was being observed, such as brushing his teeth in the morning or eating lunch, were highly disorganized. It is of interest that he was aware of his praxic difficulty, and on one occasion gave the following description of his eating: "I don't eat organized . . . If I have a spoon I don't use another item. It's a good thing I haven't got company." In general, bimanual coordination was adroit, as well as object manipulation, such that failures with objects could be attributed to either of the following major problems:

1. Difficulty with spatial orientation of the object. For example, in smoking a pipe, the pipe was held properly but brought to the mouth in the wrong plane, the stem advancing horizontally rotated 180° in the frontal plane. Given a nail in a board and a hammer, he secured the board properly, and then, holding the hammer in an appropriate manner, waved it, at right angles to the nail, in the air.

2. Perseveration of movement and inability to shift from one sequence to another. This is complementary to the visual simultanagnosia, and can be conceptualized as a simultanagnosia for movement. In this case, perseveration of one movement is a re-

flection of inability to go on to the next, and in itself does not appear to have specific import.

It should be emphasized that the patient was able to name, describe and properly hold objects which were incorrectly used, and that he was aware of the insufficiency of his response. There was no evidence, apart from the simultanagnosic component, that visual agnosia played any role in the apraxia. Nor could one account for such performance on the basis of a dementia, since transitive movements without objects were better than the same movements with objects, the latter being the simpler and more concrete task. Finally, the finger agnosia and mild autotopagnosia probably played some role in praxic errors, but again, why these should influence object-movements, or object-sequences, more than non-object transitive or intransitive movements is not clear.

Case 9

This patient with "apperceptive visual agnosia" is discussed elsewhere with regard to the agnosic picture (Chap. 19). Examination of praxis revealed normal facial and whole body movements to command and, at times, to imitation. Nonrepresentational movements were done well, but right-left confusions were present. Most limb transitive movements were adequately performed, though very slow and cautious, whether toward or away from the body. Considerable time elapsed before initiation of most actions; wrong movements were usually corrected; no definite improvement occurred with imitation. Transitive actions, on or away from the body, were fairly good. There was no tendency for substitutions of body part for object. Inadequate movements were notable mainly for their slow, coarse, abbreviated quality. Actions with objects were possible, showing more errors than without objects. These were of two types: uncertainty by vision or touch as to the nature of the object, the action improving greatly on supplying the name; and performance which remained impaired, whether the patient gave the name spontaneously, or was given the name. Many actions were done well, such as using a toothbrush, a hairbrush, throwing a ball, and even more demanding tasks such as putting a key in a lock. Other actions were impaired. For example, given paper and envelope, and asked to seal a letter (object names given), the patient spent many minutes trying to fold the paper, in abnormal planes, and never achieved the stage of letter insertion. Again, when told to dial the operator on the telephone, the patient picked up the receiver, and simply rotated it in his hand. He seemed uncertain which end should go to his ear, manipulated the cord and finally held the receiver to his ear correctly. After a further delay, he was encouraged to continue, and attempted to dial. The limitation appeared largely visual, with groping about for the hole. Finally, he was told to take a cigarette from a pack and light it. He removed the cigarette properly, but very slowly; felt either end to locate the filter, and then placed the cigarette in his mouth properly. He did not proceed until given the matches, then removed a match (assisted), and attempted to light it on the wrong end. He made no attempt to ascertain the striking end of the match. The patient was next fitted with a mask, and object sequences were carried out with no visual cues. If anything, a deterioration occurred in performance, all movements becoming very slow and groping.

By way of general comment, the following points can be made. Movements without objects were generally superior to movements with objects, and bimanual coordination was excellent. There was little if any improvement to imitation, and the movements deteriorated with eyes covered. This tends to cast doubt on a purely visual or recognitive basis for this disorder. According to the patient's family, he managed very well at home, eating, bathing, and in toilet and other daily activities.

Errors could be characterized in the following way:

1. Actions were slow and hesitant, the patient appearing to think out each movement along the way. He required encouragement in action sequences to pass on to next stage. Object recognition facilitated many actions, but did not facilitate others; his performance was considerably worse than that of a blind man.

2. Some actions were carried out in the wrong plane, consistent with the severe spatial and constructional difficulties on testing.

3. Perseverative tendencies were quite marked. It appeared that the lassitude of action, the perseveration of normal or abnormal movements, and the spatial disorientation of the movement sequence, were sufficient to account for the apraxic picture.

4. There seemed also to be an amnesic element, as in the cessation of movements midway in a sequence, and the necessity to be reminded of the latter part of an action. An attentional problem could also account for this, and clear separation was not possible.

These two cases illustrate the range of disability seen within the ideational category. The cases are of particular interest since one occurred with apperceptive agnosia (Case #9), and the other with

simultanagnosia or Balint's syndrome (Case #8). In both, the difficulty settles mainly 'on two, possibly three, major factors. These
consist of spatial disorientation, perseveration and an amnesic disorder. In the simultanagnosic, both the spatial and the perseveratory
elements were marked, as was the apraxia, but object recognition was
quite good. In the visual agnosic, these elements were not so apparent,
nor was the apraxia very severe, but visual recognition was profoundly
altered. This fact, plus the failure, in many instances, of object recognition to facilitate the use of the object, leads to the conclusion that
object recognition per se does not play a vital role in the genesis of
the apraxia. In this regard, it is of interest that in one case of "associative" agnosia (Benson and Rubens, 1971), personal examination
revealed no evidence of ideational (or other) apraxia. Further, regarding the perseveration, it cannot easily be separated from an
inability to proceed, and this in turn may simply reflect a "motor
amnesia." This may also be true of confabulation, the confabulatory
response being only a "random" perseveration, and therefore, an indication that the patient cannot move on to the next step. This is not
an amnesia for specific units; rather, the movement sequence seems
to "run down," terminating at almost any point in the sequence rather
than at critical junctures.

We are left then with a spatial disorder and an amnesia for the
units of an action sequence. This action sequence issues out of an
abstract structuralized representation within which, as within the
speech system, two major processes are brought to bear, a conceptual
organization, determining the ordering and the calling up of units
of the action sequence, and a function, comparable perhaps to the
syntactical aspect of language, by which the interrelationships of
those units are established and maintained. The processes combine to
produce a smoothly flowing motor sequence. The syntactical element
provides for the hierarchical unfolding of well-fitting partial movements, the conceptual or semantic element brings up the partial movements and fits them into the movement skeleton.

The defect in ideational apraxia is similar, therefore, to that in the
deep expressive speech system. There we see disturbances in both
word meaning and processes of verbal memory. In ideational apraxia,
the disruption of the organization of the action, the appearance of
partial movements at the wrong time in the movement sequence,
parapraxias and perseverations, substitutions into conceptually or
morphologically related actions, and the failure to evoke a movement
at the moment of its need, all recall the deficits which are found at

the corresponding aphasic level. Thus, we may almost speak of ideational apraxia as a "fluent" apraxia, contrasting it with "nonfluent" apraxias of anterior origin. In ideational apraxia there is an abundance of partial movements, each normal in itself, and the overall movement sequence, though disorganized, has an ease and an effortless quality as is seen in the speech of the posterior aphasic.

Just as the earliest stages of the expressive speech system are coextensive with auditory perceptual functions, there is a bond between the motor action and the visual perception. Speech issues out of an organization common to speech perception, and action develops out of an organization common to visual perception. In ideational apraxia there is always some balance between injury to the system through which the action unfolds, and the system for visual perception, though ordinarily there is an emphasis more in one direction than another. That is why patients can show severe agnosia and a mild apraxic component, or severe ideational apraxia with mild disturbances of visual recognition. In the latter case, however, where the action system is more heavily involved, so also will be parieto-occipital mechanisms concerned with eye movements. This may lead to the spurious conclusion that the recognition defect is secondary to an eye movement disorder, and the apraxia secondary to both, though, in fact, ocular apraxia (Balint's syndrome and/or simultanagnosia) and the visual recognition defects are manifestations of the same disturbance which leads to ideational apraxia. It is unknown whether ocular apraxia can appear without ideational apraxia, though the reverse, ideational apraxia without ocular apraxia certainly does occur.

From this discussion, it is clear that to consider ideational apraxia as only a more severe form of ideo-motor apraxia is comparable to holding that posterior aphasias are deteriorated intermediate forms, a view that is wholly contradicted by the facts. Moreover, it is important to note that there are some ways in which object movements can achieve a greater degree of complexity than those without objects. This may come about by way of the command situation itself. For example, telling a patient "Brush your teeth" without the object, and giving him an object and asking him to show how it is used (i.e. toothbrush) are not at all comparable tasks. In this instance, the action with the object may for some patients be more complex, for it demands a recognition factor in addition to the action, and the exact nature of the action to be performed with the object, though implicit, is not verbally specified.

Finally, the phenomenon which is a central characteristic of this disorder, greater difficulty with than without objects, is also to be seen as analogous to certain aphasic states. The object impairment in ideational apraxia, and the facilitation by objects in the anterior apraxias, are features similar to the effect of cues on the word-finding of posterior and anterior aphasics, or as has been discussed, the inverse direction of word loss in parietal and frontal anomia.

Chapter 11

IDEO-MOTOR APRAXIA

IT IS IN LIEPMANN'S case report of 1900 (Regierungsrat) that we find the first detailed description of motor (ideo-motor; ideo-kinetic) apraxia. Some twenty years later, Liepmann attempted to relate this disorder to other apraxic forms and to the physiology of voluntary movement in general. He emphasized the preservation of both the kinetic engram and the ideational scheme of the movement, for the action could take place, as in his first case, in one hand but not the other, and actions which were impossible to command could be performed spontaneously with object use. The substratum of the engram was thought to be dissociated from the rest of the brain. That the patient could not imitate the simplest motions, nor carry them out to command, nor fully utilize kinesthetic information about the object or the movement to be performed, indicated that the motor engram was separated from the acoustic, the optic and the kinesthetic components. With regard to the engram itself, Liepmann had a dynamic conception, and stressed the fact that it was not localized to specific cells or small loci, but rather consisted of patterns of neural activity corresponding to certain motor events. With regard to the concept of the movement, it was for the most part a concept of the goal of the action rather than a conscious movement plan. Liepmann noted, in fact, that it was in the unfolding of the movement, in the succession of its partial movements, that the concept first became clearly conscious. In sighted persons, this conceptual organization was, he believed, grounded in the optical, whereas in the blind, the kinesthetic element was dominant. Though Liepmann pointed out that overlap occurred between ideo-motor apraxia and the ideational and limb-kinetic forms, and related this overlap to posterior or anterior extension of the lesion, he did not, in terms of the pattern of motor disintegration, distinguish ideo-motor apraxia from the "sympathetic" or "callosal" varieties. The errors in ideo-motor apraxia were largely in the way of conceptual substitutions, motoric diversions, and amorphous or mutilated actions. Of particular importance in pathogenesis were lesions in the area of supramarginal gyrus, a localization later affirmed by von Monakow, Lange, Schilder, Morlaas, and others. Such lesions produced bilateral limb and facial apraxia through interruption of fibers from temporal and occipital lobes to the pre-Rolandic area. Apraxia of this type was either equal in both arms, or more severe on the right side. Qualitative differences in the performance of each arm were not described at that time, nor have they been described since.

Following this series of papers, Liepmann's description of apraxia became the standard by which all studies were gauged. Even such critics as Sittig and Brun were silenced when major writers with a marked functional orientation, such as Goldstein and Schilder, saw in this work a confirmation of their own more psychological views. Thus, Schilder (1935) ignored Liepmann's speculations about a pathway from concept to engram and seized upon his allusions to functional change within a broad axis across the hemisphere. Apraxia was held to be a disturbance at various levels within a developing sequence. The sequence passes, as Schilder clearly pointed out, from an optically-grounded stage confluent with the postural model of the body, through successive stages on the way toward the final action form. Indeed, it is not hard to see the germ of such a theory in Liepmann's writings, for he was invariably most careful to qualify and broaden any statement that might have suggested too particulate a view of these processes. His notion of the engram, of the concept, are insightful and surprisingly modern, and his pathological map (Fig. 5) suggests immediately the kind of processes of which Schilder spoke.

Subsequent workers have shown little tendency to deviate from Liepmann's early description, embracing either its psychological or anatomical aspects. Ajuriaguerra *et al.* (1960) and Hecaen (1968) adapt Liepmann's classification mainly for its heuristic and psychological value. There is emphasis on the conservation in ideo-motor apraxia of an ideatory plan and it is suggested that the alteration concerns the partial movements only, these being out of harmony with the whole. The defect may occur in spontaneous activity, but ordinarily appears in the situation of the examination. Movements to command are affected most severely, and particularly transitive gestures without objects. In addition to the error types mentioned by Liepmann, synkinetic movements and confusions with older or more automatic movements may occur. The disorder follows left-sided (or bilateral) retro-Rolandic lesions. This classification is extended to ontogenetic data by Hecaen.

The anatomical aspects of ideo-motor apraxia were discussed by Nielsen (1941), who, after a review of cases with bilateral supramarginal gyrus involvement, concluded in basic agreement with the above localization. Nielsen offered the unusual suggestion that spontaneous acts were better than those to command because of the "shorter course of the intercortical impulses in the former." Geschwind (1965) accepted Liepmann's localization, and elaborated upon the anatomical aspects of the typology. Though psychological terminology is carefully avoided, it is implicit in the anatomical account. Thus, lesions in supramarginal gyrus are held to interrupt acoustic-motor (arcuate or superior longitudinal fasciculus) and visual-motor pathways passing deep to the gyrus, thereby separating the various modality components of the ideational scheme from the more anterior motor engrams. Geschwind does not distinguish qualitatively between supramarginal gyrus apraxia, "sympathetic" apraxia and "callosal" apraxia, rather stressing the uniformity in each of the command, imitation, object-use, hierarchy. According to Liepmann's account, the three forms which constitute ideo-kinetic apraxia should not differ markedly from one another, and because of this theoretical attitude, no attempt to separately characterize them has yet been made.

APRAXIA OF THE SUPRAMARGINAL GYRUS

In his case of the Regierungsrat (1900), Liepmann attempted to correlate apraxia with lesion in the dominant supramarginal gyrus, and his schema of overlapping apraxic zones (Fig. 5) clearly indicates the importance which Liepmann attached to this region. A lesion in this area was thought to produce apraxia of both arms, equal bilaterally or more severe on the right side. An accompanying lesion of the callosum, in addition to producing left-sided apraxia, could have an additive effect on the impairment of the right side. Support for this localization was also provided by Kleist (1911), and good anatomical cases were provided by Strohmayer (1903) and Kroll (1910). In 1941, Nielsen discussed the problem of supramarginal gyrus apraxia, and some of the problems attendent to this localization. He pointed out that clinical and pathological studies of left middle cerebral artery thrombosis demonstrated that a lesion of this region and its subjacent white matter did not necessarily result in ideo-kinetic apraxia. Nor in fact did the destruction of both supramarginal gyri, but rather a bilateral "ataxia" with difficulty in fine finger movements.

Hecaen (1962) supported the left parietal localization for bilateral ideo-kinetic apraxia. In those cases in which left-sided apraxia has been attributed to right parietal lesion, two underlying elements are noted, constructional apraxia and apraxia for dressing. According to Hecaen, the occurrence of a restricted left-sided ideo-kinetic apraxia from right parietal lesion remains in some doubt.

Geschwind (1965) has discussed this condition at length. The clinical picture is one of bilateral apraxia, either equal in both hands or worse in the right hand, and otherwise similar in its pattern of disability to that seen in the other ideo-kinetic forms, i.e. poor performance to verbal command, only slight if any improvement with imitation and superior object handling. The lesion is presumed to interrupt a pathway from Wernicke's area and the visual region to the motor area, the arcuate or superior longitudinal fasciculus. This accounts for the failure of praxis to verbal command and imitation, while preserved object use is attributed to minor hemispheric processing or conditions of kinesthetic facilitation. The disorder is frequently associated with conduction aphasia, the localization of which is also thought to be supramarginal gyrus, as well as with facial apraxia. In my experience, however, there is no obligatory bond between these three associated states, for the conduction aphasic may present with little or no apraxia, or with facial or limb apraxia independently. The converse, limb apraxia secondary to parietal lesion without aphasia, has not been described. In fact, it is unlikely, except for callosal syndromes, that apraxia can occur in the absence of aphasia. The reverse, however, is seen frequently enough.

One must admit that the clinical description of this syndrome has in several respects been wanting. Most observers have simply noted the presence or absence of apraxia under different test conditions, without devoting much attention to the nature of the performance itself within each condition of testing. Such a study is needed in this area. Certainly, in supramarginal gyrus apraxia we no longer see the spheric substitutions of the ideational apraxic, as in brushing the shoes with a toothbrush, or using a pair of scissors like a screwdriver. The motor pattern has begun to break down such that derailments, anticipations, perseverations, etc. become more evident. The goal of the movement, however, in contrast to the ideational apraxic, can be discerned in the faulty performance. Yet the patient is not yet at the stage of the anterior apraxic, the sympathetic dyspraxic and limb-kinetic apraxic, for whom maladroitness and clumsiness are the rule.

CALLOSAL SYNDROMES

In his discussion of callosal disorders, Liepmann postulated four possible forms. Types 1 and 2 in his diagram (Fig. 6) are char-

acteristic of "sympathetic" apraxia. This condition, described originally by Liepmann, consists of apraxia of the left arm and leg in a
patient with Broca's aphasia and right hemiparesis. The left-sided
apraxia is presumably due to involvement of the left limb-control area,
with or without callosal extension, resulting in an isolation of the
corresponding region in the right hemisphere. If the left hemisphere
is dominant for movement, the left limbs, deprived of guidance by the
left hemisphere, become apraxic while an obligatory apraxia of the
right side is obscured by the overlying right hemiparesis. The para-
digmatic study of this form has to be the case of Liepmann and Maas
(Ochs) discussed above. Though objections can be raised against this
case, viz.: the apparent dementia, the occurrence of an ideational
apraxia and disturbed object use, and the postulation, by Liepmann,
of an isolated agraphia in the left hand in a severe Broca's aphasic
who, no doubt, would have been agraphic in the right hand also
were it not hemiparetic, the case remains an important one in view of
Liepmann's fine analysis and his discussion of the role of callosal
pathology. Concurrent with this report, Liepmann (1905) published
a controlled study of a group of patients with right hemiparesis,
showing that slightly over two-thirds of those with motor aphasia also
had an associated left-sided apraxia. In spite of this high incidence, the
disorder has not since been the subject of careful study. This may be
because of the common assumption that left-sided apraxia, or for that
matter ideo-motor apraxia in general, is identical to that seen in
restricted lesions or section of the corpus callosum, the latter being
the purer and therefore more suitable disorder for investigation. This
argument, that "sympathetic" apraxia is a callosal apraxia contami-
nated by right hemiparesis, will be discussed shortly.

Liepmann's type 4, left-sided apraxia due to callosal lesion, is seen
clinically most often with pathology in the distribution of the anterior cerebral artery. Characteristically, there is apraxia of the left arm
and leg, left-sided agraphia and, commonly, astereognosis in the left
hand. The first clear example with pathology, recorded by van
Vleuten (1907), was a fifty-five-year-old man with general paresis who
was found to have mild paraphasia, word-finding difficulty and
tremulousness and grasping of the right hand. In spite of these motor
defects, the right arm was judged to be eupraxic, while the left arm,
affected with only a fine tremor, was severely apraxic. This was true
for movements to command and to imitation. Postmortem revealed a
large sarcoma of left hemisphere, destroying cingulate gyrus and the
left half, and right genu of corpus callosum. The existence of this

disorder was subsequently verified by other cases, and most recently by the remarkable case of Geschwind and Kaplan (1962). This patient was a forty-one-year-old man, operated on for a left frontal glioma, with mild paraphasia, moderate right hemiparesis and mild sensory changes on the right side. The discovery that he was able to write with his right hand but not with the left initiated a series of studies to evaluate the function in that extremity. He was able to name objects held in the right hand but not in the left, although drawing and object manipulation were correct. He could select an object held in the left hand visually from a group of objects before him. He was unable to select an object held in the left hand with his right hand. Movements to verbal command were impaired in the left hand, but adequate to imitation and object use; whereas, movements in the right hand were, given the hemiparesis, normal. Postmortem examination revealed massive involvement of left hemisphere by tumor, and infarction of the anterior two-thirds of corpus callosum. The right hemisphere was normal. This case, which should serve as a model for the future study of such patients, indicates that earlier reports demonstrating sensory or stereognostic impairment in the left hand as a sign of right parietal disease need thorough reassessment. It is probable that cases of this type were responsible for the idea that unilateral left apraxia could be produced by a right parietal lesion. Certainly, a diagnosis of parietal involvement could not now be made without appropriate nonverbal tests of sensory function. Moreover, those cases in which right parietal and callosal damage were judged to have a summative effect on left-sided apraxia (Klein and Ingram, 1958) must, in light of our recent understanding of callosal syndromes, be interpreted with care.

In spite of the fact that two of the most important cases concerned tumor, the incidence of this syndrome with isolated callosal tumor is very low. Similarly, callosal degeneration has not been documented to produce the picture, and it is absent in callosal agenesis. The more common clinical variety, right crural monoplegia and left apraxia through infarction of left superior frontal lobe and anterior callosum (anterior cerebral artery syndrome) is felt, by Ajuriaguerra and Hecaen (1964) to be less common than generally supposed. The authors point out that the anterior cerebral artery also supplies part of the internal region of parietal lobe, which is known to be associated with apraxia. The purest group of patients in whom this question might be resolved are undoubtedly those with commissurotomy. Gazzaniga *et al.* (1967) have described in these cases some difficulty

on verbal commands and imitation with the distal left-sided musculature, though object use was apparently preserved, as well as movements utilizing proximal groups, such as pointing and drawing.
Unfortunately, a description of the kinds of praxic errors seen was not
provided. When single printed words were flashed tachistoscopically
to the left hemisphere, they could generally be written out with the
left hand, and simple hand positions could similarly be imitated. Such
findings indicate a surprising degree of ipsilateral control, leading the
authors to suggest that it is the impairment in this control system
rather than the callosal disconnection per se that accounts for cases
such as those reported by Liepmann and Geschwind. They suggest
that the callosal syndrome should be approached, not from the standpoint of a guiding left hemisphere and a passively responding right,
but rather from an understanding of the equilibrium existing *between*
the hemispheres.

With regard to Type 5 of Liepmann, left-sided apraxia from subcortical lesion catching commissural fibers from the left side, this disorder has, to my knowledge, not yet been adequately documented.

To summarize, the callosal syndromes fall mainly into three groups:
1) pure callosal lesion; 2) callosal lesion plus left frontal lesion, right
arm nonapraxic; and 3) Broca's aphasia, right hemiparesis and left-
sided apraxia, with or without a callosal lesion. Whether group 2 is
different from the pure callosal case is uncertain, but there are suggestive, though not carefully investigated, differences between groups
1 and 3. This is not surprising, since it is hardly to be expected that
lesion of an association area (e.g. Broca's area) would produce a
condition identical to combined or independent lesion of the callosum. It is my impression that patients with sympathetic apraxia tend
to use the left hand clumsily, the movements being coarse but approximating the desired action. As with speech in the Broca's aphasic,
the target movement can be seen in the altered performance. Thus,
asked to flip a coin, such a patient might open and close his hand, or
clasp his thumb tightly against a clenched fist, or rub thumb and fore-
finger together as if feeling a piece of fabric. In two patients with
restricted left-sided apraxia and presumed callosal lesion (one case of
trauma; one degenerative condition thought to be Marchiafava-
Bignami disease), the left-sided movements were of a totally different
nature. Movements were fluid and dextrous, and errors were often
wholly unrelated to the demanded task. Thus, such a patient when
asked to flip a coin might point his finger to his forehead, or wave his
hand in the air. In the first instance, therefore, movements are coarse

but directed toward the goal; in the second, dextrous but often wholly unrelated to the movement requested. If this difference proves to be correct, a reappraisal of Liepmann's account of ideo-kinetic apraxia would be required.

In this regard, another problem requiring study is the role of imitation in the facilitation of certain movements. Most patients with sympathetic apraxia perform poorly to imitation, though some improve greatly. Callosal apractics also imitate poorly, unless the movement to be imitated is presented only to right hemisphere. Performing a movement with the right hand first was said, by Liepmann, to facilitate some performances in the left hand, presumably on an "imitative" basis, but whether this corresponds to the ability to carry out imitative gestures generally is not known. The necessity for presentation to right hemisphere of the movement to be imitated only emphasizes the complex nature of hemispheric interaction. There appears to be a competitive aspect of hemispheric function accounting for many of the effects of callosal section, rather than failure to get information across to the right side. It is of interest in this regard that even Liepmann wondered whether a callosal lesion could not aggravate preexisting right-sided apraxia, a possibility not envisioned in his diagrammatic account.

Chapter 12

LIMB-KINETIC APRAXIA

T HIS CONDITION WAS first postulated by Liepmann (1900) on a case of Westphal (1882; see Westphal, 1907), a patient with impaired position sense and spasticity of the right hand with clumsiness and difficulty on simple purposeful movements. Westphal interpreted the disorder as a loss of kinesthetic memories. According to Liepmann (1920), the clinical picture consists of coarse, mutilated simple movements, while more complex motions such as sewing may not even get started. Errors resemble those of ataxia, and are not diminished by imitative or transitive movements with objects. Subsequently, Heilbronner (1905) designated the condition as "cortical apraxia," noting that it was related to slight monoparesis of the arm, and including "instrumental" and facial apraxia in this group.

Under the term "innervatory apraxia," Kleist (1907) described the case of a forty-four-year-old syphilitic man who, following bilateral strokes, demonstrated a motor aphasia, considerable bilateral spasticity, and slowness and awkwardness of movements in the left hand. On the strength of this case, which is certainly far from ideal, Kleist argued that innervatory apraxia especially affects movements of the hand, fingers and face, with slowness and stiffening of the muscles involved. There are no sensory defects, nor is there necessarily a reduction or poverty of motion in the involved limb. The difficulty appears particularly in isolated movements, with loss of fine movements, or partial movements of a sequence. There is disturbance in the simultaneous action of separate muscle groups, as well as in the smoothness of the overall sequence. The impairment is proportional to the motor complexity, and appears to have a relationship with, though independent of, both paresis and the "kinetic memory." There is no disorder of ideation, for the correct movement always appears in the deficient performance.

This description was accepted by Lange (1936) who pointed to the fact that limb-kinetic apraxia occurred largely as a digital disorder, occasionally limited to individual fingers. He suggested a pathogenesis intermediate between the mnestic and the paretic, emphasizing that the memory function was intact and that strength was not necessarily impaired.

In the years following Lange's monograph, the disorder received only scattered attention in the literature. Under the heading of "kinetic apraxia," Denny-Brown (1938) described a frontal form secondary to perseveration of contactual reactions which he termed magnetic apraxia. This formulation has not achieved wide support, for the lack of strong perseveratory tendencies and grasping in frontal apractics. Certainly, the degree to which these occur cannot account for the clinical picture. In 1941, Nielsen discussed the disorder as "cortical motor pattern apraxia," and suggested a loss of kinetic engrams in area 4, as well perhaps as area 6. With Friedman (1941), he described a case in which there was weakness of finger movement and wrist extension as the predominant findings in a recovering hemiparesis. This case, however, fails to be convincing in a differentiation from paresis, though it is likely that an isolated impairment of wrist extension can occur. Thus, in a personal case, a seventy-four-year-old right-handed man developed weakness of the left arm and face lasting approximately three hours, then gradually clearing. When seen six hours after onset, the only finding was complete inability to extend the wrist above the horizontal, though extensor strength of fingers and wrist in the horizontal position was normal. This finding also gradually disappeared, and the diagnosis was presumed to be transient cerebral ischemia. This case confirms the fact that isolated movements can be abolished in the absence of true paresis.

More recently, Ajuriaguerra and Hecaen (1964) have devoted some attention to this problem. They point out the distal and contralateral predilection, the impairment of automatic as well as volitional movements, and the resemblance to ataxia, and follow Kleist in attributing difficulty in the execution of an act to the intricacy of its motor form, and not to its psychic complexity. However, the localization is uncertain, and there is disagreement as to the autonomy of the syndrome.

Finally, Luria (1966) has noted a disturbance similar to limb-kinetic apraxia in patients with premotor lesions. These patients have normal strength, and can perform simple isolated movements well. The difficulty appears in a series of individual movements, in the loss of ". . . kinetic schemes that provide the afferent organization" of the motor series. The result is that highly organized movements become isolated actions involving the appropriate muscle groups. Thus, deficits appear in highly skilled movements such as typing, musical instrumentation and handwriting, and in one of Luria's own cases, in tapping Morse code. In developing his formulation, Luria has relied heavily on the work of Foerster (1936). This author studied patients with lesions in areas 3, 1 and 2, and sensory deficits in contralateral limbs. In these patients, an "afferent paresis" was described in which demanded movements could not be carried out, the action resulting in a diffuse contraction of agonist and antagonist groups. Thus, Luria concluded that the post-central area is responsible for directing motor impulses to definite groups of muscles, and for giving precision to the motor act. Pathology in the post-central region results in "kinesthetic apraxia," a disorder related directly to Liepmann's ideomotor form. The premotor zone, on the other hand, is then responsible for the kinetic organization of the movements, insuring the inhibition of movements once initiated, and the smooth transition from one movement to the next. A disturbance in these mechanisms results in limb-kinetic apraxia.

However appealing this formulation may seem, it runs into difficulty immediately as one looks at the various tests of motor sequencing that Luria used to demonstrate the deficient performance. Such tests as the reproduction of a series of hand positions (e.g. palm-fist-edge), tapping tests, and so on, far from being specific to premotor lesions, are impaired to some extent in almost all aphasic and/or apraxic patients, and are associated with pathology well beyond the frontal lobes. Motor sequencing or, for that matter, rapid or responsive limb movement is, in fact, one of the most difficult of tasks for the brain-injured patient.

The defect in limb-kinetic apraxia falls, perhaps, into two major groups. There are cases, like the one briefly described above, with normal strength and sensation, but loss of one or more isolated movements, the distal extensors appearing to be the most sensitive. These cases conform to Hughlings Jackson's principle of "loss of movements rather than individual muscles." A second group, which appears to be the type that the early workers had in mind, concerns the patient with normal or relatively normal strength, tone and sensation, and difficulty with complex motor performances. The more complex the movement, the greater the difficulty. Movements such as writing, typing, playing the piano or even dialing on the telephone may be quite impaired, and corresponding abnormalities are seen in rapid and fine movements on routine neurological testing. This condition is essentially an akinesia of the distal part of the limb, appearing as the first sign of a developing hemiparesis, or the remnant of one in abeyance. Certainly, if one examines a large number of recovered motor hemiparetics, an akinetic stage involving the hand can often be seen at a time when strength has returned.

Chapter 13

FACIAL APRAXIA

FACIAL APRAXIA WAS first described by Hughlings Jackson (1878), on noting that some aphasics were unable to protrude the tongue on command, while able to move it well under spontaneous conditions such as licking the lips. Jackson stressed the similarity of this voluntary-automatic dissociation to that seen in aphasia. Subsequent papers by Liepmann (1920), Lange (1936), and others, helped to further define the condition. The problem was recently reviewed by De Renzi *et al.* (1966), who give an incidence for facial apraxia of 90 per cent in Broca's aphasia and 33 per cent in conduction aphasia, and note that facial apraxia is frequently independent of limb-apraxia.

Geschwind (1965) has discussed the anatomy of the disorder, concluding that lesions which involve a pathway anywhere from posterior speech area to association cortex anterior to the face area (via arcuate fasciculus) will result in facial apraxia. The most common lesions, those in or around Broca's area, presumably cut off connections to the left face area (rostral to inferior precentral gyrus) as well as fibers which pass via corpus callosum to the right face area. If the left face area alone is involved, sparing callosal fibers, the corresponding region on the right can mediate bilateral facial movements. Geschwind holds that the association cortex involved in facial praxis is not the same as Broca's area, and he is critical of views which maintain that Broca's aphasia is a form of (bucco-facial) apraxia. Thus, Broca's aphasia and facial apraxia may vary independently, some Broca's aphasics may repeat well what cannot be said spontaneously, and conduction aphasics with facial apraxia show a different picture than Broca's aphasics, particularly in the lack of dysarthria. This problem was also discussed by De Renzi *et al.* (1966) who noted the occurrence of facial apraxia in nonaphasic left brain-damaged patients, and concluded that all intentional oral movements, both verbal and nonverbal, are controlled by a common "key-board."

The clinical picture is similar to that of other praxic disorders, with the most severe difficulty to command, some improvement to imitation, and facilitation with objects. It is of interest that object facilitation is so superior to imitation, even without actual contact between object and patient. In the case where the patient is asked to blow out a match, for example, the visual cue on imitation does not, to a simple anatomical approach, seem so different from the visual object cue, i.e. a lighted match. In neither case can one speak of success through the use of alternate pathways. Rather, it would appear that the improved performance is a result of a reduction in the abstract and artificial nature of the test situation. In most cases, errors consist of complete failures, substituted movements, perseverations or distortions of correct movements. The disorder affects not only facial movements but other bilaterally innervated movements, apart from those of the trunk, such as coughing, or breathing rhythmically to command. There is no obvious correlation between spontaneous facial expression and degrees of apraxia, nor with the presence or absence of facial paresis. While patients with severe facial weakness may tend to be more dysarthric in speech, neither dysarthria nor weakness is a constant feature of facial apraxia. Also it is worth noting that both anterior lesions (as in the Broca's aphasic) and posterior lesions (as in the conduction aphasic) can produce bucco-facial apraxia, with or without articulatory defect. Whether these are identical forms of apraxia, or differ in the manner of the "ideokinetic" and "limb-kinetic" types, is not known.

Though single movements are rarely if ever affected in isolation, cases of a restricted lid apraxia have been described. Lewandowsky (1907) recorded the case of a cerebral diplegic with loss of voluntary closure of the eyelids either singly or together, though closure could be approximated by following movements and closure was achieved in sleep. Schilder and Lange have also discussed this disorder. It should be noted that while patients with facial apraxia will invariably have normal eye movements, some degree of lid apraxia is not at all uncommon. In patients with mild or resolving right facial weakness and minimal or no facial apraxia, there is often a greater difficulty in winking on the right side, though bilateral closure is normal. Occasionally, patients will show exaggerated synkinesias in some directions of gaze. For example, on looking upward to command, a patient may show contraction of frontalis muscle and exaggerated lid retraction preceding or accompanying otherwise normal eye movements, whereas spontaneous and following movements will be unaffected. In this instance, the "apraxia" seems clearly to be the residual of a resolving facial weakness, and comparable to at least one form of limb-kinetic apraxia.

Chapter 14

TRUNCAL APRAXIA

TRUNCAL APRAXIA WAS the subject of a lengthy treatment by Sittig (1931) who explained it on the Jacksonian principle that the more automatic functions have a lower and more generalized localization, and are therefore, less likely to be damaged by a restricted pathology. Lange (1936) reviewed a few cases and suggested the possibility that the corpus callosum might be particularly related to this disorder, though he hesitated to affirm that truncal apraxia could appear as an isolated defect. The problem of truncal apraxia has not since been widely discussed, except in so far as these movements are preserved in patients with otherwise severe apraxia. Geschwind (1965) has discussed them as "whole body movements," noting that their preservation in callosal cases would disallow a role for the callosum in the integration of this type of bodily movement. Following Flechsig (1901), he postulated that whole body movements to command are mediated through a temporopontine pathway, the bundle of Türck, passing, at least in macaque, from posterior temporal region to the dorsolateral nuclei of the pons. Geschwind speculated that involvement of this pathway should produce an apraxia for whole body movement, although no cases have thus far been reported.

Clinically, there are cases in which the preservation of whole body movements is quite striking. One may have instances in which there is severe limb and facial apraxia, but truncal movements are excellent, and cases in which there is little apraxia but comprehension is so poor that the only commands which the patient can carry out are those involving truncal movements. Patients of the first type, unable to "make a fist" or "salute" to command, will carry out a command such as "take three steps backward, turn around, bow and then sit down." In a personal case of word deafness, nothing could be understood but whole body commands, and these were carried out flawlessly. In fact, the patient muttered "What was that, what did you say?", and looked quite puzzled as he performed the demanded movement. It would seem that in such cases the order must be comprehended, and the movement carried out, through the agency of right hemisphere. That this is at least a possibility is suggested by the fact that in a patient with total left hemispherectomy (Smith, 1966), whole body movements were still possible, a fact explainable only through right hemispheric mediation. In the case where comprehension is reasonably good, however, a different explanation is demanded. It has been suggested, in the discussion on ideational apraxia, that voluntary movement issues out of an optical-spatial organization in which the postural model of the body forms a central part. There is differentiation out of this organization into finer and more highly individuated movements, a differentiation which, at least through inferences made from pathological localization, appears to take place over a postero-anterior axis superior to the classical speech area. Disturbance at rostral levels in this process will leave actions induced by the deeper organization intact. The fact that the right hemisphere can comprehend and apparently carry out truncal movements, but not isolated movements of the left side, indicates that the depth structure which is responsible for truncal movements has a representation in each hemisphere, while those distal stages in the process concerned with the more highly individuated movements are mediated through left hemisphere. At least the "volitional" aspect of praxis, as with speech, requires processing the full range of the motor development in dominant hemisphere.

Of related interest is the so-called "apraxia of gait," first described by Gerstmann and Schilder (1926) as a disorder of walking in the absence of limb weakness, ataxia or sensory impairment. There is loss of initiative, clumsiness and an impairment in voluntary control. Projections of superior frontal gyrus were thought to be implicated. Van Bogaert and Martin (1929) pointed out that gait disturbance, "frontal disequilibrium," might be produced by many factors such as loss of initiative or postural tone, arrest of voluntary activity or apraxic movements, and correlated the disturbance with subcortical lesions in the pre-frontal region. Bell (1934) reviewed the subject in relation to lesions of corpus callosum, his descriptions suggesting the gait disorder seen with callosal tumors or degenerations to be of the "apraxic" type. For Delmas-Marsalet (1936), gait apraxia was a true apraxic disorder and was correlated with lesions in F1. The condition has been discussed by Denny-Brown (1938) in relation to his frontal kinetic apraxias, and designated "magnetic apraxia." Meyer and Barron (1960) contributed a scholarly review in which the following "frontal" gait disorders were defined: (1) ataxia and cerebellar signs secondary to expanding lesions of the frontal lobes, with cerebello-medullary compression; (2) ataxia secondary to functional interference of the eighth cranial nerve, resulting from expanding frontal lesions; and (3) apraxia of gait secondary to localized frontal lobe pathology without displacement. These authors clearly distinguished frontal ataxia from apraxia of gait, noting the inertia of movement, perseveration of posture, rigidity, and "magnetic" character of the latter. More recently, Petrovici (1968) has confirmed the lack of initiative and motor spontaneity in these cases, and noted the improvement of performances *once initiated,* and the facilitation by rhythmic commands or by music. Moreover, separate movements with one leg are better performed than simultaneous movements with both legs. The condition was aligned with innervatory (limb-kinetic) apraxia, with disturbance in the postural set necessary for the initiation of movement.

However, the disorder does not conform to a true apraxia. Normal strength and coordination are insufficient for such a diagnosis in the absence of volitional movement, for apraxia has to be considered inappropriate, not uninitiated, movement. In my experience, patients with gait apraxia as, for example, that seen in normal pressure hydrocephalus, show marked inertia in getting up and walking similar to that seen in Parkinson's disease, while specific movements of the legs and feet to command, such as crossing either leg, kicking, tapping, crushing a cigarette, etc., are often performed quite well. In severe cases, such movements may not be possible when the patient is standing, though they can sometimes be carried out in the sitting or supine position. Whatever resemblance to apraxia there is suggests the limb-kinetic form, and this category, as mentioned above, appears to be transitional to paresis.

Chapter 15

DRESSING APRAXIA

AMONG THE EARLIEST descriptions of this disorder is a report by Marie *et al.* (1922) of two patients who, in the absence of other signs of apraxia, had great difficulty in dressing themselves. The authors noted what appeared to be a disorientation as to the correct procedure for putting on clothes rather than a maladroitness in the act of dressing, and attributed the condition to a defect in spatial representation. In the following years, other case reports appeared (Alajouanine *et al.*, 1934; Kroll, 1910; Garcin *et al.*, 1938), but it was not until the paper of Brain (1941) that wide attention was drawn to this disorder. In Brain's cases, there was inability to put on garments properly, either spontaneously or to command, without other signs of apraxia. His patients, like those of the previous authors, appeared aware of their difficulty in dressing, and complained of it. Brain also discussed a patient of Wendenburg, which must be the earliest account on record, who did not know which was the inside or outside of his coat, put his clothes on upside down and his legs into the coat sleeves. The disorder was noted to be independent of right-left disorientation and constructional apraxia, but rather had a close relation to disorders to the body scheme.

Subsequently, dressing apraxia was extensively studied by Hecaen and Ajuriaguerra (1942, 1951). They pointed out that patients may eventually manage to dress themselves correctly, but that the act of dressing is not carried in its usual automatic fashion, in contrast to the usual case in apraxia where automatic acts are less severely affected. They distinguished two principal aspects to the syndrome, one in association with troubles of right-left orientation and, frequently, acalculia and visual-constructive defects, and another in association with disorders of body scheme. In a recent study by Hecaen *et al.* (1962), dressing apraxia occurred in 22 per cent of right, and 4 per cent of left hemispheric cases, establishing a strong correlation between this syndrome and nondominant hemisphere.

The condition was also studied by Hemphill and Klein (1948), who pointed to an underlying visual-spatial disorganization. Denny-

Brown (1938) discussed the form as an example of unilateral neglect, and aligned it with other syndromes of hemispatial "amorphosynthesis." While there is a group of patients who do not dress themselves on the neglected side, there are also cases with either no left-sided neglect, or difficulty in dressing on the presumably unimpaired side. Thus, the patient who puts his arm in his pants-leg or tries to put his shirt on backwards, making errors in both the limb-sleeve relationship as well as right-left and inversion errors, does not clearly conform to Denny-Brown's analysis.

Since its description, the exact position of dressing apraxia with respect to the apraxias generally and to disturbances of visual-spatial organization has been uncertain. It is not, in Liepmann's sense, a true apraxia for patients do not appear to understand how to proceed, whether able to do so or not, and the voluntary-automatic, or command-object dissociations are not in evidence. A possible relationship in this regard to ideational apraxia can be discounted on the independent occurrence of the two disorders, and their contrasting hemispheric localization. The one thing most authors seem to agree on is that the disorder does not retain a high degree of specificity, but rather reflects one or more underlying conditions, whether right-left disorientation, visual-spatial agnosia, or ideational apraxia. Evidently, further study of case material will be necessary before a more thorough classification can be attempted.

Chapter 16

BIMANUAL APRAXIA

FINALLY, WE WISH TO call attention to a form of apraxia which may warrant a degree of independence from those discussed. Occasionally patients have been observed to have particular difficulty in bimanual coordination, though this is usually in the presence of other apraxic manifestations. Schilder, in particular, stressed the difficulty some patients have in bimanual movements, and movements about, or across, the projected spatial midline. Other authors have commented on the possible role of corpus callosum in bimanual activities, although callosal or callosal-sectioned patients do not show such impairments. The following case appears to be an example of this condition.

Case 10

A forty-eight-year-old right-handed man was readmitted to the Aphasia Unit for study in April, 1970. The problem began in 1960, with increasing confusion over a two-month period, and led to a diagnosis of "diffuse degenerative disease." When first seen in 1963, the principal finding was generalized apraxia, with some indication of slow progression over the intervening years. Between 1963 and 1970, little change occurred. Neurological testing revealed normal cranial nerve functions with certain exceptions (see below), mild increased reflexes on left side, absent Babinski's, broad-based gait with short steps but no ataxia; sensation was normal.

Speech was nil, only a few sounds being possible, e.g. "jin . . . jin." These were uttered in rapid, perseverated and explosive fashion. On counting, he could say "one . . . te . . . the . . . ," but could go no farther. He was unable to whistle, or hum. He could not imitate tongue or lip positions necessary for certain speech sounds. The problem appeared secondary to apraxia, i.e. a "true" speech apraxia.

Comprehension was good for pointing to objects, objects described and yes/no questions. More complex material was tested through multiple choice responses, by shaking his head yes or no. Responses

192

were difficult to evaluate because of the optic, verbal and limb apraxia. Identification of sounds and music was intact.

Naming was similar to speech. He was able to get the first sound of a word out, e.g. for cork: "c, cok"; for pencil: "pa." Performances were similar in all modalities, and for all item classes named. He could select the correct name from a group well. *Repetition* was identical to naming. *Spelling* and comprehension of spelled words was nil; *calculation* was possible through multiple choice tests, but impaired. *Reading* was fair; he was able to match some difficult words with objects, as well as to spoken words. There was facilitation by moving the paper before him, or writing the word before his eyes. *Writing* and drawing were impossible.

Praxis

There was severe facial apraxia, not helped by imitation. Optic apraxia was present with tonic fixation, inability to look to the right, left or upward without first turning his head, and following movements were poor. Diversion of gaze was not helped by blinking. Nonrepresentational movements were severely deficient, and whole body movements were also apraxic.

Regarding limb praxis, intransitive movements, both toward and away from the body, were severely impaired, nor were they helped by imitation. Transitive actions on and away from the body were equally impaired to command and imitation, but remarkably facilitated by object-use. For example, asked to brush his teeth, he first showed his teeth, then after some wandering movements, tapped his index finger to his incisors. There was no improvement to imitation. Given a toothbrush, he brushed his teeth promptly and correctly.

Thus far the difficulty is inexceptional; severe impairment of all movements to command and imitation, and marked facilitation by object use. Yet a striking thing is seen when he is given movements to perform that require bimanual coordination. Thus, given a key and a lock (two objects), a hand-drill (one object), a screw and bolt, or a pair of scissors and paper, he is unable to perform any movement sequence to completion. At times, one hand will desist and the other will carry out appropriate movements on the object or object-part concerned; then, the situation will reverse itself, the active hand becoming quiet and the other hand manipulating the object correctly. The total movement cannot proceed, for only one hand can act at a time. Occasionally, mirror movements are seen, but this is infrequent. If the examiner holds one of the objects in a set, e.g. the bolt or the paper, he is able to carry out the action quite well with either hand. Clearly, the difficulty is in bimanual coordination, in the carrying out of two different movement patterns simultaneously in each hand. That sequencing per se is not at fault here is seen in his ability to perform sequential tasks with either hand alone. Thus, given a pitcher of coffee, a cup and a spoon, and instructed to pour some coffee, stir it and have a drink, he carries out the full movement accurately with either hand alone. Asked to hold the cup in one hand and pour with the other, he is unable to proceed. Similarly, asked to call the operator on the telephone, he is unable to hold the receiver and dial at the same time, and can only carry the movement out by placing the receiver on the table, dialing, and then lifting the receiver up again. One hand, either hand, cannot hold the receiver while the other hand dials. We may summarize the difficulty as follows:

1. Generalized facial-optic-verbal and limb apraxia, with impairment for command and imitation, facilitation with object use. The correct action can be selected from a group.

2. Impairment with objects in those sequences requiring simultaneous bimanual activity, either with two objects, or with one object on which both hands carry out separate movements. Mirror movements were occasionally seen. Sequences were possible with either hand alone.

It must be emphasized that the impairment with objects was *not* comparable to that seen in ideational apraxia. In the latter, movements are affected in either hand, even though bimanual actions may be worse. In this patient, simple or complex movements with objects in either hand were done well and were markedly superior to movements without objects. The deterioration occurred only when different movements (or postures) of both hands simultaneously on an object were required. Even in actions requiring mirror movements such as wringing out a wet towel, there was difficulty, though identical simultaneous movements of each hand, with or without objects, could at times be carried out, e.g. vague movements of "playing" a piano, tapping index fingers for a brief period in unison, or the hand position of praying.

Chapter 17

DISCUSSION

THE APRAXIAS ARE not separate entities related only incidentally through anatomical connections, but are the result of
interference in the genesis of voluntary movement. In this process,
the movement complex passes from a conceptual to a motoric form,
undergoing a progressive differentiation comparable to that which
occurs in the speech system. Liepmann's localization of the different
sub-types at successive points over the cortical mantle reflects this
relationship. In fact, there is a striking similarity between Liepmann's
extended region of voluntary movement and the classical speech area
just beneath it. The implication is, of course, that disorders of movement, like those of speech, are distributed in a postero-anterior
fashion. This distribution may correspond to a process of development over this axis, one that proceeds out of a bond that is forged
primarily with one perceptual system, the acoustic for speech, the
optical for movement.

Accordingly, it should be possible to define, in praxis as in speech,
a series of hierarchically-related pathological levels corresponding to
the different apraxic syndromes. Up to now the problem has not been
studied in this way, most authors relying on the voluntary-involuntary
or command-object use dissociation, rather than on careful observation of each separate apraxic form. Yet, some general patterns of
breakdown can be seen. In ideational apraxia, for example, there appears to be involvement of structures underlying conceptual organizations which are grounded in an optical frame. Most patients will
show visual agnosic and/or visual-spatial difficulties. The disorder
is most apparent in serial movements, not because of a disturbance in
serial ordering but because these actions place a greater demand on
the capacity to maintain a constant correspondence between impaired
deep, and intact surface, mechanisms. The frequent derailment and
substitution, and the aspontaneity of acts in sequence, reflect an
incapacity in this regard. The movement complex, developing out
of optical strata and confluent with the postural model of the body
(Schilder, 1935), is insufficient to guarantee an accurate sequential

unraveling of constituent items. The frequent preservation in this
and other forms of apraxia of whole body movements is explained by
their "proximity" to this initial stage, being rather more a condensation of the act in the postural system. The difficulty in performance
of an act will generally parallel its degree of somatic restrictiveness as
well as its complexity. Along these lines, one can explain the dissociation between object-use and command. In ideational apraxia, the act
is possible to command for the conditions require working in the
confines of the body sphere alone. The act is carried out—usually,
perhaps invariably, with body-part substitution—as a performance
within the postural model itself. The introduction of an object adds
complexity to the intrapersonal referent. Now body-part must act on
object, and the object must act on another body-part or another
object. The object brings about a loss of the immediacy of the act.
Besides this, other contaminations occur with objects. There is a
greater frequency of spatial dislocation, objects being used in the
wrong place or advanced in directions that are not appropriate to the
action. Even with the patient's eyes closed, objects place demands
on the visual perceptual system—if only through inner visualization—
and in this way influence some performances. Finally, acts with
objects are, for certain patients, more demanding than acts in pantomime. If the patient has knowledge of the act, the object will facilitate
motor control. This does not have to be a conscious knowledge, as
seen in the example of tieing a necktie in pantomime. If however, the
knowledge of the act is not wholly sufficient to its performance, with
or without objects, the object will require even greater precision with
regard to digital manipulation and actual use, for movements without
objects will be accepted as adequate that would be completely un-
acceptable were they to be performed with objects. The command-
object use dissociation is analogous in some respects to the situation
in anomic and conduction aphasia where differentiation also depends
on the response to a concrete cue, i.e. the whole word cue of repetition. There is, however, another point of similarity between ideational apraxia and the posterior aphasias. This we have referred to
through use of the term fluency to describe those movements which
are retained, meaning by this the ease, smoothness and dexterity of
otherwise erroneous motor performances. This indicates a certain independence of those levels in the hierarchy close to the motor side.
If we stretch the analogy a little further, the possibility appears that
the manifest component units in a simple motor sequence might
reflect derangement in a fashion comparable to that of paraphasia.

Even though praxic differentiations are scarcely so refined as those of speech, except in the case of the sign language of the deaf, this nevertheless constitutes a most interesting line of inquiry.

In ideo-motor apraxia, the defect is at an intermediate stage in the development of the motor performance. There is a stage of parapraxis with spheric substitution of total movement patterns (semantic parapraxis) leading to one in which the action is conceptually determined but faulty in the execution of its parts. Here the partial movement is affected, with substitution, deletion, anticipation, perseveration, etc. There is a similarity between the change in parapraxis and that of paraphasia, both having conceptual or semantic, and unit, components. With the exception of callosal cases, this may well follow a distribution across the hemisphere, with semantic parapraxia the more posterior, and unit parapraxia the more rostral manifestation. With frontal lesions, one then finds disturbances in the activation and implementation of adequate motor patterns (limb-kinetic apraxia) .

At the intermediate level, object use is facilitating. This is effected by the act of manipulating the object, through a reduction in the opportunities for unit parapraxia. Object use also eliminates body part substitution, diminishes contamination from grasping, and aids in the comprehension of the task. Probably there is little facilitation through purely visual means or through kinesthesis, for performance is unaffected by wearing a heavy glove, and deteriorates minimally with both a glove and a mask. Further, some actions are improved without object contact. Thus, patients will often demonstrate the action of an imaginary key much better when a lock is held up before them or, failing to blow out a match to command and imitation, they will carry out the correct action to a lighted match. In such cases it is not strictly the visual presentation that affects the proper action, but rather the setting in which the visual presentation occurs. Thus, an unlit match, or a lock not positioned for opening, may fail to elicit the correct movement. In such cases one cannot speak of cueing the other hemisphere, for there is no reason to think that imitative cues and cues in the object situation involve different perceptual systems. This indicates that there is a further, and perhaps more fundamental, aspect to object facilitation, that of bringing about a more concrete (i.e. less volitional) setting for the desired movement. In this sense, movements with objects are comparable to performance in conversational speech. This may be particularly well seen if patients are presented a group of objects and asked to demonstrate their actions. On the other hand, requests for specific movements through imitation or command are comparable to repetition and naming (especially, naming to description) tests in aphasics. It is not surprising, therefore, that a disorder which concerns the latter two tasks especially, such as conduction aphasia, is so often, though not invariably, associated with ideomotor apraxia. What this indicates is not necessarily the interruption of adjacent pathways, but the interference at comparable stages in the microgenesis of speech and movement.

Supramarginal gyrus (ideomotor) apraxia is distinguished largely by unit parapraxia, occasional semantic parapraxia and relatively fluent movements. If semantic parapraxia becomes the dominant feature then a more posterior lesion or a pure callosal syndrome is to be suspected. With more anterior localization, movements become increasingly slow and clumsy (one might say, nonfluent), and unit parapraxia, though still in evidence, gradually begins to disappear. The reduction in semantic parapraxia allows the target movement to be more clearly discerned in the disordered performance. This is the usual picture of sympathetic apraxia. When those elements accounting for the slowness and clumsiness of movement become the major feature, then limb-kinetic apraxia is seen. Here the difficulties concern largely paretic and "dystonic" features, and a comparison to the syndrome of phonetic disintegration is not altogether unwarranted. With regard to facial apraxia, there is a suggestive progress from semantic to unit substitution and eventually to sloppy facial movements which appears to parallel the change in limb praxis.

Finally, there are two further points to be made. First, the apraxia of the callosal syndrome will, as mentioned, be marked largely by semantic parapraxia. The conceptual relationship of substituted to correct movement may not be as clear as in the semantic parapraxia of posterior dominant hemisphere disease. It may well be a general rule that closeness to the target movement in left-sided apraxia is a reflection of interhemispheric sharing. That is why sympathetic apraxia is not a true callosal syndrome, for the target movement is always clear in the clumsy or inappropriate performance. Secondly, it is of interest that in ideational apraxia the impaired performance follows the sequence: object-no-use-imitation-command, while in ideomotor apraxia, the impairment occurs in the exact opposite fashion. This reciprocity we have encountered is repeatedly in the speech-expressive and perceptual systems, and is of fundamental importance in psychopathology.

III. AGNOSIA

Chapter 18

INTRODUCTION

THE TERM PSYCHIC blindness (Seelenblindheit) derived from findings by Munk (1877) that dogs with extirpation of the caudal poles of the occipital lobes, though able to avoid or jump over obstacles without difficulty, behaved indifferently in the presence of food, other dogs, or dangerous situations such as fire. In analogy with these experimental studies, visual agnosia was interpreted as a form of "psychic blindness" in which there was retention of vision with loss of recognition, or loss of the signs or symbols through which visual recognition took place. The distinction between a purely visual awareness of an object and the conceptual identification of the object, though made by Wernicke as early as 1874, did not receive much attention until the case report of Lissauer (1889). In this paper, Lissauer recognized three forms of agnosia: *the apperceptive** with distortion of the sensory impression of the object in consciousness; *the associative* with intact vision but impairment of the pathways leading from sensory impressions to memory images; and *a mixed form* containing elements of the other types. Liepmann (1900) was responsible for the separation from agnosia of disorders of the motor-executive system, and later distinguished between dissolutive and disjunctive types of visual agnosia, similar in theory to those of Wernicke and Lissauer.

Following this early account, the study of agnosia passed into a period of healthy uncertainty. Von Monakow (1905) discounted this entity as an effect of diaschisis within the visual system, and as late as 1914, von Stauffenberg could comment that no adequate case of

---

*In early philosophical writings, apperception implied a conscious state in which the object of the perception stood in relation to the cognitive store. For Wündt, the apperceptive process acted to fuse into whole objects (i.e. foveal images) the many details of sensation which were unresolved in the total visual field. This fusion was an active process and took place through cognitive mechanisms. The term was then used by Lissauer to designate the (impaired) activity through which this fusion comes about, elementary perception presumably being normal. Because the apperception had been considered a higher form of perception with a special relation to memory, Lissauer's distinction is somewhat unorthodox.

apperceptive agnosia had yet been described. This seemed to be supported by Poppelreuter's (1914–1917) extensive study of traumatic cases, in which no classical instances of agnosia were to be found, those few cases with failure to recognize some simple objects or familiar persons occurring largely during the acute pre-surgical or post-surgical state and, therefore, tending to support von Monakow's notion of diaschisis. Accordingly, Poppelreuter held that visual agnosia was not a definable clinical picture, but rather a disintegration of the complex perceptual process into a multiplicity of individual defects.

The case of Goldstein and Gelb (1918) was of importance in re-awakening clinical interest in agnosic phenomena. This twenty-four-year-old man, wounded in the occipital region, with some reduction in temporal fields but good acuity (R 5/10, L 5/15), intelligent and nonaphasic, was found to have severe visual recognition problems. Reading was accomplished only through a letter-by-letter technique, utilizing cues from finger tracing and head movements, while obscuration of the letters with cross-hatches or tachystoscopic presentation, abolished reading altogether. There was impaired recognition of line drawings and contour figures, and physical objects were said to be inferred from single characteristics, e.g. dice from black dots on a white surface. Visual imagery was presumed lost in spite of the fact that some excellent drawings were produced from memory. There was said to be no difficulty in walking about and in other daily activities. The case was interpreted, in accordance with gestalt theory, as a loss of the ability to experience compactly organized visual impressions, a failure to grasp the whole, and was aligned with the apperceptive agnosias of Lissauer. This case has received a good deal of criticism. Poppelreuter argued that constricted visual fields were responsible for the symptoms, an assertion denied later by Goldstein (1943), and Lange (1936) and more recently Bay, considered the patient an hysteric. In spite of these criticisms, however, the thorough clinical testing and trenchant analysis have made the case a model for all subsequent investigations.

In the years following, a great variety of interrelated subtypes were sifted out of the agnosia category, such as prosopagnosia and color agnosia, and articles dealing with specialized forms appeared. With regard to visual *object* agnosia, three major lines of study have emerged. Continuing the classical doctrines of Lissauer and Liepmann, Geschwind (1965) maintains that there is a disruption, through callosal and cortical pathology, of modality specific sensoriverbal linkages. This leads to the isolation from the speech area of visual perceptions. Poppelreuter's views on the importance of field constriction and the adequacy of the perimacular zone, have been championed by Bay (1953) who holds that in all cases there are, coexisting with reduced intellectual capacities, important defects in that system of spatiotemporal transformations which the simulus goes through on its way to perception (Funktionswandel); that is, that agnosia is primarily a low-level visual defect. Combining the gestaltist position with comtemporary physiology, Luria (1966) speaks of a defect in ". . . the synthesis of isolated elements of visual perception, and of the integration of these elements into simultaneously perceived groups." Here the disturbance lies within the perceptual sphere alone, in the building up of perceptions, while a distinction between this building-up process and the recognition of the perception is not drawn.

Chapter 19

APPERCEPTIVE VISUAL AGNOSIA

USUALLY NOTED DURING the recovery of cortical blindness, apperceptive visual agnosia may either persist for extended periods or undergo, after several weeks, a modest continuing improvement. Patients may have intact fields to perimetric testing, and visual acuity may be normal or nearly so, this usually evaluated, in the presence of alexia, through dot or line discrimination. Disturbances of gaze with random wandering eye movements are common though perhaps not invariable, and are related to bilateral occipito-parietal lesions. Visual evoked potentials may be normal. Patients may be able to detect hue differences, at least to 7–10μ, and differences in luminescence to 0.1 log units. Tests of spatial summation, and flicker fusion thresholds may show only minor deviations from normal (Efron, 1968). Though previous studies have indicated that subtle disorders in functional ability may play a role (Bay, 1953), such as impaired local adaptation (fading time) and inadequacy of the perimacular field, these have not proved to be present in all patients and occur in the absence of visual agnosia (Ettlinger, 1956). Further, in a personal series of dysphasic young men with left hemisphere lesions, no impairment on an object identification task was found while wearing a mask which limited vision to a central 3 degrees. Similar findings were described some years ago by Goldstein (1943). Thus, a defect in "primary" visual function of the type noted by Bay, with dysphasia and/or mental reduction, even if present in agnosic patients, would not be a sufficient cause for the condition.

The principal clinical findings are those of failure to identify, describe or copy the simplest objects or line-drawings on visual presentation, inability to select objects on command, and impaired performance on matching tests. Tracing an object may be impaired; showing and then withdrawing an object, or having the patient draw with eyes closed, does not facilitate performance. Patients can ordinarily trace a simple outline but, in contrast to the case of Goldstein and Gelb (1918) who was able to read and identify drawings in this way, this does not generally appear to facilitate identification. In contrast, identification and description of the object or its use may be possible upon touching it or perceiving it through another modality. While auditory naming is generally excellent, tactile identification is usually impaired. Patients cannot draw objects or geometrical figures held in one hand, and cross-matching simple objects, or blocks, from one hand to another, or making relative distinctions on two blocks in one hand, such as larger or heavier, is also mildly to moderately impaired. The defect may be so severe that simple geometric figures or even straight and curved lines cannot be distinguished. At times, relative distinctions are possible such as the larger, more intense, or more deeply colored of two objects. Motion is ordinarily perceived and will assist in recognition. Placing hatch marks in letters, or overlapping two figures, will easily produce derailments and indicates that the patient is following only that portion of the line immediately perceived. Single dots can often be localized on paper, often after a period of search, but multiple dots cannot be counted. There is difficulty in bisecting single lines, much less indicating multiple lines drawn on paper. Small objects are often perceived better than large ones, and picture interpretation—or even description—is impossible. Patients can often give good estimates of spaces over which they have walked, and can at times estimate the distance of moving objects with fair accuracy. Patients may confabulate the names of objects visually presented, and persist in their confabulation even after palpation. An inattention to visually-presented objects was noted by Pick, and compares to similar phenomena in patients with word-deafness.

The behavior of these patients is of some interest. Similar to patients with cortical blindness, their daily activity does not altogether reflect the severity of the visual handicap. They will often walk about quite confidently, only occasionally bumping into obstacles, and though not denying their difficulty, will usually treat it somewhat indifferently. A sluggish apathy, probably identical to what was termed Willenlosigkeit by the German school is very common. In recognition tasks, the patient will peer at or around an object, giving the impression of a myope, or he will search for an object directly before him, at times identifying it when it falls in his peripheral field, at other times, when viewed centrally. As Critchley (1964) has emphasized, performance is variable, and fatigue will play an important role. Responses are usually more accurate to simple isolated objects than to complex or multiple objects, though placing an object in a familiar setting is said to have a facilitating effect.

Alexia is perhaps an invariable accompaniment of this form, and corresponds to agnosic alexia in type. Tactile reading with block letters or numbers is also impaired. Constructional performance is poor and visual-spatial defects are often the residuum of recovered object recognition. There are also errors suggestive of ideational apraxia. Though color naming and recognition defects occur, in most cases there is a stage in the dissolution of form where color persists. Similarly in recovery, color recognition precedes the recognition of objects. Visual imagery may be impaired, to some extent perhaps independently of dream, while visual hallucinations are characteristic of the initial stages of the disorder. With loss of visual dreams, R.E.M. activity persists and dreams may take on a purely auditory flavor. In one patient personally studied, there was no evidence that waking visual perceptions reappeared as dream residues. On tests of after-imagery in one case, only a red color was described on repeated trials with a bright light, and with a lighted square, only a simple straight line could be seen. This was comparable to performance on direct perception. The only possible abnormalities were a (described) lack of definition of the image, a diffuseness and a briefer than normal duration.

The localization of "apperceptive" visual agnosia is agreed by most workers to be occipital or occipito-parietal, with bilateral lesions mandatory. As the visual fields are normal, striate cortex must be relatively preserved, although good correlative cases are lacking.

Case 11

A thirty-seven-year-old man was transferred to the Aphasia Unit in October, 1969. He had been in good health until June, 1969, when he suffered a myocardial infarction with ventricular fibrillation resulting in a coma of ten days duration. On regaining consciousness, he was described as dysphasic and cortically blind. At the time of transfer he was alert and well-oriented; there was minimal bilateral dysmetria but no ataxia, a variable extinction pattern to double simultaneous stimulation and some difficulty in sensory localization. He was found to have some deficiency in recent and remote memory, proverbs were concrete, calculation ability was nil. His speech was fluent without paraphasia, comprehension and repetition were intact, reading and writing were impossible. There was dressing apraxia and a suggestion of ideational apraxia, though other limb and facial movements were normal.

The most striking disturbance was in the visual sphere, where in spite of relatively good acuity, as measured by his ability to detect an 8 mm white object at 10 feet, normal visual fields on tangent screen testing, and ability to discriminate luminosities to .03 log units, he was almost wholly incapable of recognizing any object or drawing by vision alone. On a series of 20 objects, only 2 (a pen and a pair of glasses) were correctly named, whereas 15 were thereafter named correctly by touch. He was unable to recognize a simple geometrical shape unless it was drawn in front of his eyes, and even then his response was erratic (for a triangle he said "a line," on drawing it for him, "three lines"). He could differentiate a curved from a straight line, but failed on line bisection. He was unable to copy or trace objects before him, or objects presented and then withdrawn; drawing from memory was slightly better. He was unfailingly correct on auditory naming; there was no word-finding difficulty in sentence completion or in giving the name of an object described to him. Color naming was 50 per cent correct, matching 50 per cent, selecting a color named for him 100 per cent correct, color imagery (e.g. rabbits . . . "white") 80 per cent correct, and he was able to pick the darker of two dissimilar shades. He was able to spell simple words, but made errors on longer ones. He was somewhat better on words spelled to him.

Visual imagery was not normal, but that it was present to a moderate degree was ascertained by the following tests. He was asked to describe his living room and replied, ". . . a T.V., two orange chairs, a fold-away which can roll into a bed . . . one chair on the right . . . facing toward the T.V., the couch is right beside it and the other chair . . . there is a stereo . . . (rug?) . . . yes, greenish-brown . . . solid . . . a picture of a ship on the wall." Asked if he could picture the room in his mind, he said "Yes, I can see it real plain." He remarked that he day-dreamed frequently; described an elephant as having ". . . a long nose . . . picks up food and water with his nose . . . is big and brown, has tusks." A sugar cube was described as having four sides; he was told to mentally bisect an apple, then bisect the parts again, and was unable to count the pieces. He was able to judge textures correctly by touch, but could not identify or match raised letters held in either hand. Solid blocks were matched and cross-matched with about 75 per cent accuracy, with slight improvement if vision and touch were employed together. He was only minimally able to describe or draw geometrical shapes held in either hand. On tactile matching of meaningless patterns (Butters and

Brody, 1968) * he was able to match and cross-match fairly well if given one pattern at a time from which to select. If given a group of three or more patterns, he was unable to select the one most appropriate. He was able to tap out auditorily presented sequences.

He demonstrated after-imagery with eyes closed though described only a red color. With his eyes open, he reported that the red after-image completely filled out the examiner's face, making everything that he looked at that color. The duration of after-imagery was judged to be less than normal, and he described a "dull" red color with hazy outlines. He was then shown a luminous 2-inch square which he saw only as a "light." In after-imagery, he described seeing a horizontal red line (presumably the upper rim of the square). Guiding his eyes over the contour of the square during presentation made no difference in the imagery report.

During the immediate post-coma period, he reported having a series of nightmares, these having a definite visual character. Subsequently, the nightmares disappeared, and he offered that he had some decline in dream recall. Two evenings were spent in recording the patient's dreams. On the first, visual dreams were sketchily described in 6 of 11 (normal) R.E.M. periods; on the second night, dreams occurred in 5 of 6 R.E.M. periods, though only two of these dreams were of a visual character.

Other tests for imagery included the following. He was able to draw a map of the ward and corridor which, though extremely fragmentary, was surprisingly accurate as to general relationships, and he correctly estimated distances walked. He was unable to make up a story upon request. He was asked to pretend that a football game was taking place before him and with his eyes follow the action in a narrative provided by the examiner. His performance on this test was quite poor. Finally, he mentioned that his previous ability to play the guitar had greatly deteriorated, owing to his inability to play the desired chords. This was thought to possibly be due to a defect in visualization.

Case 12

A seventy-one-year-old left-handed post-operative lung cancer patient, while in the hospital for evaluation, awoke one morning blind. Initially, only light perception remained, corneal reflexes were present but there was no reaction to visual threat; an EEG a few days afterward revealed bilateral posterior slowing. On examination,

---

*Test kindly performed by Dr. Butters.

he was alert with fluent nonaphasic speech and normal comprehension. He did not seem to show much concern about his visual difficulty, but that he was aware of it was beyond doubt. Initially, he was unable to read, write or draw, had mild disturbances of limb praxis bilaterally, could not calculate, spell or name words spelled for him. As gradual improvement took place, he could discern movement in the left hemi-field, with alloesthesia of objects presented to the densely hemianopic right side. Visual acuity gradually improved but at no point in the course of his disorder was it testable. At times he could see very small objects at quite a distance, suggesting fair acuity, but for the most part was unable to fixate on points of light or objects. In spite of this severe visual handicap, however, he was able to accurately steer himself around an obstacle course of chairs and tables set in his path. When asked what he saw, he said ". . . it all runs together" and on one occasion exclaimed, "I'm blind!" He was unable to name objects visually, draw them or describe their use, nor could he identify simple geometrical shapes drawn before him. He was able to indicate colors with about 80 per cent accuracy; color and tactile namings were about 60 per cent correct. He was able to draw a solid geometrical object held in his hand slightly better than one before his eyes, but his performance here was still quite poor. Over a two to three week period, his performance on all tests improved to the point where he was able to read numbers and a few letters, write simple sentences and identify objects fairly well.

Of special interest, however, is his performance on visual imagery tests when his condition was rather severe. He reported that around the time of onset of blindness, and for the following week or so, he was having terrifying nightmares. On questioning, it appeared that these were of a striking visual character, and they were vividly described by him. Clinically at this time he was unable to describe his home, his wife, any animals, nor could he draw anything from memory. It was impossible to obtain from him any descriptive information pointing to the presence of visual imagery. As his vision improved, so did the clinical tests of imagery, his dreams continuing to have a strong visual character though no longer terrifying.

Case 13

A twenty-five-year-old man, reported previously (Benson and Greenberg, 1969; Efron, 1968) went into decerebrate coma following prolonged exposure to carbon monoxide. Gradual improvement took place over the next seven months, at which time he was transferred

to the Aphasia Unit, Boston V.A. Hospital. He was alert and cooperative, but there was evidence of a mild generalized memory impairment, and performance on proverb testing was quite concrete. Except
for some hesitancy and occasional pauses in word-finding, speech was
normal. Comprehension and repetition were also reasonably normal.
Color naming and matching were normal, reading was abolished, as
was writing; spelling was poor as were verbal and written calculations.
There was left dyspraxia, minimal on the right side; right-left orientation and finger gnosis were normal. Impairments in the visual and
spatial sphere are described in the published case report and will
not be recounted here. Of special interest is the marked disturbance
in visual imagery. His descriptions of common objects were severely
impoverished. For example, the flag was described as ". . . cloth,
rectangular in shape, many bright colors, blows in the breeze and
sometimes makes flapping sounds as it is blown"; a dog as having
". . . a tail and body . . . good company in the house . . . loves people
that feed him." There was only slight difficulty in tactile naming,
but tactile identification of block letters or geometrical figures was
impaired. He was able to draw a square from memory much better
than visually. His ability to trace geometrical objects was superior to
drawing them. A R.E.M. study was normal in character but revealed
absence of visual elements in his dreams.

Comment

In all three cases, the patients were strikingly apathetic about their
disorder, though in no case was frank denial present. Their ability
to walk about the ward without bumping into objects was better than
anticipated from clinical tests of visual capacity. There was no clear
difference in recognition of small or large objects, though in all cases
movement facilitated identification. Again in all cases, color recognition was superior to object recognition, and tactile naming, though
much better than visual naming, was also somewhat impaired. That
involvement of tactile naming should occur is of some interest,
for it may reflect the state of inner visualization. Lange (1936) found
tactile identification to be commonly affected and attributed this to
failure of the internal optic sense. Critchley (1965) has also commented on the frequent impairment of tactile naming. Correlation
with other tests of visual imagery would appear to be of compelling
interest. In Case 8, the poor tactile performance on block letters and
geometrical shapes, and the inability to describe or draw solid geometrical shapes palpated, contrasts with the performance on tactile

cross-matching and tactile naming of objects and textures. This is consistent with a moderate impairment in tactile revisualization, with greatest difficulty in tasks requiring greater effort in revisualization. However, the relatively good tactile naming in Case 13, with severe visualization defect, tends to throw some doubt on a revisualization hypothesis. Evidently, more work is needed in this area before any conclusion can be reached.

Concerning visual imagery, there were obvious deficiencies in all patients though not of the same magnitude. In Case 11, visual as well as dream imagery was present; in Case 12, visual imagery was abolished though dreams were present; in Case 13, both visual imagery and visual dreams were markedly reduced or lost. It is striking that in Case 12, where waking visual images only were lost, there were nightmarish visual dreams. This suggests that the waking image is less resistant than the dream image, and that its abolition reflects a slight encroachment upon the visual image function, resulting in excessive image activity in dream. In all cases there were nightmares at the time of onset of the agnosia, suggesting a similar explanation. In Case 13, however, the nightmares were a stage of excess on the way toward an eradication of dream imagery altogether. Taken together, these cases suggest that there is a continuum of involvement, from agnosia with relative sparing of visual imagery, to agnosia with loss of waking imagery and preservation, and in some instances hyperactivity, of visual dream imagery, to loss of both waking and dream images. Though it is difficult to quantify such things, it is also my impression that the mental state of these patients was affected in a general way consistent with this progression.

The problem of visual imagery was a major concern of early writers on the subject. Claparede (1900) thought that one day it would be possible to clearly distinguish two categories: asymbolia with and without memory images. Pick also insisted on this distinction (Asymbolie mit Erhaltung der Erinnerungsbilder un gestorter Identification verursacht durch Leitungsunterbrechung, im Gegenteil zur Asymbolie mit Ausfall der Erinnerungsbilder). In the cases presented here, three overlapping forms can be distinguished, one with *preserved* mental and dream imagery, another with impaired imagery but retained dreams, and a third with loss of all imagery, this appearing only as a more severe variant of the second form. The delineation of these separate forms introduces the question of an isolated irreminiscence.

This condition, first described by Charcot (1887), consists of loss of visual imagery and dream in the presence of normal speech and perception. On the face of it, that visual imagery should be impaired while perception is normal, seems as unlikely as loss of verbal imagery (inner speech) with normal verbal expression. Probably we are dealing here, not with an organic syndrome but with cases of psychoneurosis. Indeed, Schilder (1951a) remarked that Freud, who had the opportunity to speak with Charcot's patient, suspected a neurosis. Of the two cases of Brain (1954), one was considered a neurotic depression by Zangwill, the other received hospitalization, E.C.T. and insulin treatment for a depressive reaction. Considering these two cases, and the aforementioned case of Charcot, it is surprising that Brain suggests a lesion in the parastriate region. Loss of visual dreams with cerebral lesions has been described by Humphrey and Zangwill (1951), but these cases, though intriguing from the standpoint of right parietal susceptibility for this disorder, were extremely complex examples with many other disturbances, notably in the visual-spatial sphere, and R.E.M. studies were not done.

Further discussion of apperceptive visual agnosia is included in the next chapter.

Chapter 20

ASSOCIATIVE VISUAL AGNOSIA

THIS DISORDER WAS originally described by Lissauer (1889), and characterized as an inability to name, describe or give the use of objects visually perceived in the presence of good ability to draw the object or identify it through other sensory channels. Subsequently, it was noted that patients failed to select the object named from a group, or the correct name when offered. In theory, matching of objects should also be spared, though defects appear when objects similar in size and shape are employed. The capacity to draw the object without identification is crucial to the diagnosis and has been considered a sign that perception is intact. In some cases, once an object or drawing has been named by the examiner, the patient can point out its component parts.

In the majority of cases, there is right homonymous hemianopia. Patients appear to have reasonably good acuity, as inferred from their drawings, and their ability to follow complex visual mazes or trace a line through a tangle. Depth perception, color vision and apprehension of direction may be excellent, and patients can distinguish the longer, wider, etc., of two objects. Line bisection, counting of dots on paper, and completion of geometrical patterns, as tests of visual acuity, may be performed without great difficulty. The major difference between associative and apperceptive agnosia concerns the presumably intact shape or form perception in the former.

Performance is characteristically fluctuant. Lissauer's patient, and the cases of von Stauffenberg could at times recognize single objects, or even series of objects, while at other times no objects at all could be identified. Most errors contain either circumlocutory descriptions, or morphological approximations. Thus, one case said, "It's a squarish structure sitting on top of a roundish structure" for a top-hat, or "a dog or cat or something like that" for a picture of a pig. Objects are occasionally "negatively" identified, as in the patient of von Stauffenberg who said of a picture of a rooster, "That's not a rooster." Negative recognition within sphere, as in "It isn't a cat" for a picture of a mouse, or general categorical impressions, e.g. fruit for apple, may occur. Prolonged attention to the object may at times facilitate recognition but more often has a detrimental effect. Infrequently, misidentifications will result from contaminations of preceding unidentified items, as in the response of a case seen by Pötzl. This patient was shown a bouquet of red roses with a stalk of asparagus protruding from the center. Having identified the roses only, he was next asked to name the color on the collar of an officer present in the room. After some effort, the patient stated that he saw a "green tie pin," apparently a delayed impression of the unidentified asparagus stalk. Perseveration of preceding items which have been identified, whether correctly or not, is however the more common occurrence.

Drawing is fairly good, but errors of proportion are common. Particularly in drawing faces, there may be bizarre mislocations of eyes or ears, elongation of the neck or confusion of frontal and profile views. Drawings may have elements superimposed, or even deleted. Simple two and three dimensional figures can be drawn and copied without too much difficulty, though drawing is tedious and slow, and with slavish attention to the model. Copying is superior to drawing from memory, though copying a figure does not ordinarily aid in its recognition. Copying of nonsense designs, drawing simple nonsense figures from memory after a short exposure, or recognizing in a group a design previously seen, may be quite good. There does not appear to be a difference in drawing with right or left hand. Patients may be unable to group pictures to categories, or indicate a picture inappropriate to a group. Showing both object and drawing does not facilitate recognition, nor are objects matched well to pictures. Identification of three-dimensional objects is superior to identification of the same object in a drawing or photograph.

In contrast to apperceptive visual agnosia, tactile identification may be intact to naming, matching and cross-matching tasks, and may perhaps correlate with the degree of preservation of inner visualization. This is generally spared, though deficits or loss of imagery may occur. Dream imagery and after-imagery have not been studied. Disorders of spatial ability and orientation are not uncommon, especially in the acute stages, but may be rather mild even in the severe agnosic. Mild amnesic aphasia may also be present. Reading is commonly involved, though there are cases in the literature without alexia.

The condition of optic aphasia may be a source of possible confusion, particularly as concerns the unilateral case. Postulated by Freund (1889) as a disorder of naming limited to visual perception, with retained ability to draw or describe the object, or give an account of its use, the existence of this form was doubted by most earlier workers. Pötzl thought it a ". . . weakened degree of the same basic disorder which results in optical agnosia" and Lange noted that it preceded object agnosia, or remained when the agnosia resolved. He considered it an exhaustion of identification after the stage of concept formation, the process not quite reaching the point of naming. The transitional nature of the disorder appears fairly certain, considering that it occurs in the early stages of agnosic alexia, and may occur side by side with the complete misidentifications of the associative visual agnosic. It may also appear as a stage in the recovery of visual recognition.

The anatomy of associative visual agnosia, though not precisely understood, is, in so far as what little is known at all, agreed upon by most workers. Nielsen (1937) summarized a series of cases in the literature and concluded that unilateral lesions of second and third occipital convolution in the dominant hemisphere, in association with lesion of posterior corpus callosum, were responsible. In support of this localization, Geschwind (1965) recently suggested that such pathology, including and extending rostral to splenium, would isolate perceptual contents to minor hemisphere, while the preservation of tactile recognition would be explained by its more anterior crossing. However, this formulation does not account for the preservation of object drawing, which is the critical distinction separating this from the apperceptive form. According to Geschwind, most cases show bilateral parietal lesions.

Case 14

A forty-seven-year-old physician first developed flaccid left hemiparesis of a few days duration in April, 1968 (from Rubens and Benson, 1971). In September, 1968 he was briefly hospitalized for depression, and was noted to have slightly increased tendon reflexes on the right side. From October, 1968 to January, 1969 he was in a psychiatric hospital for excessive drinking and suicidal depression. In March, 1969, he was admitted to hospital in coma, presumably from an overdose of chloral hydrate. On arousing, difficulty with recent memory and poor object identification were noted. There were accentuated reflexes on the right with Babinski on that side, as well as right homonymous hemianopia. A pneumoencephalogram showed mild ventricular enlargement, greater on the left side; carotid arteriography was normal.

Examination on the Aphasia Unit confirmed the presence of right

homonymous hemianopia with slight macular sparing. Visual acuity
was 20/30 corrected and OKN was normal bilaterally. Careful testing
revealed the following. There was normal speech, verbal comprehension, writing and spelling. Naming was impaired only to visual
presentation. Praxis, right-left orientation, topographic orientation
and clock-setting were normal. Drawing and copying of geometrical
forms and line drawings of objects was accurate though slavish. Color
naming and pointing to colors on command was impaired, though
matching and naming colors to description was intact. He was unable
to recognize familiar faces, those of his family and even his own face
in the mirror (see page 225). He was unable to name, describe or
demonstrate the use of many common objects. There was slight improvement on pointing to objects named. If he confabulated the
name, his description of its use would correspond to the confabulated
name. He could match identical objects and draw their outlines without identifying them. Pictures of objects were also named poorly in
spite of accurate copies of line drawings. When pictures or objects
were named for him, he was often able to then point out various
parts of the previously unrecognized item. Reading was greatly
limited, and proceeded through literal analysis. Letters were read
slowly and with morphological confusion. Visual memory and depth
perception were good. WAIS testing done in September, 1968 showed
113/130, and in May, 1969 86/125 (performance/verbal).

By way of general comment on this case, it is to be emphasized
that the measured visual acuity 20/30 should not be taken to imply
that visual perception was intact. The patient described alteration in
color perception, and remarked of his difficulty in recognizing faces
that they seemed ". . . out of focus, almost as though a haze were in
front of them." Further, misidentifications were characteristically
morphological, e.g. violin for key (picture), spool for cork (object),
suggesting some degree of perceptual disturbance. Morphological confusion of letters also suggested a perceptual defect, and relates the
disorder to agnosic alexia. Furthermore, in agreement with this, copying of line drawings, though fairly accurate, was slavish. Over time
there was improvement to a stage where most objects and colors were
recognized, while those misnamed could in general be selected correctly. This occurred only on visual naming, and appeared consistent
with the "optic aphasia" of Freund.

DISCUSSION

". . . in optic agnosia the issue is an interference with the process of cognition as it develops in hierarchical layers, and not the loss of some elements" (Schilder).

Earlier, we distinguished two major steps in the perceptual process, an initial formative stage (I), prior to awareness, in which the signal is transformed to an (abstract) spatial representation, and a secondary phase (II) in which this representation is matched to a trace system, and analyzed into private space and awareness. The stimulus-complex is held to exert a driving or determining influence on the perceptual image rather than providing a substrate upon which, through a linking up of other stimuli, the perception will be built.

Disorders of the initial stage will have a "sensory" character. This, one might say, is the negative side of Stage I disorders, and appears in tests such as those of Bay (1963). The positive side relates to cognitive processes no longer guided by adequate signals. This takes the form of internally structured perceptions which then come to the fore. Imaginal contents will intrude upon the perception. Pötzl studied this phenomenon, and found a strong relationship between dream imagery and agnosic visual experiences. This has also been discussed in relation to word-deafness where hallucinations frequently appear as the initial phase. Both vision and audition make use of constructive mechanisms in the Stage I process. The former begins with a complex signal reconstructed through a process of shape specification. This reconstruction is matched to memory, the traces of which are presumably distributed in the space-coordinate system (Lashley, 1951), and is then articulated into abstract (mental) space. In analogous fashion, audition requires the "simultaneous synthesis" of temporally patterned signals to an abstract spatial representation, which combines with memory prior to resequentialization. In vision, there is facilitation of Stage I disorders ("apperceptive agnosia") with simple uniform stimuli on recognition tasks. On the other hand, in Stage II defects ("associative agnosia") discrimination of similar objects is impaired and patients will deteriorate with simplification of the test stimulus. Stage II defects are aided by signal diversity which for Stage I acts only to increase the complexity of the signal. Thus, the apperceptive agnosic is aided by a line drawing, the associative agnosic by the real object. Conversely, in audition, Stage I defects ("sound agnosia") are worsened by homogeneous signals and helped by signal diversity, while Stage II patients ("word-deafness") deteriorate almost as a function of the degree of differentiation of the signal.

Both Stages I and II are active systems, the one "receptive" and synthetic, the other "expressive" and analytical. They are neither

parallel nor *sensu stricto* hierarchical. From the point of view of the
real object or signal, Stage I is prior to Stage II, but from the point of
view of the perception, Stage II has priority. However, within each
stage, sublevels can be defined which follow the pattern of hierarchical
organization. Moreover, there is reason to believe that the "minor"
hemisphere has a special role in Stage I, and the "major" hemisphere
in Stage II processing.

Regarding the anatomical substrates of Stage I and II processes,
there is not a great deal that can be said. Stage I concerns the primary
sensory cortices (e.g. visual, auditory). The work of Hubel and Weisel
(1965) indicates that the process of visual shape specification occurs
over striate and prestriate zones. This corresponds to the deficit in
"apperceptive visual agnosia," characterized by Teuber (1968) as a
premature termination of just such an hierarchic feature-extracting
process. Concerning Stage II, there is, in the visual system, evidence
that occipital lobes are necessary for visual imagery and dream, as
these are abolished with bilateral occipital lobectomy (Alajouanine
and Lhermitte, 1963). Some workers have been led to prematurely
conclude from data of this type that the prestriate area is the site of
the visual memory store. Other work, reviewed in Weiskrantz (1968)
indicates that somehow in this process temporoparietal cortex is involved. Certainly, the occurrence of formed visual hallucination on
temporal lobe stimulation is consistent with this interpretation. Most
of the experimental work stresses a motoric or sensing function for
this region, a conventional way of describing Stage II function. This
stresses the "expressive" aspect of the process. It seems likely that the
parasensory areas are not the sites of the modality-specific stores, but
are essential to the elaboration of that store into imagery or veridical
perception.

If we consider the patient with visual object agnosia, we find
striking confirmation of this account in the clinical presentation. In
"apperceptive agnosia" there is damage to those mechanisms for shape
and angle detection which provide for stimulus modeling. It is not
surprising, therefore, that the patient has great difficulty in the discrimination of visually complex and disparate objects. In severe cases,
the patient can discriminate little more than between a straight and
curved line. Identification of faces may, in fact, return prior to objects, and objects prior to written words, though letter and object
identification may recover at about the same time. Moreover, simple
symmetrical objects and letters are the first to be recognized. Visuo-
sensory defects are present (Bay, 1953) and severe impairments in

contour and shape perception (Efron, 1968) can be demonstrated. The disturbance radiates into tactile identification, which is frequently—if not invariably—impaired, and spatial constructional tasks such as drawing from memory. This accompanying visual-spatial agnosia (*quod vide*) persists as a residual in the recovered apperceptive agnosic, and is a sign that the damaged visual "feature-extracting" system is identical or contiguous to that involved in primary constructional disability.

In "associative agnosia" there is interruption at a later phase in perception. The signal has completed the greater part of the process and so the patient has an improved perceptual world. The matching of signal to trace establishes the degree of recognition (in some patients, the sense of familiarity without identification). Matching also involves a delineative function. This has to do with signal analysis and the articulation of the content into mental space. Thus, in "associative agnosia," the patient has great difficulty in distinguishing items which are visually similar, particularly items within a single class such as faces. The cognitive element need not be of primary importance, and errors tend to show morphological rather than conceptual links to the correct item. Here words may return prior to objects, and objects prior to faces, the progression being from the visually complex (i.e. unique) to the visually simple. Thus, in the severe case, the patient cannot identify objects, faces or writing; in the less severe case, object recognition returns and prosopagnosia may exist in relative isolation (present case). The concept of prosopagnosia (*quod vide*) as a mild form of associative agnosia is also consistent with the comparable frequency of incidence, and the anatomy of the two disorders.

The question of preserved drawing in "associative agnosia" deserves some comment. The fact that drawing from immediate memory is so much worse, suggests copying in these patients to be largely an imitative action. In this respect, it is similar to echolalia, especially since both occur in the absence of signal comprehension. Echolalia has been shown to represent incomplete participation by the content in the full process of speech formation. If copying is at all similar in this respect, it may well have to do with the parallel between speech, as the action system of auditory perception, and praxis as the action system of vision. Finally, regarding optic aphasia, this appears to be the mildest form of "associative agnosia." It corresponds to a stage in recovery after object recognition has returned, and may coexist with prosopagnosia. The disorder is transitional to anomia.

Chapter 21

VISUAL-SPATIAL AGNOSIA

IN VISUAL-SPATIAL agnosia (apractagnosia), as Critchley (1953) has pointed out, it is largely the conceptualization of relationships in extrapersonal space that is disordered. There is "a difficulty in putting together one-dimensional units so as to form two-dimensional figures or patterns." At the core of the syndrome are the visual-constructive disabilities, such that the patient is unable to apprehend or reproduce all but the simplest visual-spatial relationships. Neglect for left visual space is a frequent accompaniment and this, together with the visual-constructive defect, probably accounts for the findings of right-left spatial disorientation, dressing apraxia, and perhaps, topographagnosia (disturbed map reading and route finding), all of which are seen in a considerable number of cases.

The condition was first described by Kleist (1911, 1934) as "optic apraxia," later "constructional apraxia," an executive disorder distinct from other apraxias, in which the spatial component is missing. Other reports by Poppelreuter (1917), Seelert (1920) and Strauss (1924) helped to further define the syndrome, and it has been thoroughly discussed in recent reviews by Critchley (1953) and Warrington (1969). A range of disturbance has been observed, from mild cases who complain of difficulty in the use of tools or tying knots, to more severe cases with lack of insight, and disorganization on tests of spatial ability. The defect is apparent in the copying of simple geometrical figures (e.g. circle, cube, Rey figure), in free drawing (e.g. house, clock, bicycle), in stick patterns, mannikin assembly and three-dimensional block constructions. Critchley has reviewed the characteristics of drawing in these patients and has noted: crowding of the drawing into the corner of the page; a copy generally smaller than the model; tremulous wavy lines with occasional mirror reversals; and a tendency to draw vertical lines oblique, or to persist in one dimension. Also impaired are block designs (Kohs blocks) with faulty reproduction of either design, block outline or both. Some findings of Kaplan (personal communication) suggest the usefulness of this test in distinguishing right from left hemispheric cases, the latter tending to retain the block outline but failing on the design, the former failing even the outline. Difficulty on tests requiring little active participation, such as counting the component blocks in a cube, or judgments as to correct or incorrect patterning, have led some workers to maintain the importance of perceptual over praxic defects. In addition to left spatial neglect, right-left and topographical disorientation, one occasionally sees, in right hemispheric cases, difficulty in written calculation and reading due largely to gaze instability and spatial neglect. Writing may also show the effects of spatial disorganization, and patients may have difficulty on clock setting, jigsaw puzzles and other games.

The localization of the syndrome has been the subject of much lively discussion over the years. Originally thought due to major hemisphere damage, the pendulum began to swing the other way with the papers of McFie and Zangwill (1960), Piercy *et al.* (1960) and Piercy and Smyth (1962). At present, it is generally agreed that visual-spatial agnosia is more common and more extensive with minor side lesions, but whether this is simply a matter of severity or reflects some qualitative difference in hemispheric organization is not yet clear. Some investigators, notably Zangwill and co-workers, believe that qualitative differences exist in the performance of right- and left-lesioned patients. They noted that drawings of right hemispheric cases were piecemeal and fragmented with energetic superimposed strokes, while those of left-sided cases retained accurate spatial relationships, but were simplified and drawn slowly. Piercy *et al.* (1960) noted superior copying in the left-sided group. Warrington summarized her findings as showing right hemispheric cases, ". . . better able to analyze the model (cube, star) in terms of its constituent parts. The left-sided cases found difficulty in making this analysis, but might still produce an acceptable copy by slavishly reproducing the various lines without logical sequence." Bogen (1970) has discussed the impairment in drawing with the right hand in commissurotomy patients, and supports the notion of hemispheric specialization. Recently, Benson and Barton (1970) found constructional deficits with widely distributed cortical pathology, more severe with posterior than anterior lesions, and more consistently present with right than left hemispheric pathology, but by no means so specific or restricted as implied by other workers. Finally, an added problem in the interpretation and localization of constructional difficulties is the finding of visual-spatial disorganization in subcortical dementia (progressive supranuclear palsy). This disorganization is quite severe, and does not appear to be a consequence of gaze paralysis.

In sum, the visual-spatial syndrome of the major side appears to be either a weaker or less complete form of the minor side expression, or an executive or praxic disorder, i.e. constructional apraxia, properly called. This problem has been reviewed in an excellent paper by Benton (1967) who concludes that ". . . in some sense, the right hemisphere plays a 'dominant' role in the mediation of visuoconstructive activity in man . . . (and that) this 'dominance" is relative, not absolute."

One of the earliest theories as to the nature of the disorder was Lhermitte's (1928) suggestion of a disturbance in spatial thought interrupting the connection of spatial perceptions with the faculty of their motor utilization. Subsequently, Meyer-Gross (1935) described a disturbance in what he called "activity space" (Wirkraum), an inability to utilize the personal-spatial referent, e.g. the hand, for action in extrapersonal (visual) space. Since then, authors have emphasized this dual character of the disturbance, the perceptual and the motor difficulties, either of these usually held to be the primary factor. One approach of particular appeal, in that it recognizes the essential unity of the perceptual and motor elements, emphasizes a disturbance in spatial concepts. Van der Horst (1932) argued that "both in our actions and in our perceptions the *spatial sense* acts as a psychic *category*, by means of which *gnostic* and *practic functions* are *connected* together by one and the same *direction radical* (his italics)." More recently, Ettlinger *et al.* (1957), have taken a somewhat similar view. The authors stressed a deficiency in spatial thought, with the perceptual process itself involved in the breakdown of spatial concepts, and they aligned the disorder with apperceptive agnosias of Lissauer.

It is not surprising that impairments in visual space and action occur, for as we have argued, both perception and movement issue out of a common level in the cognitive process. The milder constructional disability with left hemisphere lesion is an indication that the opposite hemisphere plays the larger role, i.e. has a priority, in visual-spatial function. On the major side, cognition is directed toward a further verbal stage; on the minor side, there appears to be a kind of proficiency at that level of thought development for which the minor hemisphere is most specialized.

In some respects the disorder appears to be a milder form of the visual-spatial defect than in apperceptive agnosia. The unilateral spatial disorganization may be thought of as sufficient to disrupt only the more advanced stages of the visual synthetic process while sparing the apprehension of form and pattern. Thus, in Adler's case (1944) of carbon monoxide poisoning, there was recovery of object recognition while the visual constructive defect remained. Moreover, the experience with patients having cortical blindness suggests the visuo-sensory and visual-spatial to be contiguous if not coextensive processes. These processes appear to be more selectively involved with right hemispheric pathology. Certainly, we have seen repeatedly, in the discussion of sound-agnosia, of autotopagnosia and of the apraxias, the suggestion of a preferential right-hemispheric concern with Stage I processing, i.e. with sensory-constructive mechanisms, and left-hemispheric role in Stage II perceptuo-motor mechanisms. There is no rigid separation of function, however, for bilateral lesions often act to compound the unilateral defect. This is particularly true for Stage I defects (e.g. apperceptive agnosia, autotopagnosia) but may also have application in apraxia and aphasia.

Chapter 22

PROSOPAGNOSIA

A LTHOUGH MENTIONED from time to time in the early literature, prosopagnosia or inability to recognize faces was first systematically described and discussed by Bodamer (1947) on the basis of three personal cases, all post-traumatic with severe visual defects. Drawing attention to studies of "inborn" infantile smiling responses and maternal recognition (see Brown, 1967), in which a strategic function for the ocular zone, or Ocula, was advanced, Bodamer postulated a pathological fixation within the ocular element of this primordial capacity. Thus, patients returned to an infantile state in which only the eyes were clearly perceived. Though this explanation has not received wide acceptance, Bodamer's case descriptions, and subsequent publications by Hecaen *et al.* (1952), Pötzl (1953), Pallis (1955) and Bornstein and Kidron (1959) helped to establish the authenticity of the syndrome.

Clinically, prosopagnosia may exist in the absence of a defect in object recognition, or rarely, facial recognition may be preserved in some cases of object agnosia (Hecaen and Angelergues, 1962). According to Bornstein, true prosopagnosia is not usually connected with a visual-object agnosia, nor does it appear with visual-spatial agnosia. While the coexistence of prosopagnosia with defects in object recognition is not surprising (all three of the cases of apperceptive agnosia here reported have shown this impairment), preservation of facial recognition with object agnosia is not so easily explained, and in view of its rarity certainly requires further study. Ordinarily, there is good visual acuity, stereoscopy and depth perception, and the estimation of distance and direction may be quite well preserved. Metamorphopsia may interefere with facial recognition, but this does not appear to be the usual mechanism. Defects in visual fields are commonly, if not invariably, present. Faust (1947) has emphasized the frequency of superior quadranopic defects, a finding supported by Hecaen and Angelergues (1962). Although perceptual function has not been demonstrated to be normal in a single case, it is usually held, as with other agnosic disturbances, that the perceptual impairment is not sufficient to account for the severity of the defect. Patients are unable to identify human faces or photographs of family, close friends, well-known people, or even themselves in the mirror. There is usually a lack of familiarity with the unidentified face, although some instances are described where patients were aware that they had previously seen faces which could not be identified. This problem suggests more an anomia than a perceptual defect. Not only are patients unable to name the face, but no account can be given of the individual represented. Depending on the severity, there may be inability to distinguish young or old faces, male and female, or even between human and animal faces. Recognition of facial expression may also suffer. What facial identification occurs, is usually accomplished by specific characteristics such as birth marks, glasses, hair style, or more often by dress, voice or the sound of the individual walking. Patients may be able to indicate errors in drawings of faces, add elements which have been deleted, or embellish a drawing with glasses, a moustache, etc. though performance here may be far from normal. Ability to identify facial parts in isolation is said to be good, though ambiguous items (moustache versus eyebrows) are easily confused. There is difficulty in learning new faces, and in some cases, in matching very similar photographs. Revisualization of faces may or may not be spared. Topographical memory may also be impaired (Hecaen and Angelergues, 1962). If revisualization is affected, and faces cannot be described or recollected from memory, visual memory for other objects or animals may be impaired, as in Brain's (1941) case who visualized all animals as having only four legs and a tail. Recognition of individuals in a dream, with or without impairment of waking imagery, has not yet been studied. The difficulty is not limited to human faces. There may be errors with other perceptually similar items such as animals, flowers, fruits or automobiles. Faust's case had difficulty with pieces of furniture, De Renzi's with wine bottles, and a patient of Bornstein's lost the ability to identify previously well-known birds, complaining that they all looked the same.

The localization of prosopagnosia is uncertain. The condition may occur with pathology clinically localized to either right or left hemisphere. In the six cases to come to autopsy, there have either been bilateral lesions or unilateral lesions with involvement of corpus callosum (Gloning *et al.*, 1970).

Case 14

A highly intelligent physician with visual agnosia and agnosic alexia (discussed in Chap. 20), examined after the object agnosia cleared. The disorder in facial recognition had persisted unchanged throughout the course of his condition. Although not overtly troubled by it, he was aware and concerned about the difficulty in recognizing his wife and children, and indicated that he believed it to be primarily a matter of disturbed perception. He was able to find his way around the city and the hospital quite well, though verbal description of familiar areas was perhaps slightly deficient. He reported that faces were somewhat fuzzy and stated that he could not clearly tell them apart. He denied memory impairment, and denied also a feeling of familiarity with faces poorly or uncertainly identified. Prominent facial features could be described, though with occasional errors, as in "horn-rimmed glasses" for round spectacles. There was a tendency to see people as more slender than they actually were. As mentioned, he was unable to recognize members of his family, the hospital staff or his own face in the mirror. He could recognize a smile or frown on a human face or drawing, respond to a smile spontaneously, imitate facial movements and accurately identify facial and limb movements such as blowing out a match, kissing and flipping a coin. There was hesitancy in differentiating photographs of men and women, particularly if other cues, e.g. dress, hair length, were obscured, but he usually made the correct choice, basing it on such aspects as "skin texture" or amount of "wrinkles." He was generally able to guess the age of a face within a ten-year range, though performance was well below the normal on this test and there were times when completely erroneous responses occurred. He could tell when a photograph of a face was upside down or sideways, was able to draw simplified line-drawings of faces, frontal and profile (Fig. 7), could detect and correct deleted parts in drawings given him, and could add elements on command, such as a moustache or eyebrows. Churchill's face was described from memory as "round faced and pudgy" but a Yalta portrait was rejected as being too young. Lincoln's face was excellently described from memory as "tall, angular with a small beard, large nose and tasselled hair," but he was uncertain about a standard portrait fitting this description quite perfectly. After obtaining this description, Lincoln's face was then drawn from memory, and thereafter copied from a standard portrait photograph (Fig. 7). The disorganization of the drawing from memory is apparent, and contrasts with the copy, and with his drawing of a schematized face. When shown pictures of well-known people, he was unable to name them, or select the correct name from a group, and often rejected the correct name when offered.

The patient was given a test of animal naming and sorting. Three pictures (e.g. leopard, tiger and zebra) were shown, and he was asked

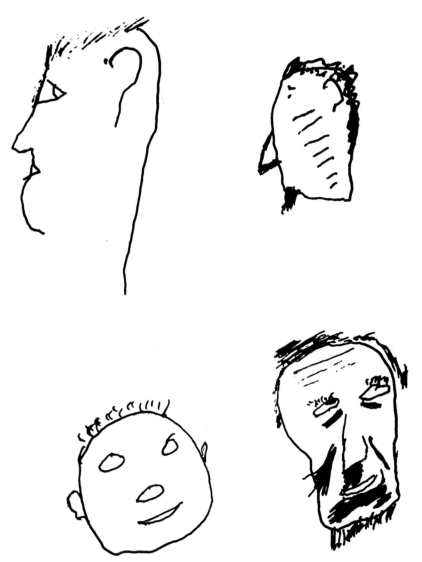

Figure 7. Case 14. Left: drawing of face in profile and frontal view. Right: *above*, Lincoln's face from memory, *below*, copy from photograph.

to group the two related animals. On this test, categorization was invariably dependent on morphological features, rather than on animal class. Thus, a zebra and tiger were placed together, excluding a leopard, because of the similar striped pattern. Other groupings were made on general configuration, posture, position of the tail, etc. When given animal names, there was no difficulty in categorizing them appropriately, using terms such as bovines, canines and so on. On naming animal pictures, errors reflected morphological confusion. Thus, a sitting bear was called a rabbit because of a physiognomic similarity. At times, the correct class was apparent, as in "German shepard" for terrier, or a "water bird of some kind" for ostrich. Animal faces seen head-on gave more difficulty than whole-body profiles, and animal pictures presented in isolation were easier than with a natural background. Naming animals to description was excellent.

The patient was then shown a series of seven photographs of well-known people (Lincoln, Eisenhower, Eleanor Roosevelt, Jackie Kennedy, Nixon, Churchill and Danny Kaye). He was unable to identify any of the photographs, or select a specific picture on command with consistent accuracy. Correct matches were explained by "Well, this one has a beard and so did Lincoln." Then he was shown a single unidentified picture which was then replaced, the pictures mixed, and he was asked to find it. This was accomplished readily. Then shown a photograph (Eisenhower) and given the name, he was able to find the picture on command a few moments later. This contrasted with his earlier performance on the more demanding Benton-Van Allen test, but there is little doubt that specific features played a part in the improved performance, e.g. Eisenhower's garrison cap. Then, shown each of the seven pictures, and at the same time given the correct name, he was able to select the correct picture on command by name in six of seven instances. The only error, a striking one, was selecting Danny Kaye's picture for Lincoln. When told he was mistaken, he said "I didn't remember the beard," and explained his other successes by "I just associated the name to the picture." He denied recognizing any of the faces shown him, and simply accepted the correct name on faith when offered. On retesting a few days later, he was given the photographs all at once and asked to name as many as possible. He correctly named Churchill ("the bald head"), Eisenhower ("the cap"), Nixon ("it's a sideways view"), and then gave Danny Kaye as Eleanor Roosevelt, and produced the rest of the names, unable to match them to the appropriate pictures. This indicates good retention of the names, and of matching characteristics of some pictures, but no recognition of the picture *qua* individual.

During World War II, the patient was an Air Force pilot, and flew over 50 missions in a P51 Mustang. He was shown pictures of various planes of that period, but was able to identify only 1 of 20 planes, failing on obvious models such as a Messerschmitt, which he flew against in combat, a Japanese zero-sen, and even his own P51. In spite of this, he was able to give a fair description of the pictures before him, and could recount the salient features of many of these planes from memory.

Performance on the Benton-Van Allen test of facial recognition was extremely poor (administered April, 1969). He was in the third percentile of normals, and 33rd percentile of the right hemispheric group. On Raven's matrices, overall performance was poor, with deterioration on the "cognitive" items, and good ability on initial perceptually-challenging material. Performance was very poor on hidden figures, and grossly deficient on Poppelreuter's figures. Finally, if a piece of paper was presented to him containing 3–6 dots, each 3 mm in size and scattered randomly over the page, and exposed for 0.25–0.5 seconds, he was generally able to report the correct number of dots.

DISCUSSION

There are almost as many theories of prosopagnosia as there are reported cases. In addition to the account of Bodamer which has been discussed, Bay (1953) has observed a sensory defect in combination with an intellectual decline, and explains all agnosic forms on this basis. Pallis (1955) suggested a relation to spatial thinking, and a failure of incorporation in memory due to lack of salient perceptual features. Bornstein (1963) emphasized a disturbance in Gestalt formation, and Hecaen and Angelergues (1962) a disturbance in perceptual discrimination. It is the latter hypothesis that seems presently to have most support. Thus, Beyn and Knyazeva (1962) have noted that ". . . generic recognition may be intact but individual recognition grossly impaired," indicating, they believed, ". . . a failure in recognition at its most specific and highly individual level." De Renzi *et al.* (1968) discussed the subtle differentiations necessary for facial identification, and concluded that the difficulty was ". . . not because of unfamiliarity or because of lack of verbal labels, but because they (faces) are very similar to one another and, therefore, their identification requires the ability to detect small formal differences." This argument is very appealing, and helps to relate the disorder to other visual agnosias. A parallel can be seen in everyday behavior, as when the

Westerner says, "All Chinamen look alike," testifying to the greater difficulty for him in isolating the particular from a relatively invariant class. Further support of this idea comes from studies in patients with right hemispheric damage demonstrating increased difficulty in matching or identifying faces. It is worth emphasizing, however, that in one study prosopagnosic patients performed quite normally on these tests (Tzavaris, personal communication).

One inference from this body of experimental work is that right hemispheric pathology is related to the difficulty in facial identification, and that this defect occurs in the most highly differentiated perceptual performance, namely identifying a specific human face. This receives some support from the finding that prosopagnosic patients also have difficulty with equally challenging discriminations, as in the identification of animal faces, fruits, furniture, etc. The one problem with this interpretation, as Russell has emphasized, is that if prosopagnosia occurred with unilateral disease, particularly, as a subtle manifestation of that disease, it would be a much more common finding.

There is some evidence, reported by Milner (1967), that the right temporal lobe may play a preferential role in facial identification. Thus, patients with surgical lesions of this lobe have increased difficulty on facial recognition tasks, whereas left temporal patients perform considerably better. While there is as yet little clinical support for this localization, the high incidence of superior quadrantanopias in prosopagnosia, and one study demonstrating some correlation between left superior quadrantanopias and impaired facial recognition (Newcombe and Russell, 1969), makes this possibility worthy of further study. Related to this is the difficulty in facial recognition seen in patients with bilateral surgical resection of anterior temporal lobes. The defect, of course, is not confined to facial recognition, and is limited to acquaintances made during the period affected by the memory loss. In one personal case of post-herpes encephalitis, the patient had difficulty in recognizing his own wife whom he had married shortly after the illness, and could identify no individuals met during the period in question.

Finally, in a personal exploratory study designed to evaluate the contention that prosopagnosia is the result of a combination of visual impairment with aphasia, a group of young soldiers with gunshot wounds restricted to left hemisphere, aphasic and right-handed, were fitted with a mask reducing visual field to a central 3 degrees only. Subjects were then requested to identify (match) at 1 meter distance,

objects, object-pictures and two sets of pictures of faces, one set 9″ ×
12″ which required scanning to be seen in entirety, and another set 2″
× 3″ which fell within the visual field and could be seen as a whole.
In preliminary studies, no errors on objects or object-pictures occurred, and there was only minimal difficulty with small or large
facial pictures.

In attempting to explain this disorder, we may first turn to the
case which has been discussed. On the one hand, there is strong evidence for a perceptual defect, as in the morphological confusions on
face and animal identification, the difficulty in facial matching on the
Benton-Van Allen test, the patient's own descriptions of faces, the
similar errors in drawing and copying and, in fact, the subjective
accounts by the patient of his problem. Further, many pictures (for
example, animals) were recognized when presented in profile against
a white background, but not when mildly ambiguous, or in a natural
setting. Hidden figures were done poorly, and reading was of the
agnosic type. However, other tests of perceptual ability suggested at
least adequate perceptions. Routine testing disclosed fairly good
ability to perceive lines and geometrical configurations, to match nonsense figures either directly or from memory, and to copy drawings of
simple objects. Raven's matrices were done poorly, but in a manner
that reflected the logical rather than the visual complexity of the item.
The ability to rapidly count dots presented simultaneously before him
suggests that the entire field was perceived, and argues against a
failure in Gestalt formation. Naming does not seem to be specifically
impaired, though it may be the subtlest form of a memory defect
reflected in the speech system. Thus, optic aphasia appeared not infrequently in object identification, but only occasionally in face identification. Difficulty with names of faces otherwise recognized should,
therefore, appears as a transitory stage in recovery of prosopagnosia.

It seems, therefore, that the disorder in this case must be approached from the same standpoint as that in "associative" visual
agnosia, for the failure to identify common objects resolved, leaving
an inability to identify more restricted object groups, such as faces
and animals. Certainly, linking prosopagnosia to visual agnosia would
help to explain a number of problems. Thus, the rarity of the one
disorder is paralleled by the rarity of the other, and the clinical
association with visual agnosia, which is of striking frequency, would
be taken to indicate a functional relationship between the two forms.
Those cases of prosopagnosia without associative visual agnosia would
be milder forms of the latter, while it is conceivable that apperceptive

agnosia could improve to the point where faces might be recognizable but not objects. To understand this is to understand the complex nature of perception. This process, we have argued, is essentially a two-stage affair, the first stage having to do with constructive, the second with discriminative mechanisms. Apperceptive agnosia is a disorder of the first system, that of shape specification and the preparatory stages of perception. This involves the spatial organization proper, and so defects of spatial performance are always present. Impairments in facial recognition in this disorder are always strictly *visual*. There may, however, be a stage in recovery where sufficient information about a face is extracted so that it is recognizable, while objects continue to present difficulty. Perhaps this owes to the two-dimensional nature of faces, or possibly at this stage the uniformity of the object aids in its identification. At any rate, when prosopagnosia co-exists with apperceptive agnosia, it is of a fundamentally different type than in the case here described. In disorders of the second system, "associative" agnosia, there is a disturbance of the stimulus complex at or beyond the stage of its assimilation to memory. The constructive process has proceeded farther along, and so the patient has an improved perceptual world, though it is still abnormal. Failure of the complex to achieve that degree of structure such that mnemic traces are appropriately called-up, results in vague perceptual experiences and morphological confusions on identification tests. This stage operates, we have seen, on a different basis than the first, for here object similarities confer a disadvantage on further processing. The mechanism is one of selection and individuation of a discrete percept, a process which is complicated by physical uniformity. Prosopagnosia will result from the fact that "faces," having passed through the constructive process, that part of the process disordered in apperceptive agnosia, present too few individual features to facilitate passage through a delineative stage. Thus, we see that the same syndrome, prosopagnosia, can result from two opposite conditions. This conforms to enlightened clinical opinion which has all but conceded that there are two, possibly three, separate forms of this disorder. In the one form, however, it is the end-stage of the pathology, in the other, the first to appear.

Chapter 23

ANOSOGNOSIA

A NOSOGNOSIA, OR LACK OF awareness of disease, was first described by von Monakow in 1885 in two cases of cortical blindness, and a short while later, by Pick (1898) in a case of left hemiparesis. The following year, Anton (1899) took up the problem in some detail, with observations on a case of demonstrated cortical blindness and a case of presumed cortical deafness. Denial of hemiplegia was first specifically discussed in a brief paper by Babinski (1914) who coined the terms *anosognosia* for unawareness of paralysis, and *anosodiaphorie* for those instances where the disabled limb was recognized as such, but appeared to give little concern. On the strength of these two cases, Babinski raised the possibility of a right hemispheric preference, and correctly argued that the sensory impairment, present in both of his cases, was of critical importance in the genesis of the syndrome.*

DENIAL OF BLINDNESS

Following Anton's description, the syndrome came to be recognized as a frequent accompaniment of cortical blindness. Soon after, cases of denial with peripheral blindness were described, as in a patient of Stertz (1920) with optic atrophy, Stengel's (1946) case of peripheral blindness with frontal lesion, and cases of Redlich and Dorsey (1945), though in all such patients some degree of mental reduction or confusion was present. Thus, blindness of central or peripheral origin, in combination with some disturbance of consciousness came to be accepted as the *sine qua non* of the disorder. These dynamic aspects were stressed by Redlich and Bonvicini (1911) who pointed to the influence of diffuse effects, and the apathetic nature of the patient's behavior. Though considered independent of dementia and hallucination, anosognosia was found to bear resemblance to the Korsakoff state. This was emphasized by other writers, notably Schilder, who argued that even in ordinary cases of Korsakoff's psychosis, there was

---

*Anosognosia for speech is discussed separately with the aphasic disorders in which it appears.

Aphasia, Apraxia and Agnosia

a selective memory deficit pertaining to traumatic events. In the recent series of Gloning *et al.* (1968), however, only one of eleven patients with denial had a Korsakoff's psychosis though a tendency to confabulate was noted in all.

Other opinions were not lacking. In his original paper, Anton described an "amputation" of the visual lobes from the rest of the brain, and approached the problem from the standpoint of the integrity of the concept of the self. Pötzl (1928) proposed a dissociation between perceptual and kinesthetic functions, and related this to thalamocortical interruption. Consistent with this view, were suggestions that denial was secondary to substitution of visual images for sensations. In the case of Lagrange *et al.* (1929), denial occurred during periods of visual hallucination, indicating that the hallucinations may have been interpreted as real images. This was accepted by Morax (1960) and Alajouanine and Lhermitte (1957) who noted the role of confabulation in the false interpretation of hallucinatory or memory images. As Redlich and Dorsey (1945) point out, however, patients can be blind and hallucinate without having denial, nor do a majority of patients with Anton's syndrome hallucinate. A further point is that complete blindness is usually required for denial to appear. This is well illustrated by Stengel's (1946) case of denial with peripheral blindness and frontal lesion. This patient had absolute denial in the right totally blind field, but would occasionally admit visual loss on the left side where some function, viz.: ability to see light and at times count fingers, was preserved. The suggestion of Gloning *et al.* (1968) that denial may arise through preservation of islets of vision appears contrary to most experience. Too little information exists, however, to be definite on this point. There is then a complex of factors necessary for Anton's syndrome: complete blindness; confabulatory trends, at least within the affected perceptual sphere; and coincident with the confabulation, some alteration of mentation. The following case is an example of the interplay of these factors.

This was a seventy-year-old man seen in 1967 with greatly reduced vision and a Korsakoff's psychosis due to a suprasellar cyst. The patient could at times count fingers and recognize some objects, and could walk only by groping his way along, frequently bumping into objects. Because of a marked Korsakoff's state, vision could not be adequately tested, but it was evident that, in spite of severe memory loss and confabulation, there was recognition and concern over his considerable visual difficulty. Following a diagnostic vertebral angiogram, there developed what appeared to be complete blindness, presumably secondary to spasm of posterior cerebral arteries. Mental state was otherwise not greatly changed, but at this time a definite Anton's syndrome appeared. After a few hours, vision seemed to improve slightly to the previous state, and anosognosia disappeared. In this case, near-total blindness and a marked Korsakoff's psychosis did not produce denial until blindness became complete.

In a second case, the importance of complete blindness is again seen. Here also, the Korsakoff state appeared insufficient to produce the denial. In this case, the lack of correspondence between hemiplegic denial and denial of blindness, reported previously by Gloning *et al.* (1968), serves to emphasize the limitation of those accounts which depend on general aspects, intellectual reduction or memory loss to the exclusion of other factors.

This forty-nine-year-old professional artist was seen in 1970 with a history of right homonymous hemianopia since 1968, presumed secondary to vascular disease, and recent onset of blindness (i.e. left hemianopia) and left hemiplegia. There was a past history of alcoholism and Korsakoff's psychosis. On examination, there was complete blindness, the patient responding only to strong light in his eyes. Otherwise, he could not distinguish night and day; there was no response to visual threat. Blindness was denied, at times vigorously, at other times in an indefinite way, as in "There has been something wrong with it (vision), I don't know what, but I think it's alright now." There was also denial of left hemiplegia. Visual imagery was impaired, with bizarre responses. Thus, he was unable to describe a giraffe, and when asked to describe a zebra, said, "A zebra is like a giraffe having a nightmare." Objects were described through confabulations. A marked Korsakoff's state was present. At times, he was seen talking to himself, suggesting hallucinatory phenomena, but hallucinations were denied. Nightmares occurred at the time of onset, but for only a brief duration. Over a two-week period, there was slight improvement of vision, such that brightness and occasionally some movement could be discerned. At this time, he readily admitted that he was blind, and became despondent about this problem. The left hemiplegia continued to be denied, and the mental state, characteristic of Korsakoff's psychosis, remained unchanged.

Thus, it appears that Anton's syndrome requires a combination of complete blindness, at least complete in that part of the field subject to denial, and confabulation within the visual sphere. Clinically, denial of blindness occurs in from 30 to 50 per cent of patients with cortical blindness. Transient blindness, as in eclampsia or migraine, is ordinarily not denied, whereas blindness from massive bioccipital lesion generally is denied (Morax, 1960). Patients may deny that they are blind, report visual experiences which are obviously confabulated, and act as if they could see quite well. They may walk confidently, though repeatedly bumping into walls and furniture; confabulations may occur on naming tests utilizing vision, and perhaps touch as well. Often patients will give unrealistic explanations for their difficulty, as in "It's too dark in the room" or "I don't have my glasses." At times there is fluctuation in the occurrence of denial. This may correlate with visual hallucinations, as in the already cited case of Lagrange *et al.* (1929) or perhaps with visual acuity or mental state, though the problem needs further work. Hallucinations and metamorphopsias may intervene, though not with great frequency. Other symptoms include those found in association with cortical blindness. In addition to the general mental impairment or Korsakoff state, an amnesic aphasia may be present. Finally, patients are generally apathetic and slow in their responses, but euphoria has been occasionally reported.

DENIAL OF HEMIPARESIS

Most authors accept Gerstmann's (1942) classification, in which three forms are recognized; partial to total unawareness of hemiplegia; amnesia, imperception or denial of the affected limbs; and distortion or other illusory phenomena referable to the hemiparetic side. In an excellent review, Critchley (1953) noted the progression from unawareness, to denial of paralysis, to denial of the limb, whether or not hemiparetic. This continuum between the different forms is linked to the normal tendency to forget the left side of the body. From this, Schilder argued for the presence of an "organic repression" through which the varieties of anosognosia would appear as stages in a pathological decompensation. Weinstein and Kahn (1955) have stressed the denial for other illness-related topics, and the amnesia for the anosognosic period after recovery. These authors distinguish explicit and implicit denial, recognizing within these categories, most of the different forms.

Clinically, the syndrome is ordinarily present in the acute stage of a hemiplegia, and is associated with some confusion and disorientation. Occasional long-standing cases have been reported, but this is exceptional. Neglect of the hemiparetic limbs may appear in spite of normal strength; in the lack of use, in poor hygiene, as well as in a failure to comb the hair, shave, or apply cosmetics on the affected side. Critchley has emphasized that the neglect seems to be sensorily-conditioned, for there is no hesitancy to use the limb in such tasks as putting a glove on the unimpaired hand, or scrubbing the intact side of the body. Difficulty in crossing the projected midline should be noted. Ordinarily, the disorder appears in the absence of aphasia. Patients may admit the defect but seem unconcerned, they may attribute weakness to unrealistic problems such as arthritis, fatigue, or to the fact that the other hand is generally used for the requested performance. Hemispatial inattention and/or deviation of head, eyes and body to the opposite side may be present. Weinstein and Cole (1963) noted the frequency of metaphoric explanations, as in a patient who referred to his good side as "sweetheart" and his paretic side as "wife." A tendency for joking and facetious misnaming was also observed in their series. Most often, however, patients are said to appear apathetic. Ajuriaguerra and Hecaen (1964) comment that in such patients, "At times one can also notice a state of indifference to the outside world, of inertia, apathy and disinterest." On direct questioning, patients may deny any difficulty with the limb at all. The relationship between degree of hemiparesis (especially sensory impairment) and frankness of denial has not been studied, but is deserving of attention.

The observations of Weinstein *et al.* (1955) that denial may extend to the intact limbs if these are tied down also demands closer study. I have not found this to be a common occurrence in anosognosic patients. According to Weinstein, patients may also deny or avoid discussing hospital-related material, but whether this represents a general anosognosic trend, or reflects an impairment in recent memory, of which illness-related material forms the major part, is not yet established. Thus, one personal case denied blindness, but admitted to diplopia from a third nerve palsy which had been present for the preceding two years. Another, denied paralysis of the left arm (total) but admitted weakness in the paretic left leg. This patient related the history of an amputation of the first two fingers of the left hand, and discussed his past phantom experiences freely. Asked to make a "V" sign on the left, he explained his failure on the obvious fact of the amputation. Asked to move his left little finger, he refused to admit that it was paralyzed. Thus, denial may spare a less recent disorder in the same system, may involve one of two (usually the most severely involved) paretic limbs on the same side, and may spare deficient *performances* in the same body part depending on the reason for the deficiency. Some patients with or without severe paralysis, will deny the *existence* of the disabled limb. The patient may refuse to admit the presence of the limb, attribute it to the examiner or some other person, or in a state of hemidepersonalization ask where the limb is, say that it has "taken a trip" or search for it elsewhere in the room. Illusory movements of the immobile limb, often disappearing when the latter is touched, or passively moved to the illusory position, and supernumerary or distorted limbs may occur.

Associated with this picture at times is hemispatial neglect and denial of a visual field disorder. It would be of interest to know whether patients with hemiplegic denial would recognize a field defect on the same side, but cases relevant to this question are lacking. One must also distinguish in such patients between a true field defect, and one simulated by hemispatial neglect. Further, it should be emphasized that it is not the neglected field defect that gives rise to limb denial, for as Kramer (1915) originally showed, patients continue to deny even if the hand is placed in the intact field. Finally, patients may express the anosognosia indirectly, through deletion of the appropriate side in drawing a clock or a human figure, in ignoring activity to that side, in auditory inattention and so on.

The condition affects left hemiplegics well out of proportion to those, with or without aphasia, with paresis of the opposite side. For Weinstein and Kahn (1955) it is not the aphasia of the left hemispherics that obscures the anosognosia, but the greater ability of right hemispheric patients to conceptualize the difficulty in terms of metaphor, idiom and synonym. Other authors hold that limb neglect is of equal frequency in either group, but denial more common with right-lesioned patients, while some argue that sidedness is an artifact of aphasic contamination, and that no true predominance exists. The notion that the right hemisphere is the repository of the body-image is acceptable to but a few contemporary writers. Most theories posit a specific sensory defect in combination with some degree of mental reduction. A dissociation between perceptual and kinesthetic functions was suggested by Pötzl (1928), and Campbell first noted the relation to confabulation. Subsequent authors have commented on the Korsakoff-like state of such patients.

Barkman (1925) reviewed the autopsied cases to date, and concluded that right thalamus was involved in all. Nielsen (1939) confirmed the relation to thalamus, suggesting that anosognosia derived from intrathalamic lesion or thalamic isolation from cortex, while imperception of limbs required lesion of thalamoparietal peduncle. Gerstmann (1942) agreed that right optic thalamus, thalamoparietal radiation, or right parietal cortex were of particular importance, and that ". . . lesions of the cortex about or below the right interparietal fissure are most apt to induce the psychologically complex manifestations of the condition than those farther away from it or closer to thalamus. . . ." Finally, based on this localization, Pötzl and Hoff (1931) reproduced the clinical picture with intravenous injection of atophanyl, thought to paralyze the thalamus, while at the same time icing, with ethylchloride, the left and right centroparietal region of cortex in patients with postoperative cranial defects. They were unable to produce the syndrome with only one of the above conditions.

DISCUSSION

The essential components of Anton's syndrome are complete blindness and a confabulatory trend. The latter is taken for, or identified with, a state of confusion, although it may be confined to a single modality. It is probable that the less complete the blindness, or the more peripheral its origin, the more important are the confabulations, whereas, if the blindness is absolute, and cortical in origin, the degree of confusion and confabulation does not necessarily have to be severe.

Confabulations are a sign of an interruption or impedance of some sort in the perceptual process, and do not point to a superimposed disorder, i.e. Korsakoff's syndrome. Thus, patients with anterior callosal syndromes will not only confabulate on tactile naming in the left hand, but will act in such a way as to support their confabulations. This is an important clue to those processes involved in the building up of perceptions. Geschwind (1965) has speculated that confabulations may indicate disease of association areas. While there is little real evidence one way or another on this point, one opposing argument would be the role of hallucinatory or memory images in sustaining a confabulatory trend, since there is some indication that imagery demands intact parasensory areas. In any case, the view of intramodal confabulation as a result of interruption, probably *complete* interruption, of perceptual development within that modality leads to the following tentative formulation.

With regard to neglect of hemiplegia, kinesthetic information from the sensory paretic limb fails to undergo a normal development. If awareness is otherwise normal (i.e. there is no confusion) the existence of the limb in visual awareness guarantees its survival as a part of the "body scheme," the neglect arising because of the priority of the kinesthetic sense in the organization of body (personal) space. If now, there is an overall reduction in awareness (i.e. some degree of general confusion), there will be a failure of the percept, *disabled limb,* to overcome the effects of kinesthetic loss. This will lead to one of two different but analogous responses, denial of the existence of the disability, i.e. *denial of a change in state,* or denial of the existence of the limb, i.e. *admission of the change in state.* If visual correction does not suffice, how is the individual to interpret the lack of sensory information about the limb? Clearly, the absence of information is judged to mean either the absence of impairment or the absence of the limb. One may ask on what basis the patient makes his response. The difference seems to be that in the first instance, lack of sensory information is just that, a deprival of new information about the body, whereas in the second instance, lack of information is utilized *qua* information, and the patient is led to conclude that the body part does not exist. Hallucinatory substitutions represent the intrusion of visual and/or kinesthetic images into awareness when the influence of the cortical projection zone is lost. As such, there is a direct parallel with the auditory hallucinations which appear in cortical and word-deafness, and with the visual hallucinations which are commonly seen in cortical blindness and apperceptive visual agnosia (*quod vide*). The pathological localization in minor hemisphere (see Gainotti, 1968) reflects again the special relation of that hemisphere to visual-spatial processing.

There is ample evidence that the kinesthetic sense has a priority in the organization of personal (bodily) space. Nielsen (1938) describes patients as saying that ". . . they felt as though their limbs were no longer there, and that, while their limbs looked like theirs, they did not feel like them, and they must believe their feelings." For extrapersonal (visual) space, the reverse is true. Thus, Anton's syndrome presents a parallel situation. Lack of awareness of hemianopia is seen in 25 per cent of cases, a figure comparable to that in hemiplegics. Denial of blindness results from visuosensory loss, where the lack of new information permits the conviction that vision has remained unchanged. The situation in which the sensory loss leads to a denial of the existence of extrapersonal space has not, to my knowledge, been reported though may, in fact, be a possibility. Visual hallucinations represent, as in analogous states, the release of imaginal products which, in the absence of sensory data (i.e. lesion of primary sensory area) do not achieve the quality of real percepts. As in hemiplegic denial, the failure to interpret sensory loss as an impairment of that modality, i.e. as blindness, requires some degree of confusion. This confusion, in fact, may to an extent be occasioned by the blindness itself, just as disorientation can be induced by the opposite situation, homogeneity of visual fields as in snow blindness. Thus, absolute cortical blindness, confabulation and some confusion may well be indissolubly linked. In this respect then, we are surprised not by denial but by recognition of disease, for the latter demands more than just a concrete understanding of the informational level, it requires an interpretation of the information received.

Chapter 24

COLOR AGNOSIA

A MONG THE EARLIEST descriptions is that of Wilbrand (1884) who, under the term amnestic color blindness, reported a case with good color perception unable to name colors, and attributed the disorder to an aphasia. Lewandowsky (1908) discussed the topic in detail, arguing that it was not simply a result of aphasia, but of a separation of the concept of colors from that of objects. Difficulty in color sorting, and the agnostic character of the syndrome were first emphasized by Sittig (1921).

For Goldstein and Gelb (1918), the disorder was a reflection of impaired categorical behavior, as seen in characteristic defects of color-sorting, and the reduction of behavior to a more concrete level. For Pötzl (1928), there was a perceptual disorder giving rise to a defect in grouping, naming and/or comprehension, and for Critchley (1965), a combination of mild visual impairment with dysphasia. Geschwind *et al.* (1966) explained it in the manner of pure alexia, namely a disconnection, by left occipital and splenial lesion, of perceptions in right hemisphere from the left hemispheric speech area. This account was further developed by Oxbury *et al* (1969). Since anatomical data is available for but a handful of cases, lesions are usually inferred from the association with alexia, viz.: left occipital lobe and splenium of corpus callosum. In the series of Gloning *et al.* (1968), left temporo-occipital lesions predominated with regard to color agnosia, while two cases of Lenz with defective color perception without alexia are cited with bilateral lingual gyrus lesions without lesion of splenium.

There is no uniform picture of defective color recognition. In mild cases, patients will give qualified responses such as "bluish," or "somewhat greenish," or they may show a tendency to the concrete, as in "sky-blue" or "strawberry-red." Still others will fail to respond, will show verbal paraphasia as in "green" for *brown* or will give descriptive phrases such as "the Irish color" or "the color of blood." Patients who confabulate a color name will ordinarily not select the correct color name from a group, but rather, will reselect from a group the originally misnamed color. In some cases, particularly in dementia, the verbal substitutions may take the form of an even more complex response, e.g. "fuchsia" for *red*. Among aphasics, semantic and/or phonemic paraphasia for color names appears to be greater than that for objects in the more posterior cases. There may be reduced awareness for the defect in color identification, or frank denial once demonstrated. In the majority of patients, red is the most resistant color. Although congenital color blindness ordinarily does not interfere with color naming, Ishihara testing should be routinely performed.

Patients should be tested for sorting colors, for arranging shades of one color, or hues, in order of intensity. They should be required to discard nonmatching colors from a group, match colors to objects, and to written or spoken color names, and the reverse, matching objects and color names to colors. Correct color names should be selected from a group. In this respect, it should be emphasized that while naming and discrimination of colors should both be tested, these performances are by no means comparable. The normal individual is capable of discriminating literally millions of colors, but has only about a dozen or so color names, plus modifiers, in his vocabulary (Chapanis, 1965). Both ordinary (Holmgren wool skeins) and pure colors (Farnsworth, 1949) should be employed. An attempt should be made to correlate performance with different colors. For example, in cortical blindness, patients first recover colors of the long wave band (red, yellow) and lastly recover short wave lengths (blue, violet) (Gloning *et al.*, 1968). The possibility of a similar gradation in color agnosics has not yet been studied. Patients should be asked to spontaneously list color names and to list objects of a certain color. They should be asked to color a picture with crayons appropriately, or indicate pictures painted in an inappropriate manner. Color imagery should be tested through descriptions of familiar objects (flag, banana, etc.) with care to distinguish associative from nonassociative responses. Colors should be shown and then removed prior to naming, or re-presented in a group for nonverbal identification. The color progression of after-images should also be noted. According to Pötzl, the types of errors in color imagery correspond to those on direct naming, a finding which suggests that the same activity orders the material of perception and imagination. Some patients may have loss of color vision (achromatopsia), distortion of colors, or hallucinatory experiences. There are nonagnosic conditions in which dissociation between color and object occurs, as in illusory visual spread, occipital lobe stimulation, and mescal intoxication (Critchley, 1965).

Finally the association of color defects with alexia is well-known, and any evaluation should include thorough testing in this category. In Gloning's series, 70 per cent of pure alexics had some color defect. In his review, Lange (1936) concluded that the color agnosias were only variations on a common theme, but that consideration of these variations was essential to a full understanding of the problem.

Certainly, there does appear to be a wide range of expression of this disorder: 1) In one form the color defect is either a part of a larger perceptual problem, i.e. apperceptive visual agnosia, or is a stage on the way toward object imperception. In the former, the severity of the disturbance is such that color-agnosia is only a minor finding. In the case where object recognition is preserved, however, the comparison with visual object agnosia becomes more hazardous. In visual agnosia, it appears that colors are more stable than objects. However, in the recovery of cortical blindness, there is evidence that form identification returns sooner than colors. It is assumed that this would concern striate rather than parastriate pathology. The frequent observation in color agnosics that red is the most resistant color would be explained by this localization, for in the resolution of cortical blindness red is the first to reappear. 2) In the second form, the color name is qualified or given in concrete fashion. It is uncertain whether this reflects primarily a visual or linguistic deterioration. Gloning *et al.* (1968) have pointed out that this "amnestic" color defect occurs as a stage in the recovery of color agnosia. 3) A third form is that in which confabulation occurs in the face of intact non-verbal recognition testing. This appears to largely be the result of a disorder determined on the linguistic side, though minimal perceptual defects are no doubt present. 4) Color naming may be especially vulnerable in certain classes of aphasia. This is exclusively a language-based defect, occasioned perhaps by certain characteristics of the color name. 5) Impairment of color imagery probably follows the pattern of visual object agnosia, though correlation with the above categories has not been established.

The impression one gets is of a continuous process from color reception to naming, which may be interrupted at various points. This continuum is similar to that discussed with the object agnosias, where according to the locus of interruption, either the visual or the verbal segment of the process will be the predominant clinical element. The incompatibility of this account with that of the disconnection theorists, in which the distal limbs of the process are implied to be functionally discontinuous should be readily evident. The resistance which such views offer to a more dynamic approach stems largely from the application of unique single case studies to problems which require the integration of cases of wide as well as marginal diversity.

Chapter 25

AUTOTOPAGNOSIA

THIS REFERS TO THE inability of some patients, noted by Pick (1922), to indicate the various parts of their body. Pick's patient, when asked to point to her left ear, searched about on the table and said, "I don't know, I must have lost it." In Pick's cases, diffuse brain disease was ordinarily present, and the disorder was correlated with bilateral parietal lesions. Subsequently, reports seemed to confirm this localization, although occasional cases with left parietal pathology have been reported. Schilder (1932) discussed the problem and accepted a lesion in the inferior parietal lobe.

The disorder appears in naming body parts, indicating them on command, matching body parts to pictures, to the examiner or a doll, and matching from self to examiner or from one side of the body to another. There is commonly some fluctuation in performance, and patients often seem bewildered by their difficulty, with little awareness of the magnitude of impairment. They may deny knowledge of the body part, admit ignorance, mislocate parts, or give bizarre responses. Thus, one case, asked to show his elbow, said "My elbow, an elbow would be over there (pointing to the door)." A moment later, however, he was able to match the body part (elbow) to the correct name. Next asked to point to his forehead, he motioned in the air in front of him saying, "It should be to the right of the door." Asked what he was looking for, he replied, "a forehead." When asked what a forehead was, he said, "I should know that," and apologized for his poor performance. Patients may indicate through their response that they understand the command, as in De Renzi's case who, in connection with the word "wrist," said, "there is the wristwatch," or to "ankle" spoke of his children breaking their ankles, though still unable to point correctly.

Fragments of this disorder are not uncommon in posterior aphasics, particularly verbal confusions of proximal joints, though the bizarre responses of the more typical cases are not seen. More often, the patient is not truly aphasic, though mild anomia and dementia are generally present. Also found are disorientation for right and left, constructional defects, ideational and/or optic apraxia, and disorders of writing and calculation. With regard to the central defect, the difficulty with body parts, patients no longer seem to apprehend their individual semantic properties. This may affect even those divisions of the body which one would expect to be highly resistant, e.g. head, leg. In this respect the disorder compares with ideational apraxia where the object-concept is lost. To what extent these disturbances parallel each other, viz.: in body-part concepts and object-concepts, is not known. The evidence from aphasia suggests that object and body part naming may dissociate, but whether this occurs at the deeper level of ideational apraxia and autotopagnosia is a matter of future investigation.

According to De Renzi and Scotti (1970), autotopagnosia is not restricted to body parts, but may appear on pointing to parts of inanimate objects, e.g. the fender or hood of a car. The authors draw a relation to ideational apraxia, consistent with the above formulation, and suggest the basic defect to be one of analyzing a whole to its parts. In this respect the condition recalls that of "associative visual agnosia" where the reverse situation often occurs, namely the better ability to name parts of an object once the object itself is named.

While bilateral parietal disease is associated with autotopagnosia, unilateral (left) parietal lesions are more closely identified with the Gerstmann syndrome. This disorder (Fingeragnosie) was first described by Gerstmann (1924) in a fifty-two-year-old woman unable to recognize, indicate on command, name or select the separate fingers of her own hands or those of other people. Also demonstrated were right-left disorientation, acalculia and agraphia, a complex of findings which Gerstmann later demonstrated to occur in discrete fashion, and which he correlated with a lesion between angular gyrus and second occipital convolution in the left hemisphere. After his later papers (Gerstmann 1927, 1930), reports appeared by Lange (1930), Schilder (1932) and others, all tending to confirm Gerstmann's description. Most cases had left parieto-occipital lesions, except the ambidextrous patient of Herrmann and Pötzl (1926) with a right parietal tumor. The disorder was generally understood as an impairment of the body scheme, affected in its most highly differentiated part.

Strauss and Werner (1938) extended this interpretation as to be consistent with the finding that the little fingers, which are most highly differentiated, are the most vulnerable. Other theories include Lange's notion of a loss of "direction in space" and of a deautomatization of the transition, in the use of the hand, from personal to extrapersonal space. Stengel (1948) also discussed the factor of spatial disorientation, and Ajuriaguerra and Hecaen (1964) have noted the suggestively high correlation between finger agnosia and constructional apraxia. Regarding the localization, Gerstmann's original finding of lesions in dominant angular gyrus, or between that gyrus and second occipital convolution is most generally accepted.

The work of Benton (1961; see Critchley, 1966) and others, which is critical of localizing attempts, must be interpreted with caution. Their finding that large extraparietal lesions or nonlocalizing decompensations can produce the syndrome does not refute the fact that the syndrome can also occur with relatively small angular gyrus lesions.

The clinical picture is that of finger agnosia in combination with any of three elements, acalculia, agraphia and right-left disorientation. Frequently associated are constructional defects, alexia, apraxic phenomena, color agnosia, hemianopia and pain asymbolia. Apart from the mild anomia, the patient is not aphasic. Though generally not noticed till it is revealed in testing, the difficulty with fingers is the principal defect, and concerns a failure to point to, or present, the individual fingers on command, to name fingers, and to match from hand to hand, from a map to the hand, and vice versa. The defect is constant for both the patient's hands and those of other people, a mannequin, a drawing, or the fingers of a glove, and is present on both verbal and nonverbal testing. Difficulty imitating finger postures may occur, and according to Schilder, impairment of fine finger movement as well, though Schilder believed this to be on a cognitive rather than apraxic basis. The disorder need not involve finger praxis as such, however, for Gerstmann's case could sew and thread a needle, and a patient of Lange could play the piano. Patients should be tested with eyes opened and closed, and mild cases with the so-called Japanese illusion (interwining the fingers and inverting the hands). Partial cases may show preservation of the thumb and little finger, with only the middle fingers involved. Finger agnosia is ordinarily bilateral, rarely if ever unilateral, and may in some cases involve the toes. Right-left disorientation, agraphia and acalculia are the weakest constituents for unlike finger agnosia, these are often early and poorly localizing signs of nonspecific brain damage. The agraphia, however, may be severe and occur in the absence of alexia though it is probably the same as that seen in agraphic alexia. Copying and transliteration are preserved.

DISCUSSION

Our understanding of autotopagnosia, and its partial expression, finger agnosia, are rooted in the concept of the "body-image." While some workers interpret this model quite literally, we understand by it an abstract patterning of information relevant to personal (somatic) and extrapersonal (visual-auditory) space. The body image, therefore, is a system of spatial analysis. Processes referable to this system occur as preparatory levels in movement and perhaps also in language, and as with movement and language, undergo a series of transformations from deep to surface stages. These transformations take the form of a progressive individuation of content, and are directed toward the attainment of levels which are qualitatively unique. A parallel in the microgenetic development of all three systems—the kinesthetic-motor, the acoustic-linguistic and the optic-tactual-spatial can be seen. Accordingly, the *knowledge of the hand is to the body concept as speech is to language competence.*

This view, that the hand is the most highly differentiated body segment, suggests the possibility of planes of involvement. Not only deep (autotopagnosia) and surface (finger agnosia), but intermediate defects should occur. Further, as with prosopagnosia, the defect in finger recognition should prove to be one of specificity, not selectivity, i.e. there should be other category difficulties. For example, testing may disclose impairment in the identification of the teeth (incisors, molars, etc.), the toes, the components of the eye (lids, lashes, eyebrows, iris), etc.

There is no reason to search for subtle bonds between the Gerstmann elements. Even the occurrence of a "developmental Gerstmann's syndrome" does not argue for the functional interrelatedness of the components, for calculation, writing, right-left orientation and finger discrimination are all learned about the same age. In the child, this may simply reflect the disparate effects of a maturation lag. Certainly in the adult, defects in calculation and right-left orientation have, at least at the present stage of knowledge, little or no value in localization. The agraphia appears more closely related to the condition of agraphic alexia (*quod vide*) than to finger agnosia, and is at any rate a symptom common to lesions of wide distribution. It would appear that Gerstmann, in the title of his initial paper—*Fingeragnosie* —defined the principal and, in fact, only characteristic finding in the disorder.

IV. ALEXIA

Chapter 26

AGNOSIC ALEXIA

THE FIRST DESCRIPTION is generally attributed to Kussmaul (1877), who distinguished between verbal and literal alexia, and offered the term word-blindness. Accepted by Wernicke as "subcortical alexia," and presumed secondary to separation of the central terminations of the optic nerve from the visual image center, the syndrome did not receive much attention until the paper of Dejerine in 1892. Dejerine's case, studied over a four-year period until death, was a sixty-eight-year-old man of high intelligence who suddenly developed right hemianopia, complete literal and verbal alexia and inability to read musical notation. His writing, both spontaneous and to dictation, was essentially normal though he was unable to read what he had written. Copying was slow and defective; recognition of objects and numbers was intact. At postmortem, the pertinent lesions were found to involve the lingual and fusiform lobules, the cuneus, and the occipital tip, all on the left side, and the splenium of the corpus callosum. Dejerine's conclusion was that the left occipital lesion, in combination with the splenial lesion interrupting fibers from right to left visual cortex, blocked the passage of written material to the dominant visual word memory center in left angular gyrus. That this center was still intact was shown by the retained ability to write. Accepting this argument in principle, Bastian (1898) commented that the lesion would also have to interrupt callosal fibers from right to left angular gyrus, since the pathway: right visual cortex to right angular gyrus to left angular gyrus, would form a natural bypass around the lesion postulated by Dejerine.

This theory has formed the basis for an important line of alexia study, and as seen in papers by Trescher and Ford (1937), Maspes (1948), Geschwind (1965) and Mouren *et al.* (1967), has proved a fertile and imaginative conception. In its present form, the theory holds that impressions of written material in the undamaged right visual cortex are unable to reach the dominant parietal association cortex via homologous callosal pathways. This results in an interruption of visuoverbal transfer for letters and colors, while numbers and objects, because of their kinesthetic associations, circumvent the posterior callosal lesion. The weakness of the theory is that it does not adequately account for the involvement of musical notation and relative sparing of numbers, since musical reading is learned through instrumentation, and has an equally strong kinesthetic component; the functional differences within alexic categories, with letter sparing and "word-blindness," partial alexia, alexia in only one of two languages, and so on; the lack of permanent alexia with left occipital lobectomy, presumably intercepting terminations of right callosal fibers to left visual association area; and lastly, the fact that qualitatively, the *character of the alexia* is very different in the pure and aphasic forms, a difference hard to explain since lesion of the conducting pathway should not, theoretically, produce an alexia different than lesion of the center to which it leads. Finally, there is another problem which, at the present time, is not yet clearly defined. It appears that the left-visual field alexia of restricted callosal cases, differs from the left-visual field alexia in the patient with callosal *and* left-occipital lesion, the former being more on the order of a paralexia, the latter, a primary visual impairment.

In contrast, however, to the associationist view, a different orientation gradually emerged, developing with the work of von Monakow (1905) and Goldstein (1918). This approach stressed the relation of pure alexia to other forms of visual agnosia, emphasizing the similar patterns of functional deterioration within what was held to be an essentially unitary system. Goldstein, for example, believed that pure alexia was a partial form of visual agnosia, but differing on account of the different functional value (funktionelle Wertigkeit) of the stimulus concerned as well as for localization factors. This formulation was adopted by von Woerkom, and by Bouman and Grunbaum (Bouman, 1928). These authors held that such cases represented a deterioration to an earlier phase of that same process through which the differentiation of isolated forms out of diffuse amorphous organizations comes about. Pick (1931) emphasized that alexia involved a disorder of a specialized function acquired later in life, and therefore, more vulnerable. He noted a systematic deterioration within this function, from mild cases requiring tachystoscopy to demonstrate the defect, to cases with morphological confusions of letters and disturbed spatial orientation, to instances in which not even the patient's name or initials could be recognized. The latter group, he believed, was a stage in transition to the optic agnosias. This early work was discussed by Lange (1936). The argument that alexia is a mild form of agnosia was discredited by cases of severe object agnosia with good reading ability, a fatal criticism to the agnosia concept if validated (however, Lange did not specify the type of agnosia involved in these cases; not unlikely, it concerns the "associative" rather than the "apperceptive" form). Lange noted that the errors seen in alexics were similar to normals on tachystoscopy, thus corroborating Pick's argument, and he anticipated the study of Alajouanine in a discussion of the dissimilarities between the agnosic and aphasic varieties of alexia. More recently, Stengel (1948) has included the disorder with the agnosias, noting in these patients an incomplete comprehension of letter shapes. This view was endorsed to some extent by Martin (1954) who considered pure alexia a part of a larger disturbance in the sphere of spatial apprehension. The major criticisms that might be advanced against this line of reasoning are, firstly, that the conceptualization of alexia as a partial agnosia does not satisfy a need to distinguish more carefully between agnosic forms, and secondly, that there are cases in which letter perception is, on the basis of matching tests and copying, held to be quite adequate. Further, the theory does not explain why numbers are spared.

An extensive contribution to the study of alexia has been made by Alajouanine *et al.* (1960). In the "agnosic" form, the disorder is held to affect early stages in the building up of perceptions outside of the language function, such that perception is aided by reducing the amount of information relevant to the conceptual unit (e.g. a word) to be perceived. Thus, isolated letters are better perceived than strings, and letter perception is easier than word perception, the words generally being constructed analytically through a letter-by-letter process. In addition, morphological disturbances in letter identification are prominent. In contrast to this, in "aphasic" alexia, the isolated unit, the letter, is most affected and reading tends to be global, never relying on literal analysis. The authors conclude that, while the deficits are of a discontinuous type in these two forms, there is no evidence to support the postulation of different functional organizations connected by association tracts.

CLINICAL DESCRIPTION

The onset is often with dizziness and visual symptoms, with right hemianopia an almost constant, though not invariable, finding. Often, there are complaints of visual impairment within the preserved hemifield. Patients may complain that letters move, that they appear to be jumbled, or that familiar writing now seems like a foreign language. Usually anomic aphasia and difficulty in object identification are present in the early stages, and some patients will have disturbances in verbal memory. The disorder is most often due to an occlusion in the posterior cerebral artery.

Reading shows variable impairment. The defect may be mild, with fatigue, slowness and effort in reading, or distaste for reading. Patients may recognize familiar writing, or identify foreign words according to their origin, though they still may be unable to read. Usually, there is a direct relation of the alexia to the quantity and the character of the written material to be perceived. Thus, letters are read better than words, and letters in isolation better than letter strings. There is greater ease for frequently used letters, common letter groupings (e.g. U.S.A.), and letters of simple morphology (I,O). In cases with both literal and verbal alexia, letters are the first to return. Short words are better read than long words, this related to the letter-by-letter construction of the word in the presence of impaired visual span. There are errors secondary to confusion of similar forms (R and K, h, n and r), hemianopic errors (I for K, N for M), mirror errors (d for b), and inversions (M for W). Usually, there is no difference for letters arranged in vertical or horizontal fashion, or large and small letters, though the data of Alajouanine suggests more trouble with the latter. Letters presented obliquely or reversed may not be recognized at all, nor will some patients be able to reposition a letter once dislocated. They may not even note the displacement of letters within a word, to a line above or below. Some patients benefit by having the letter written before them, or moving the paper before their eyes. Tracing the letter is said to help in some instances, though copying ordinarily does not aid in reading. Facilitation by eye movements can probably be discounted. Unblocking techniques (Holmes, 1950; Kreindler and Ionasescu, 1961), which involve matching a test word to one of a group in response to an object or spoken word, have proved useful to facilitate reading in some patients. On all matching tests, whether to objects or spoken samples, the limitation is clearly related to the patient's ability to perceive letters correctly and retain them in order to spell the word. Patients will usually guess at the word, often employing devices of some ingenuity to deal with the various tests. Thus, if given a list of similar written words varying initially (e.g. construction, destruction) or terminally (e.g. promise, promises) the discrimination will depend mainly on a rapid scan of the first or last letter in the word. One can induce errors by substitution within a longer word (e.g. construction, constriction).

Similarly, patients may be able to match printed to written words with less difficulty than matching capital to lower case letters, for in the first instance there is more information on which to base their response. Ordinarily, patients of this type will have no difficulty in distinguishing between grammatical and nongrammatical sentences within a wide range, once it is established that the text has been adequately read. Similarly, these patients can perceive semantic boundaries between words presented unspaced in a sentence, their only difficulty resulting from misreading a letter and as a result going astray.

One should also test these patients with different scripts and languages. Written letters should be bidirectionally matched to other written letters, to spoken and anagram letters, and to letters written on the hand. Similar tests should be done at the word level if possible. Defects in oculomotor scanning should be noted (Poppelreuter, 1917; Warrington and Zangwill, 1957). Impairment in the perception of punctuation marks, and other signs, such as formulae, as well as in the ability to use punctuation have been described. Variability of alexia in different languages has been reported, a finding of great theoretical import. Hinshelwood (1917) described a case in which there was a gradation in the degree of alexia in four languages, being greatest in English, less in French, and least in Latin, with complete sparing of Greek, the order of loss being the opposite of that expected according to the patient's language facility. This raises the possibility that over-learned languages are more severely affected than under-learned ones, a condition the reverse of that in aphasia, and also points to the importance of educational background in determining symptomatology, a relationship first mentioned by Wernicke. Lastly, it is reported, though not without disagreement, that alexia in Japanese bilinguals may affect the syllabic Kana script preferentially, and spare the Chinese-derived ideogrammatic form.

Arabic numbers are often preserved, and at times patients will read on up into the millions, though Roman figures do not always show this degree of sparing. Explanations for this sparing of numbers include their simplified phonemic character, the smaller number vocabulary as compared to letters, and the fact that number reading is highly overlearned. This latter reason can probably be discounted in view of the above discussion on multilingual alexia. The notion that counting on the fingers establishes kinesthetic associations which allow for rerouting of number reading is untenable. Another possibility to be considered has to do with the highly spatial arrangement of numerical reading and, for that matter, numerical thought, in contrast to the linearity of words and musical notation. It is possible that the spatial capacity of minor hemisphere confers a slight advantage on number reading. Finally, numbers are read in such a way that there is constant movement toward the right side, whereas letters must coalesce into a simultaneous whole, a word. Some patients with difficulty in number reading will also have trouble in telling the time. Calculations may or may not be affected. Musical notation is often impaired, though not necessarily, and at least in one case (Proust, see Kussmaul, 1877) was disturbed selectively. Defects in color identification (*quod vide*) are common.

Spelling and spelling comprehension may be quite normal. Identification of letters or words written on the hands may also be spared.

Writing should be normal or nearly so for the diagnosis. Usually, subtle defects are present, e.g. letters are too large or too widely-spaced, there may be absence or misuse of punctuation, capitals may be disregarded, letters dropped or reduplicated. Alajouanine notes that the line is often irregular with a tendency to slope off to the right, and remarks on the similarity of writing to that of right parietal patients with constructional apraxia. Writing to dictation is as above; copying is usually poor, and at times impossible, though some patients may copy accurately and in a slow servile fashion. Ordinarily there is no difference with eyes open or closed, though in patients with simultanagnosia, it is my impression, in contradiction to an impression in the literature, that writing deteriorates on closing the eyes. The ability to copy in itself does not establish adequate perceptions, and must be augmented by such procedures as matching identical letters and words, or showing the patient a letter (e.g. A) and asking him to point to all of the A's in a paragraph. Transliteration is usually impossible in the absence of word comprehension. It is of interest that copying of geometrical figures is often better than letters, a fact not readily explained. Some patients may even show better ability to copy inverted or disguised letters, than letters presented normally. Foreign or nonsense words may be better copied than familiar words. One factor in copying which has to be taken into account is the secondary impairment that occurs when attempts to decipher a word interfere with rote copying.

Chapter 27

AGRAPHIC ALEXIA

THOUGH IT IS THE MOST meticulously described of the many clinical varieties of reading disturbance, agnosic alexia is perhaps of the least importance to aphasia theory. The more common type, *agraphic alexia* (angular gyrus alexia) was described by Dejerine (1891) in a patient with minimal aphasia but severe alexia and agraphia, and at postmortem, a lesion confined to angular gyrus. Since Dejerine's paper, the localization has been repeatedly confirmed. There is less agreement, however, on the clinical picture. Some authors emphasize the equal severity of reading words, letters and numbers, while others, such as Alajouanine *et al.* (1960), stress the relatively severe impairment of letters. In this work, however, the defect in letter identification is not clearly distinguished from the anomia by which it is often accompanied. This is of some importance, for anomics find letters particularly difficult items to name. Hecaen (1967) stressed the sparing of letter recognition over words, while Weigl and Bierwisch (1969) have noted a greater difficulty for abstract nouns, and for nouns and verbs with prefixes. According to Alajouanine, reading has a global character, without facilitation by literal analysis or letter tracing. Paralexia is present in reading aloud, especially for letters. These features distinguish this disorder from agnosic alexia, where the literal defect is the end-stage of the pathology.

Careful study of these patients fully confirms the findings of Alajouanine and his co-workers. Except in the severe case where nothing can be read at all, the dissociation between letters and words is quite striking. On reading aloud, simple words may be pronounced accurately, or paralexically (e.g. "plane" for aircraft), but rarely with phonemic distortion. Context clearly aids word recognition, and often a phrase in which a word is embedded will aid in its identification. This is particularly true for grammatical words which are very difficult in isolation. In contrast to this global reading, letters are often all but impossible. This is true even when the word incorporates a letter name. Thus, words such as: you, pea, and bee may be read well, while the letters: U, P and B are failed. Not only are letters mis-named, but patients cannot indicate or sort letters accurately to com-mand, unless first given a visual model of the letter tested, nor can they select the correct letter name from a spoken group. Matching identical or transliterated letters is often possible, and letters can be distinguished from nonsense figures. Patients will also usually recognize letters reversed or deleted in words. Series speech is or-dinarily used to aid in evoking the desired letter name, so that initial alphabet letters present the least difficulty. Capitals may be easier than cursives, and there is no improvement with the letter written before the patient's eyes. Patients are unable to match spoken letter sounds to written letters. This difficulty with letters extends also to phonetic reading. Thus, a patient able to read the word broom, or spool, may not be able to pronounce the neologism brool; or syllabic groupings will not be pronounced independent of containing words. Thus, the word *baker* may be read without hesitation, while the syllables *ba* and *ker,* spaced somewhat apart cannot be read at all. Similarly, small grammatical words present more difficulty than longer substantives. There is no clear difference for various categories of grammatical words, or for abstract or concrete nouns, though picturable nouns may prove easier.

The tendency for global reading may extend to letter groupings within the word, and lead to erroneous guesses such as "had" for chair, based on incomplete sampling. Hecaen (1967) has also noted this, and speaks of a loss of "perceptual strategy for reading." Thus, a patient of his read *chemin* as "minus," or *Le Figaro* as, successively, "ga," "le" and "o." In such cases, reading does not proceed normally from left to right, but rather, pieces of the word become the starting points of a paralexic guess. Further, reading does not always respect spaces between words, nor, in phrases in which these spaces are deleted, can the patient separate the individual words. All of this speaks for a failure to clearly identify the constituents of a word as specific formative units. In contrast to agnosic alexia, patients depend less on analysis than on a global impression of the letters before them.

In severe cases, even the recognition of English words among a set of foreign words may be impossible. In milder cases, where words are read accurately or with paralexia, matching is usually fairly good to spoken and written words, and to objects. If similar spellings are used (e.g. htread, thread, thraed, thered) or similar oral choices given (e.g. table, cable, bible, etc.) confusion will occur. Numbers are usually read better than letters, and are matched well to spoken

numbers, though difficulties will appear beyond two or three digits.
There is no striking difference between Roman and Arabic numerals.
An accompanying acalculia is common.

Much of the difficulty appears to rest with the spelling impairment.
There is inability to spell all but the simplest words, either to command or to a presented object. Spelling comprehension is but slightly
better, both orally and on matching to objects. Nevertheless, patients
can often distinguish correct from incorrect spellings of written words
which they cannot otherwise spell. There may be inability to give
the first or last letter of a simple word, accept the correct letter from
a spoken group, give the sound of a letter named, or the reverse,
give the letter of a sound offered by the examiner. Though word-lists
may otherwise be intact, patients may be unable to give a single word
beginning with a designated letter. It is important on all tests of
spelling to ascertain that digit span is not excessively impaired.
Dermographic reading will show similar impairments, usually worse
for letters than numbers. In recovered cases where the reading of
sentences is possible, difficulty appears with plurals, possessives, pronouns and tenses. There is particular trouble with Wh-type sentences.
Written commands may be understood and carried out. On phrase-
choice tests, semantic confusions are very rare, in contrast to the above
categories. If one reads the patient a simple sentence, such as "How
are you?", asking him to say what sort of punctuation is required,
or to select the appropriate mark from an oral or written group, only
periods and commas are done with reasonable consistency. Writing
is variable, but always impaired. Usually, only the patient's name and
at best a few simple words can be written. The agraphia reflects the
spelling deficiency, as well as, in severe cases, the loss of conceptualization of words as whole units. Apraxic contamination in writing should
be noted, and is a sign of wider pathology. Contrary to the view of
Benson and Geschwind (1969), there does not appear to be a definite
correspondence between writing and reading, though as mentioned
the spelling defect certainly tends to impose limitations on each.
Thus, patients cannot even write a dash for each letter in a simple
word, a performance which can be accomplished only if the word is
spelled aloud by the examiner. Patients can often write most letters
in the alphabet, numbers from 1–10, as well as many isolated letters
and digits to dictation. Copying is good, and transliteration is possible
only where letter recognition is intact. In cases where letters but no
words are recognized, there is great facility with letter-by-letter copying, in contrast to the slow, slavish style of agnosic alexics. This indi-

cates that in the latter, it is not just the failure to recognize the word
that impedes copying.

Within the category of agraphic alexia, there is a transition from
a stage where some letters, but no words, are recognized, to a stage
where words are read globally, accurately or with paralexia, with
difficulty in letter naming. This latter coincides with the presence of
anomia, which probably is responsible for both the paralexia and
defective letter reading. Further, a transition can be seen from this
stage to the alexia of Broca's aphasia. Here, letters also are more
poorly read than words, but matching and sorting tests establish that
the letter name is known. This is similar to other facets of the
posterior-anterior change in word-finding, suggesting that in angular
gyrus alexia, letter names are more or less unavailable to many different kinds of testing, whereas in the alexia of Broca's aphasia, the
letter name is generally available, but the patient's hold on it is
tenuous, and it can be pronounced only with difficulty. In the
agraphic alexic with poor word, but good letter reading, the question
arises of a relation to agnosic alexia. One may express the difference
in these terms. In the latter, letters are recognized and are built up
into words. In the former, though letters are recognized, the word is
not familiar. There is an inability to combine the letters into a
meaningful whole, a word. In the one case we are dealing with a
"sensory" defect, in which the linguistic system upon which the recognition of words as semantic entities depends is intact, whereas in
the other, perception of letter and word is normal, or nearly so,
though written words do not appear to make any sense. A final comment on agraphic alexia concerns the absence of hemianopia, which
serves to further distinguish this form from agnosic alexia. When
hemianopia occurs, it is a sign of posterior extension or subcortical
penetration with involvement of optic radiations.

Hecaen (1967) has described a form of literal alexia with ability
to read some words. Here, the capacity to read is better for substantives, particularly picturable nouns, and deteriorates dramatically
with functional words and neologisms. The paralexia takes the form
of a misreading in the semantic field of the given word. Words are
read through recognition of the general meaning of the word rather
than its specific lexical value. One of Hecaen's patients read the word
Italy as "republic," and *republic* as "Italy." A patient of Beringer
and Stein (1930) is mentioned who read *India* as "elephant." Benson
and Geschwind *et al.* (1969) describe a patient who read the word
living-room as "the place we go after dinner to watch T.V." Weigl

and Bierwisch (1969) describe a patient with this disorder, who made repeated errors of the type "trousers" for *blouse,* "sandals" for *socks,* and so on. In my experience, the syndrome has always accompanied "agraphic alexia," and is a part of the global reading present in such patients. One case, for example, read the word *zebra* as "giraffe," *hound* as "dog," *play* as "ball." He was able to match single words to pictures representing the semantic class of words which he otherwise could not pronounce. In addition to the paralexia, he produced periphrasic accountings of the word to be read which resembled his performance on naming tasks.

Semantic paralexia has also been studied by Marshall and Newcombe (1966). In their case, this occurred against a background of verbal paraphasia in object naming, and paragraphia in writing to dictation, though reading errors were the more prominent symptom. These errors, which occurred especially on reading nouns, were generally synonymic and of the type: "vase" for *antique,* "parrot" for *canary,* and "sick" for *ill.* Occasional completions, e.g. "gentleman" for *gentle,* and visual errors, "exit" for *next,* were also seen, the latter predominantly for adjectives and verbs. The symptom of semantic paralexia, the authors persuasively argue, suggests that in reading aloud the full dictionary entry of the word must be retrieved and encoded into the appropriate phonological form. Semantic paralexia points to a breakdown in the encoding process at a generic level, i.e. at the level of "distinguisher" or semantic markers.

The phenomenon may also be related to the ability of right hemisphere to extract information from the written message in an otherwise global alexic. Certainly, this is consistent with the performance of callosal patients, as well as with the occurrence of similar errors in normal and dyslexic children. The fact that it does not occur in agnosic alexia could be attributed to the impairment of right visual cortex which occurs as a consequence of left occipital and callosal lesion. In this connection, the incidence of left-handedness or ambidexterity in a personal series of such patients appears to be quite high. There may also be a relation to the degree of language proficiency prior to injury. Another consideration concerns the relation of the paralexia to the word-finding defect. The paralexia is similar to paraphasic misnaming in sphere, e.g. "comb" for *brush,* or circumlocutory descriptions, e.g. "the place where the Vatican is" for *Rome,* both common productions of anomic patients. The greater severity in reading aloud than in naming may relate to the inequality of "perceptual challenge" in the two conditions. There is also a similarity, at least in theory, to conduction aphasia that might be pointed out. In the one, there is paraphasia in spite of cueing with the written word, in the other, paraphasia with a verbal cue. The semantic paraphasia of the one and phonemic paraphasia of the other, are reflections of the stage involved, not of unique mechanisms. A further parallel to conduction aphasia lies in the general relationship of the latter to the anomias (*quod vide*) and the occasional verbal paraphasias which occur, as in the patient of Henneberg who repeated "telescope" for *microscope,* or "Xenophon" for *Hercules* (see also Isserlin, 1936). Finally, individuals who are not taught to read very fast premorbidly, may perhaps be more likely to show this kind of paralexia. Such manner of reading (i.e. globally) is, of course, the normal method of deaf-mutes, who learn to read without benefit of phonetic analysis.

Chapter 28

APHASIC ALEXIA

A LEXIA MAY ALSO OCCUR in Wernicke's aphasia (aphasic alexia) where it appears to be related to a lesion of posterior T1. The original explanation by Wernicke was that reading was acquired as an association to learned word sounds, and therefore was dependent on the stability of sound images. In highly educated sensory aphasics, this dependence is not as great and reading may be spared. The localization has been more or less confirmed by Nielsen (1939) who noted that the alexia underwent a change from a semantic to an aphasic to an agnosic form, according to whether the lesion involved T1, angular gyrus or left occipital lobe with splenium. Luria (1966) recognizes the form as occurring with lesions of T1. He notes that in severe cases, words appear as noise with only fragments of the material understood. In less severe cases, patients grasp individual words and understand their meaning, though there is difficulty in phonetic analysis. According to Hecaen (1967), the disorder in reading is parallel to that in spoken language. Letters and numbers are read better than words, the latter with paralexia. A severely paralexic reading impairs comprehension. The disorder is mild with lesions limited to temporal lobe, becoming more severe as the lesion extends posteriorly.

Though this form has not been as clearly delineated as could be wished, it does appear to differ from "agraphic alexia" in some respects other than severity or the addition of an aphasia. Patients are often able to read aloud quite well, though paralexic errors similar to those in speech are apparent. The paralexia is increased by word length and unfamiliarity, and bears no constant relation to reading comprehension. There is no dissociation between reading words and letters, as in other forms of alexia. In patients with the capacity to understand single spoken words, matching of written to spoken words will be fairly good, with difficulty relating to the length of the spoken and written word. Matching words to objects, matching written to spoken, and print to cursive letters and numbers is good. With regard to reading comprehension, patients will often perform better on simple written commands than on multiple choice sentence completions. On written commands, words read paraphasically may lead to a correct performance, while an incorrect response or complete failure may as well accompany a correct reading. Patients will also be able to separate words juxtaposed in a sentence, in contrast to the agraphic alexic, though they may be unable to read the words aloud. In mild cases with speech imperception and verbal paraphasia, the reading comprehension deficit may be quite minimal. There may be very little in the way of grammatical confusion or difficulty with plural and possessive forms, which is characteristic of most, if not all, other aphasic disorders. Spelling and comprehension of words spelled is usually impossible, though patients can often distinguish correct from incorrect written spellings. Writing, both spontaneous and to dictation, is paragraphic, though letters are usually formed well. Writing will present spelling errors similar to those seen in tests of spelling ability. Patients with severe spelling difficulty may pronounce words they are unable to write, and will not be helped by letter cueing. One patient, for example, on being shown a spoon and asked to write its name, was not able to produce anything at all. Giving the word spoon at the same time did not help, nor even after he was given the letters SPOO could he supply the final letter. This contrasted with his excellent ability to match the written word to orally given words and objects. Such cases indicate that, while the agnosic alexic with good spelling reads through literal analysis, the severe aphasic alexic with poor spelling may, if the word is not produced spontaneously, be forced to write through a kind of literal synthesis in which the spelling defect is the limiting factor. Copying is often quite good, and usually transliteration of lower case letters to capitals, or of unfamiliar and nonsense words is possible. This is not uniformly true, however, for at times transliteration of words which are not understood or read by the patient is totally lost. The situation then is opposite to that seen in normal subjects where words which cannot be read can easily be transliterated.

As mentioned, some cases show a clear dissociation between reading aloud and reading comprehension. Nielsen (1939) discussed one form of this dissociation as "word meaning blindness," emphasizing that reading was possible but without comprehension of what was read. In most patients, however, the reverse is usually seen, paraphasia in reading aloud with variable preservation of reading comprehension.

The description by Nielsen of reading aloud without comprehension brings us to the disorder of so-called *transcortical alexia*. This condition was first described by Dejerine (1880) in a patient able to read aloud and write to dictation, but unable to understand what she had read or written. Autopsy revealed a large glioma of inferior parietal lobule. Little was written about the disorder subsequent to Dejerine's paper, and one has the impression that it may have become confused with cases of alexia with good copying, also termed trans-cortical alexia by some authors. Symonds (1953) discussed the entity and suggested that it must coexist with word deafness or the patient would understand words as he read them aloud. Certainly this explanation seems a little artificial, and since the alexic cannot read aloud, and the word deaf are able to read aloud with understanding, it is hard to imagine what combination of defects Symonds had in mind. In my experience, the disorder has been accompanied by defects in speech comprehension as well as paraphasia, i.e. as a component of a Wernicke's aphasia. It affects those patients who improve to the point where reading aloud is no longer paraphasic, while expressive speech still is. Further, silent reading comprehension may, in fact, be possible if careful testing is done.

There appear to be two possible explanations for the condition. It can perhaps be accounted for by the fact that reading aloud requires the utilization, in the Wernicke aphasic, of an expressive speech system for which awareness is minimal. Thus, the patient is as little aware of what he reads aloud as of his spontaneous speech. This has the interesting implication that the Wernicke aphasic is unaware not only of his erroneous speech, but of his appropriate speech as well. A second possibility concerns the fact that ability to read aloud is, in normals, superior to reading comprehension to begin with. Thus, we all can read sentences which we do not understand, as well as foreign languages where even the function words are not recognized. Perhaps a general deterioration within the system responsible for reading could account for a lowered level of performance with maintenance of the functional imbalance between reading aloud and reading comprehension.

Chapter 29

ALEXIA IN BROCA'S APHASIA

SOME AUTHORS HAVE described alexia in Broca's aphasia. Nielsen (1939) discussed this problem and concluded that reading difficulty does occur in motor aphasics, probably because the patients concerned used, or thought of, lip movements to aid in reading comprehension. Luria (1966) has noted in such patients a failure to distinguish the separate sounds making up a word, especially the vowel sounds. He also noted the pathological inertia which affects reading performance. Some support was given to Nielsen's conclusion by the finding that having the patient hold his tongue between his teeth may accentuate the reading defect.

If one examines Broca's aphasics of mild to moderate severity, the following defects are evident. Reading aloud usually exhibits the same paralexic and agrammatic disturbances as does speech in conversation, often with a striking dissociation between ability to read whole words, which may be quite good, and inability to read letters. Numbers are read better than letters, through use of a motor series to aid in expression. Patients who have automatic use of the alphabet will do better, though even these patients will show difficulty with initial letters which fall within the compass of the series ability. There are phonemic substitutions in reading words, increased by unfamiliarity and word length, and letter substitution in reading letters. There is difficulty in reading unknown or nonsense words, for the patient is unable to construct the word phonetically, a deficiency in contrast to the agnosic alexic who reads precisely in this way (Benson *et al.*, 1971). This dissociation between literal or syllabic reading and the reading of words is not related to articulatory demand, for patients will readily read words which constitute letter sounds, e.g. pea, though unable to read the letter "p." Conversely, letters will at times be read as words, as in "zero" for z, "two" for t, "no" for n.

Though noted occasionally in the earlier literature, this finding of "letter blindness without word blindness" was first documented by Hinshelwood (1900). In his cases, however, patients were generally unable to point to letters on command, a finding not borne out in the majority of anterior aphasic patients. Most patients can match letters, point with fair success to letters on command, sort letters, identify the loci of misarranged or deleted letters, select correct letter names from a group, and so on, suggesting that the perception and identification of the letter is not at fault. Sabouraud *et al.* (1963) have also observed this phenomenon in their study of Broca's aphasics, emphasizing the difficulty in phonetic reading. Thus, their patients could read "lit" but not "li," or "fermez les yeux" but not "fermelezieu." Although a satisfactory explanation is not yet forthcoming, this dissociation of literal and phonetic reading from the reading of verbal ideograms may well account, at least in part, for the agrammatic character of reading aloud.

As in aphasic alexia, there is no clear relation between reading aloud and reading comprehension, for words are understood which cannot be pronounced, and a paralexic reading does not necessarily interfere with word comprehension. The difficulty with letter reading secondarily affects oral spelling, which is usually severely limited. Comprehension of spelled words is only slightly better, but patients will often be able to distinguish between correct and incorrect written spellings. Performance on sentence completion tests will not clearly mirror sentence comprehension since other factors are involved, and one can often obtain surer information by listening to the patient's own labored account of the material, or through yes/no responses to verbally given multiple choices. Written commands may be carried out quite well, though apraxia may intervene.

Finally, there are a number of reading errors prominent in Broca's aphasics, which seem to occur to some extent in all aphasic patients. There may be inability to add punctuation to a simple written sentence, or determine, in a set of two sentences, which is the correct punctuation. Inability to distinguish between two sentences of similar grammatical form may occur, as in sentences where the only difference is the presence or absence of a plural or a possessive "s," or an "s" in contraction form. Thus, sentences of the type: "That is my brother's dog," "That bike is the boy's," "Two boys are here," and "This boy's very good," are not consistently differentiated from a pair in which the "s" is deleted. The plural "s" returns first, possibly more readily in sentences where an "es" plural is involved (i.e. watches versus boys). When given a choice between the (correct) contracted and (incorrect) plural form, as in "That boy's afraid . . ." versus "Those boys afraid . . . ," the response will favor the plural form first in the more severe case, and only later, when the plural is secure enough to be seen as incorrect, will the patient select or guess at the contracted form. In contrast to these disorders, patients can usually select the correct form of the verb, and are sensitive to substitution of key nouns.

Chapter 30

DISCUSSION

A S IN THE DISCUSSION of visual agnosia, two stages are distinguished in the alexias, one in which the received signal undergoes a process of feature-extraction, and construction, and a second stage in which this structural complex, in relation to memory, passes into perceptual awareness. Disorders of the first stage (agnosic alexia) are characterized by the following features: the defect is proportional to the amount of data to be processed, particularly if the data is visually complex; distortions in the signal occurring at various phases of its specification will produce responses indicative of abnormal morphological configurations in perception; and the process whereby words and images are evoked by the distorted signal will be incomplete or faulty. Such a formulation is consistent with the clinical picture of agnosic alexia. The preference of letters over words, and short words over longer words apart from word meaning, the morphological confusions, and the verbal errors which reflect these confusions, all support this account. Further, the fact that the responses of normal subjects during tachystoscopy resemble those of alexics under normal conditions, that alexic patients have their disorders magnified by tachystoscopic presentation, and that severe agnosic alexics may show prolonged tachystoscopic latencies for object identification (Tomlinson, 1970, personal communication) as well as the additional clinical observation that most patients with agnosic alexia show difficulties in object identification early in their course, all tend to bring this disorder into line with the visual agnosias. It is possible, therefore, to support the views of earlier writers that agnosic alexia is the subtlest form of apperceptive agnosia. The possible objection that the disorder is restricted to left visual field is countered by the fact that the right visual cortex is probably less specialized for written information than the left. Whereas in the presence of an intact splenium the right visual cortex may serve well enough for reading, the addition of a splenial lesion makes this impossible. The suggestion is that splenium concerns rather a modulatory than a transfer capability. It is of interest that Gazzaniga and Sperry (1967), in studying reading in the left visual field of two patients with callosal section were able to demonstrate simple word-object matching in the face of loss of verbalization of words seen. While their findings are difficult to evaluate in view of the age of one case (12 years) and the IQ of the other (70–80), there is no argument with their conclusion, that ". . . the functional capacity of a unilateral cortical area with its contralateral counterpart intact may appear to be quite different from that seen in the presence of contralateral lesions." If this is the case, as seems so from the clinical material, a reinterpretation of the role of callosal function in this disorder is required. Through the postulation of a functional deterioration within right visual cortex, one can better account for the selective nature and wide range of clinical reading disturbance, from the patient for whom reading is possible but no longer pleasant, to one who can no longer read at all. It follows from this that severe alexics should have some difficulty in object identification, while those few cases of object agnosia with good reading should immediately become suspect. Certainly, of three patients personally seen with apperceptive visual agnosia none could read, and in a few patients with recovering cortical blindness, the capacity to read was not strikingly dissociated from the return of object recognition. If in some cases, reading letters does return first, it can no doubt be owed to the simpler geometric configuration of some letters (e.g. I, O) as compared to complex forms. But letters are also fairly well preserved in most patients with agnosic alexia, who read through literal analysis. In conclusion, therefore, the so-called pure alexia is an apperceptive agnosia of mild degree, affecting written material preferentially. The defect is in the order of a distortion of fine shape specification, and of the perception of complex shapes, i.e. words, as units. More severe damage within this system results in apperceptive object agnosia. Here the distortion is severe enough to obscure simple objects. In some cases, the acute stage is characterized by an accompanying optic aphasia, i.e. particular difficulty in the visual naming of objects, but this is only a mild form of visual agnosia.

Disorders of the second stage have in common the fact that reading breakdown relates to interruption within an hierarchical language-based system, and therefore, has direct affinities with the different forms of aphasia. Three separate reading defects, accompanying each of the major aphasic categories, have been distinguished, viz.: 1) agraphic alexia, with lesion in angular gyrus, usually associated with an anomia; 2) aphasic alexia, or the alexia of Wernicke's aphasia, with lesion in posterior T1; and 3) the alexia of Broca's aphasia, with lesion in or around Broca's area. These disorders can be characterized as follows:

1. In agraphic alexia there is a severe loss of reading comprehension, expressed equally in reading aloud. What reading remains is dependent upon, and facilitated by, global impressions. Words may be read only if part of a sentence, while letters, particularly in the presence of an anomia, present great difficulty unless combined into words. Spelling and writing are all but impossible.

2. In aphasic alexia, reading comprehension is often better than reading aloud, the latter often being severely paralexic and comparable to the paraphasia in speech. Comprehension appears to center mainly on the word which is the more resistant element, in contrast to agraphic alexia where words are facilitated through embedding in a phrase. The difference between letters and words is not striking.

3. The alexia of Broca's aphasia is not so much a disorder of reading comprehension as a defect in the evocation and pronunciation of letters, syllables and small grammatical words. This leads to agrammatism on reading aloud, with marked dissociation in reading words and letters. There is a similarity between the global reading of this form and the alexia of angular gyrus lesion in a stage of recovery. In the latter, however, letters are not readily identified, while words can still be read, whereas in the former, letters which are recognized (i.e. matched, sorted and selected to command) are not pronounced.

While this description of second stage reading defects is only preliminary, some relationships can be seen among the different forms. The global reading which characterizes agraphic alexia reappears in mitigated fashion in the alexia of Broca's aphasia. In both, there is a loss of phonetic reading with marked impairment in the naming of letters and the reading of small grammatical words, differing only in that Broca's alexics can still identify letters which cannot be pronounced. The similarity is further emphasized by the occurrence in both disorders, though more dramatically in agraphic alexia, of verbal paralexias within sphere. We are reminded of the situation in anomic and Broca's aphasia where a similar picture can result from quite different disturbances.

V. SUMMARY

Chapter 31

CONCLUSIONS

I T IS APPROPRIATE in the closing pages of this monograph to review briefly the major points of the preceding discussion. Our point of departure from more traditional formulations has been in the conceptualization of psychopathological disorders in terms of breakdown in hierarchic systems. Aphasia is a result of a disturbance within the linguistic phase of this hierarchy, although analogous patterns of breakdown occur within all of the functional systems discussed, e.g. language, praxis and perception. The various clinical forms of aphasia, therefore, relate to stages in normal speech production, and can be classified according to their sequence in this process.

From this point of view, a transition has been described from anomia to a group of inter-related disorders tentatively categorized as semantic aphasia. These are, in turn, preliminary to the Wernicke's aphasia complex, including transcortical sensory aphasia. In these syndromes, attuned as they are to the speech perceptive system, the disorder in expressive language has an inner bond with the impairment in speech comprehension. Both expression and comprehension undergo deterioration and recovery in molar fashion. From anomia and Wernicke's aphasia, there is a link to conduction aphasia, and from there to Broca's aphasia. The transitions appear to be as follows:

1. Within the anomias, at least two different forms can be distinguished, reflecting impairment at different levels in the sequence of word-finding. At the earliest stage, that which corresponds to the abstract store of the vocabulary item, impairment results in amnestic aphasia, *sensu stricto,* i.e. a patient who neither names objects, nor gives circumlocutions, and fails to select the correct word when offered in a group. Moreover, the patient often admits that he does not know the correct word. This form, recognized by most workers, has been correlated with lesions in the posterior portion of the middle temporal gyrus.

If the word is available, but the mechanism of its entry into the language process is impaired, the result is classical amnestic aphasia or anomia. In the mild form, there is a difficulty in evoking the correct word, which is replaced by circumlocutions and functional descriptions. The patient accepts the correct word from a group, and more often than not, behaves in such a way to suggest that at least a skeleton of the word is available.

The next stage in anomia concerns the patient who produces paraphasic misnamings. In such a case, verbal paraphasias are generally within category, as "bed" for pillow, and the patient generally self-corrects and continues to attempt to produce the precise word. The important point about this stage is that the word, or some abstract representation of the word, is available mentally and paraphasic approximations to it are recognized by the patient as imprecise.

2. From the latter form of anomia there is a transition to a stage of relatively intact lexical entry, in which the misnaming is not clearly recognized as such by the patient. That is, the patient produces a verbal paraphasia which, though tangentially related to the demanded word, is not recognized as only an approximation. The improved lexical entry is at the expense of semantic control. One variety of this disturbance is the syndrome of non-aphasic misnaming. The impairment here is largely in the sphere of referential speech.

Corresponding to non-aphasic misnaming, the syndrome of semantic aphasia derives from a comparable disorder manifested largely in expositional speech. However, in this disorder there is relative sparing of referential speech or naming. Whereas in non-aphasic misnaming, the patient might call a doctor a "butcher," identifying two disparate subjects on the basis of a shared attribute, in semantic aphasia, the defect is extended to contextual relationships (see Chap. 3). Similar errors also occur in the language of the Korsakoff state, particularly in the acute confusional prelude and in schizophrenia.

3. From these forms, there is a transition to semantic jargon. Here, the verbal paraphasia is so remote in meaning from the target word that its relationship is difficult to perceive. This is the patient who defines a spoon as, "How many schemes on your throat." According to most workers, the syndrome is a reflection of a "loss of the semantic values" of language. Thus, the condition, which began with difficulty in naming with verbal paraphasia and intact semantic control, leads finally to semantic jargon with intact lexical entry and a disruption in the semantic control of language.

4. Whereas one limb of the aphasia process extends from anomia to the semantic jargon form of Wernicke's aphasia, a second limb extends from anomia through conduction aphasia. This is clear if one considers the act of repetition, which is central to conduction aphasia.

In such patients, there is fluent and relatively intelligible speech with prominent literal paraphasia, mild deficits in speech comprehension, and impaired naming and repetition. The repetition disorder is *always* in proportion to the deficit in naming, both showing primarily literal or phonemic paraphasia. In conduction aphasia, the word has "come up" sufficiently far to the level of literal rather than verbal paraphasia. This accounts for the different speech form of the anomic and the conduction aphasic. The problem of the repetition disorder becomes clear if we consider the following example. If one asks an anomic to name an ashtray, the word is not produced but can be repeated. In the regression of the anomia, the patient first fails to cue when the examiner says "ash . . ." but repeats the word "ashtray" when offered. At a later stage, he may still fail on a long phonemic cue, such as "ashtr . . ." in which all but the final syllable of the word is given, but will still repeat the word "ashtray" when given. Ultimately, a stage is reached in which the patient neither cues nor repeats. At this point, the patient is a conduction aphasic. One observes that in this example the repetition disorder is nothing more than a failure to name, given the whole word as a cue. The transition from the anomic who fails with a cue to the penultimate syllable, and the conduction aphasic who fails given a cue including the final syllable, establishes the functional continuity between these two disorders.

5. If the picture of conduction aphasia with phonemic paraphasia is combined with that of semantic jargon, the outcome is jargon characterized by neologisms. This is confirmed by the fact that neologistic jargon improves either to conduction aphasia or Wernicke's aphasia. It has been suggested that neologistic jargon is simply phonemic paraphasia of such severity that words are no longer recognizable. This assumes that the underlying word-frame is normal. If this were the case, however, one could not account for the improvement of neologistic jargon into the semantic paraphasia of Wernicke's aphasia. It seems, therefore, that neologistic jargon must be phonemic paraphasia superimposed upon semantic paraphasia, such that the clearing of the former leads to Wernicke's aphasia (semantic paraphasia), clearing of the latter to conduction aphasia (phonemic paraphasia).

In the transition of neologistic jargon to conduction aphasia, one encounters patients quite frequently with the picture of fair comprehension, mild to moderately impaired repetition and naming, with phonemic paraphasia and many neologisms in speech. In such cases, naming and repetition may be of such quality as to exclude conduction aphasia. However, the occurrence of frequent neologisms in speech, in the presence of self-correction, is the hallmark of the transitional form.

6. The nature of the transition to Broca's aphasia is by no means clear. In conduction aphasia, all parts of speech are affected, though the small function or grammatical words may be impaired to a greater extent than substantive or content words. This suggests a relationship with agrammatism, in which the small words are lost preferentially. However, the relationship of Broca's aphasia to posterior aphasia can best be studied through a comparison with parietal anomia. In the latter condition, there is a progressive loss of nouns, verbs, and in severe cases, grammatical words. In some patients, this may reach a stage of non-fluency. In Broca's aphasia, the loss of words is in the exact reverse order, such that small words are lost first (agrammatism), followed by verbs, (stage of the "one-word utterance"), and finally, nouns are lost, such that the patient may have no speech save for a stereotypy. This reciprocity of loss is quite striking. One explanation would derive from a noun priority in the process of lexical entry, i.e. as the first to be incorporated into the sentence pattern, the nouns are therefore more vulnerable. In Broca's aphasia, the nouns have "come up" farther and are, therefore, more resistant. The small grammatical words, particularly the articles and inflections which are the last to be added to the sentence pattern, are the most sensitive in Broca's aphasia.

With regard to phonemic jargon, this form appears to be related to the phonemic jargon stereotypies which occasionally characterize Broca's aphasia. The factor of fluency in such patients can be resolved by the observation that Broca's aphasics are also fluent *within the confines of the stereotypy.*

7. The language process can be conceived as radiating in two primary directions, one culminating in articulation, the other, speech comprehension. With impairment at the most distal levels of this process, the result is either aphemia or anarthria on the one hand, or word-deafness on the other.

In a similar fashion, the apraxias and agnosias are considered as interruptions at successive stages in the emergence of voluntary movement and perception. With regard to apraxia, syndromes comparable to the aphasias can be correlated with pathology over the posterior-anterior axis of the brain. In the posterior apraxias (ideational apraxia) there is "semantic" parapraxia or substitution of entire movement patterns; in anterior apraxia (so called limb-kinetic apraxia) there is a clumsiness of fine movements (dyspraxia), while in the intermediate forms (ideo-motor apraxia), a substitution of partial movements occurs which can be analogized to phonemic paraphasia. Moreover, the order of impairment in the anterior form, viz: greatest to command, less to imitation and least to object-use, is reversed in the posterior form, a reciprocity similar to that between Broca's aphasia and anomia.

With regard to the agnosias, an attempt is made toward a microgenetic theory of these disorders, in which different patterns of impairment are viewed as referable to stages in the normal sensory (constructive) or perceptual (discriminative) process. Visual "apperceptive" agnosia concerns a deficit at a stage (I) of shape-specification and is in relation to sensory processes and physical space. Such patients may perform better in the recognition of simple uniform stimuli. In visual "associative" agnosia, the defect is on the perceptual side (Stage II) of the process, and concerns an impairment in the "articulation" of differentiated images into abstract or mental space. There will be particular difficulty with highly individuated forms, and the discrimination of similar figures. On discrimination tasks, Stage II defects are aided by signal diversity, which for Stage I acts only to increase the complexity of the signal. The converse is true of audition, where Stage I defects (e.g. sound agnosia) are worsened by homogeneous signals and helped by signal diversity, while Stage II defects (e.g. word-deafness) deteriorate almost as a function of the degree of differentiation of the signal. The various other sub-types of agnosia are discussed in relation to this model. Finally, an attempt is made toward a classification of alexia, in which the different forms are discussed in correspondence with the agnosic and the aphasic syndromes which they accompany.

In accord with this formulation, it is possible to suggest some directions for future work. Closer study of transitional or interface processes would appear to be the most pressing need, both in order to evaluate what are at this time largely theoretical relationships, as well as to obtain a more thorough description of the dynamic aspects of language pathology. Moreover, since linguistic processing is only the final stage of mentation, it is also necessary to study the sources and the patterns of emergence which give rise to linguistic events. Such an investigation would be concerned with confusional and amnesic states as well as dementia and the psychoses. Certainly, the relationship of these conditions to language disorder is a problem scarcely touched in neuropsychology.

We may ask if it is possible to say anything of those physiological processes which are involved in language, and to what extent these processes may be correlated with anatomical locale. Certainly, the evidence for such correlation is indisputable. Yet there is nothing to suggest that the regions so correlated can be identified with functions unique from those of other areas. Rather it would appear that there are certain "lines of regression" which to some extent accompany all cerebral lesions, and that those areas which are correlated with specific symptom-complexes entail not so much an interruption in the hierarchic process, but rather an intensification of the regression effect within that level.

It is possible to say but a little more about "mechanism." The old view of language and perception attributed the complexity of interaction to the diversity of processes and connections within and between the separate parts of each system. Yet in hierarchic theory, the complexity derives from the multiplicity of levels, rather than from multiple processes acting at the same level. Such an approach simplifies the search for physiological mechanisms, for these latter prove to be comprehensible in terms of reiterated effects at serial points in the transformational pattern. An attempt toward a description of such a process is made in Chapter 3. Though psychopathology gives us only a glimpse of what may be the normal mechanism, it appears to come into play at many levels. Whether this is in terms of a reduplication of mechanism at serial points, or, as is more likely, a continuous unfolding hierarchic process subject at each nodal phase to the same laws, is an open question. It is probable, at any rate, that similar mechanisms, or similar patterns in a unitary mechanism, account for such seemingly disparate phenomena as dream symbolism, perceptual formation, abstraction, grammar and word choice.

Another important area for further work concerns the role of imaginal phenomena in disorders of language, motor action and perception. We have seen that agnosic defects may be accompanied by the intrusion into perception of images of that modality. There may be a loss, a distortion or an exaggeration of imagery in agnosic states. Similarly, word-deafness and Wernicke's aphasia may be accompanied by auditory hallucinations and/or psychotic episodes, and the whole question of inner speech in aphasia is bound up with the problem of verbal imagery. The relation of the perception, the word, or the action to the image is of first importance for an understanding of psychopathological phenomena.

A final comment regarding certain subjective epiphenomena of linguistic and cognitive events. Such problems as those of awareness and volition should be the legitimate concerns of psychological research. It is my view that processes of verbal development mediate functional states related to these attitudes. This has to do with the serial or successive pattern of language production. Seriality brings to thought a state which we may describe as one of continuous penultimacy, in that language development always incorporates into itself the meaning that is sought after in expectation of a coming stage. The different manifestations of meaning experiences in simultaneous and successive systems are important clues toward an understanding of volition and awareness. There is, however, a final aspect of this that should be emphasized. This is the directedness, the affirmativeness of thought. There is a tendency in normal life toward affirmation and one manifestation of this is in the moment-to-moment development of verbal thought. In waking life, thought presses into speech in a continuous re-creation of consciousness such that thought, word and consciousness together surge into the present. The process of development of speech out of thought must be felt in this light, as a pressure towards the future. This pressure takes on the character of a drive. Consciousness is like the crystallization of this process as it actualizes in time. For this reason, consciousness seems to be a part of the matrix of the activity of thought and word. The sense of volition may be a manifestation of this process of actualization. The forward thrust of thought, the transmission of the ego state through the vehicle of inner speech, the expectant nature of verbal meaning, these are part of the idea of voluntary action.

BIBLIOGRAPHY

1. Adler, A.: Disintegration and restoration of optic recognition in visual agnosia. *Arch. Neurol. Psychiat., 51*:243–259, 1944.
2. Ajuriaguerra, J. and Hecaen, H.: Éxamen anatomique d'un cas d'aphasie de conduction. *Rev. Neurol., 94*:434–435, 1956.
3. Ajuriaguerra, J. and Hecaen, H.: *Le Cortex Cérébrale.* Masson, Paris, 1964.
4. Ajuriaguerra, J., Hecaen, H. and Angelergues, R.: Les apraxies, variétés cliniques et latéralisation lésionelle. *Rev. Neurol., 102*:566–594, 1960.
5. Alajouanine, T.: Verbal realization in aphasia. *Brain, 79*:1–28, 1956.
6. Alajouanine, T.: *L'Aphasie et le Langage Pathologique.* Bailliere, Paris, 1968.
7. Alajouanine, T., Castaigne, P., Sabouraud, O. and Contamin, F.: Palilalie paroxystique et vocalisations itératives au cours de crises épileptiques, etc. *Rev. Neurol., 101*:685–697, 1959.
8. Alajouanine, T. and Lhermitte, F.: Des anosognosies électives. *Encephale, 46*:505–519, 1957.
9. Alajouanine, T. and Lhermitte, F.: Some problems concerning the agnosias, apraxias and aphasia, in *Problems of Dynamic Neurology,* L. Halpern (Ed.). Jerusalem, pp. 201–216, 1963.
10. Alajouanine, T. and Lhermitte, F.: Aphasia and physiology of speech. *Ass. Res. Nerv. Ment. Dis., 42*:204–219, 1964.
11. Alajouanine, T., Lhermitte, F. and Riboucourt-Ducarne, B.: *Les alexies agnosiques et aphasiques, in Les grandes activités du lobe occipital.* Masson, Paris, 1960.
12. Alajouanine, T., Ombredane, A. and Durand, M.: *Le syndrome de désintegration phonetique dans l'aphasie.* Masson, Paris, 1939.
13. Alajouanine, T., Sabouraud, O. and De Ribaucourt, B.: Le jargon des aphasiques. *J. Psychol., 45*:158–180, 293–329, 1952.
14. Alajouanine, T., Thurel, T. and Ombredane, A.: Somato-agnosie et apraxie du membre superieur gauche. *Rev. Neurol., 1*:695–703, 1934.
14a. Allen, C., Turner, J. and Gadea-Ciria, M.: Investigations into speech disturbances following stereotaxic surgery for Parkinsonism. *Brit. J. Dis. Comm., 1*:55–59, 1966.
15. Anastasoupoulos, G.: Aphasic disorders and verbal hallucinations. *J. Neurol. Sci., 4*:83–93, 1967.
16. Anton, G.: Ueber die Selbstwahrnehmungen der Herderkrankungen des Gehirns durch den Kranken bei Rindenblindheit und Rindentaubheit. *Arch. Psychiat., 32*:86–127, 1899.

16a. Arieti, S.: Special logic of schizophrenic and other types of autistic thought. *Psychiatry, 11*:325–338, 1948.

16b. Arieti, S.: Some aspects of language in schizophrenia. In, *On Expressive Language*, H. Werner (Ed.), pp. 53–67, 1955.

17. Arkin, A.: Qualitative observations on sleep utterances in the laboratory, in *Psicofisiologia del Sonno e del Sogno*. Rome, 1967.

18. Arkin, A., and Brown, J.: Aphasic speech, sleepy speech and sleep-talking. *Psychophysiol.*, 1971.

19. Arnaud: Contribution à l'étude clinique de la surdite-verbale. *Arch. de Neurol., 13*:177–200, 1887.

20. Babinski, J.: Contribution à l'étude des troubles mentaux dans l'hémi-plégie organique cérébrale (anosognosie). *Rev. Neurol., 27*:845–848, 1914.

21. Barker, M. and Lawson, J.: Nominal aphasia in dementia. *Brit. J. Psychiat., 114*:1351–1356, 1968.

22. Barkman, A.: De l'anosognosie dans l'hémiplégie cérébrale. *Acta Med. Scand., 62*:235–254, 1925.

23. Barrett, A.: A case of pure word-deafness with autopsy. *J. Nerv. Ment. Dis., 37*:73–92, 1925.

24. Barton, M., Maruszewski, M. and Urrea, D.: Variation of stimulus con-text and its effects on word-finding ability in aphasics. *Cortex, 5*:351–365, 1969.

25. Bastian, H.: Some problems in connexion with aphasia and other speech defects. *Lancet, 1*:933–942, 1005–1017, 1131–1137, 1187–1194, 1897.

26. Bastian, H.: *Aphasia and Other Speech Defects*. H. K. Lewis, London, 1898.

27. Bay, E.: Disturbances of visual perception and their examination. *Brain, 76*:515–551, 1953.

28. Bay, E.: Aphasia and non-verbal disorders of language. *Brain, 85*:411–426, 1962.

29. Bay, E.: Present concepts of aphasia. *Geriatrics, 19*:319–331, 1964.

30. Bell, A.: Apraxia in corpus callosum lesions. *J. Neurol. Psychopath., 15*:137–146, 1934.

31. Benson, D. and Barton, M.: Disturbances in constructional ability. *Cortex, 6*:19–46, 1970.

32. Benson, D., Brown, J. and Tomlinson, E.: Varieties of alexia. *Neurology,* 1971.

33. Benson, D. and Geschwind, N.: The alexias, in *Handbook of Clinical Neurology*, P. Vinken and G. Bruyn (Eds.). North-Holland, Amster-dam, 1969.

34. Benson, D. and Greenberg, J.: Visual form agnosia. *Arch. Neurol., 20*: 82–89, 1969.

35. Benton, A.: The fiction of the "Gerstmann Syndrome." *J. Neurol. Neurosurg. Psychiat., 24*:176–181, 1961.

36. Benton, A.: Constructional apraxia and the minor hemisphere. *Conf. Neurol., 29:*1–16, 1967.

37. Benton, A. and Joynt, R.: Early descriptions of aphasia. *Arch. Neurol., 3:*205–222, 1960

37a. Berger, R.: Experimental modification of dream content by meaningful verbal stimuli. *Brit. J. Psychiat., 109:*722–740, 1963.

38. Bergson, H.: *Matter and Memory.* (Engl. transl. 1896 ed.), Doubleday, New York, 1959.

39. Beringer, K. and Stein, J.: Analyse eines Falles von "reiner" Alexie. *Z. Ges. Neurol. Psychiat., 123:*472–478, 1930.

40. Bertalanffy, L. von: *Organismic Psychology and Systems Theory.* Clark University Press, Massachusetts, 1968.

41. Beyn, E. and Knyazeva, G.: The problem of prosopagnosia. *J. Neurol. Neurosurg. Psychiat., 25:*154–158, 1962.

42. Bisiach, E.: Perceptual factors in the pathogenesis of anomia. *Cortex, 2:*90–95, 1966.

43. Bodamer, J.: Die Prosop-Agnosie (Die Agnosie des Physiognomieerkennens). *Arch. Psych. u. Ztschr. Neur., 179:*6–53, 1947.

44. Bogaert, L. van and Martin, P.: L'apraxie de la marche et l'atonie statique. *Encephale, 24:*11–18, 1929.

45. Bogen, J.: The other side of the brain, I and II. *Bull. Los Angeles Neurol. Soc., 34:*73–105, 135–162, 1970.

46. Boinet, M.: Aphasie (de cause traumatique). *Bull. de la Soc. de chir. de Paris, 12:*42–46, 1871.

47. Boller, F. and Vignolo, L.: Il significato dei disturbi della ripetizione nell'afasia di Wernicke. *Sist. Nerv., 18:*383–396, 1966.

48. Bonhoeffer, K.: Zur Klinik und Lokalisation des Agrammatismus und der Rechts-Links-Desorientierung. *Mschr. f. Psychiat. u. Neurol., 54:* 11–42, 1923.

49. Bornstein, B.: Prosopagnosia. In *Problems of Dynamic Neurology.,* L. Halpern (Ed.), Jerusalem, 1963.

50. Bornstein, B. and Kidron, I.: Prosopagnosia. *J. Neurol. Neurosurg. Psychiat., 22:*124–131, 1959.

51. Bornstein, B., Stoka, H. and Munitz, H.: Prosopagnosia with animal face agnosia. *Cortex, 5:*164–169, 1969.

52. Bouillaud, J.: Réchèrches cliniques propres à demontier que la perte de la parole, etc. *Arch. Gen de Medécine, 8:*25–45, 1825.

53. Bouman, L.: Cécité verbale pure. *Folia Psychiat. Neurol. Bl., 32:*328–339, 1928.

54. Bouman, L. and Grunbaum, A.: Experimentell-psychologische Untersuchungen zur Aphasie und Paraphasie. *Ztschr. f. d. ges. Neur. u. Psychiat., 96:*481–538, 1925.

55. Brain, R.: Visual-object agnosia with special reference to the gestalt theory. *Brain, 64:*43–62, 1941.

56. Brain, R.: Visual disorientation with special reference to lesions of the right cerebral hemisphere. *Brain, 64*:244–272, 1941.

57. Brain, R.: Loss of visualization. *Proc. Roy. Soc. Med., 47*:24–26, 1954.

58. Brickner, R.: A human cortical area producing repetitive phenomena when stimulated. *J. Neurophysiol., 3*:128–130, 1940.

59. Broadbent, W.: A case of peculiar affection of speech with commentary. *Brain, 1*:484–503, 1878.

60. Broadbent, D. and Gregory, M.: Accuracy of recognition for speech presented to the right and left ears. *Quart. J. Exp. Psychol., 16*:359–360, 1964.

61. Broca, P.: Rémarquès sur le siege de la faculté du langage articule, suivies d'une observation d'aphemie (perte de la parole). *Bull. Soc. Anat., 36*:330–357, 1861a.

62. Broca, P.: Nouvelle observation d'aphemie produite par une lesion de la moitie postérièure des deuxieme et troisieme circonvolutions frontales. *Bull. Soc. Anat., 36*:398–407, 1861b.

63. Broca, P.: Localisation des fonctions cérébrales siege du langage articule. *Bull. Soc. Anthropol., 4*:200–204, 1863.

64. Broca, P.: Sur le siege de la faculté du langage articule. *Bull. Soc. Anthropol., 6*:377–393, 1865.

65. Brown, J.: Physiology and phylogenesis of emotional expression. *Brain Res. (Elsevier), 5*:1–14, 1967.

66. Brown, J.: Hemispheric specialization and the corpus callosum, in *Present Concepts in Internal Medicine,* C. Gunderson (Ed.). Publ. Letterman Hospital, San Francisco, pp. 77–86, 1969.

66a. Brown, J.: Observations on language following surgical lesion of the pulvinar in man. Presented at Fulton Society Meeting, Washington, D.C., June, 1971.

66b. Brown, J., Riklan, M., Waltz, J., Jackson, S. and Cooper, I.: Preliminary studies of language and cognition following surgical lesion of the pulvinar in man. *Int. J. Neurol.,* in press, 1971–72.

67. Brown, R. and McNeill, D.: The "tip of the tongue" phenomenon. *J. Verb. Learn. and Verb. Behav., 5*:325–337, 1966.

68. Brun, R.: Klinische und anatomische Studien uber Apraxie. *Schweiz. Archiv. f. Neurol. u. Psychiat., 9*:29–64, *10*:185–210, 1921, 1922.

69. Buck, F. de: Les parakinesies. *J. de Neurol.,* 361, 1899.

70. Butters, N. and Brody, B.: The role of the left parietal lobe in the mediation of intra- and cross-modal associations. *Cortex, 4*:328–343, 1968.

71. Cameron, N.: In *Language and Thought in Schizophrenia,* J. Kasanin (Ed.). Norton, New York, 1964.

72. Cassirer, E.: The Philosophy of Symbolic Forms, I: Language. Yale University Press, New Haven, 1953.

73. Chapanis, A.: Color names for color space. *Amer. Sci., 53*:327–346, 1965.

74. Charcot, J.: Des variétés de l'aphasie. *Prog. Med., 11*:487–488, 521–523, 1883.

75. Charcot, M.: Un cas de suppression brusque isolée de la vision mentale des signes et des objects. Lecons sur les malades du systeme nerveux. Delahaye and Lacrosnie, Paris, 1887.

75a. Cheek, W. and Taveras, J.: Thalamic tumors. *J. Neurosurg., 24*:505–513, 1966.

76. Chistovich, L., Klass, I. and Kuzmin, I.: The process of speech-sound discrimination. *Voprosy Psikhologii (Psychol. Prob.), 1962, (6)* 26–39, Transl. Emanuel. College Res. Cong. Center, E-T-R-63-10, AF 19, (604) –8505, AFCRL, OAR, 1963.

77. Chusid, J., Gutierrez-Mahoney, C. and Margules-Lavergne, M.: Speech disturbances in association with parasagittal frontal lesions. *J. Neurosurg., 11*:193–204, 1954.

78. Claparede, E.: Revue generale sur l'agnosie. *Ann. Psychol., 6*:74–143, 1900.

79. Clarke, P., Wyke, M. and Zangwill, O.: Language disorder in a case of Korsakoff's Syndrome. *J. Neurol. Neurosurg. Psychiat., 21*:190–194, 1958.

80. Cohen, D., Dubois, J., Gauthier, M., Hecaen, H. and Angelergues, R.: Aspects du fonctionnement du code linguistique chez les aphasiques moteurs. *Neuropsychol., 1*:165–177, 1963.

81. Cohn, R. and Neumann, M.: Jargon aphasia. *J. Nerv. Ment. Dis., 127*: 381–399, 1958.

82. Conrad, K.: Strukturanalysen hirnpathologische Falle, I: Über Struktur und Gestaltwandel. *Dtsch. Z. Nervenheilk, 158*:344–371, 1947.

83. Conrad, K.: Strukturanalysen hirnpathologischen Fälle. Zum Problem der Leitungsaphasie. *Dtsch. Z. Nervenheilk, 159*:188–228, 1948.

83a. Cooper, I., Waltz, J., Amin, I. and Fujita, S.: Pulvinectomy: A preliminary report. *J. Amer. Ger. Soc.,* 1971.

84. Critchley, M.: On palilalia *J. Neur. Psychopath., 8*:23–32, 1927.

85. Critchley, M.: *The Parietal Lobes* (reprint 1953 ed.), Hafner, New York, 1966.

86. Critchley, M.: Verbal symbols in thought. *Trans. Med. Soc. (London), 71*:179–194, 1955.

87. Critchley, M.: The problem of visual agnosia. *J. Neurol. Sci., 1*:274–290, 1964.

88. Critchley, M: Dax's Law. *Int. J. Neurol., 4*:199–206, 1964.

89. Critchley, M.: The neurology of psychotic speech. *Brit. J. Psychiat., 110*: 353–364, 1964.

90. Critchley, M.: Acquired anomalies of colour perception of central origin. *Brain, 88*:711–724, 1965.

91. Critchley, M.: An appraisal of visual (object) agnosia. *8th. Internat. Neurol. Congr.,* Suppl. pp. 45–55, Vienna, 1965.

92. Critchley, M.: The enigma of Gerstmann's Syndrome. *Brain, 89*:183–198, 1966.

93. Curran, F. and Schilder, P.: Paraphasic signs in diffuse lesions of the brain. *J. Nerv. Ment. Dis., 82*:613–636, 1935.

93. Davidenkov, S.: Impairments of higher nervous activity. Lect. 8 and 9, *Visual Agnosia.* State Publ. House, Leningrad, 1956.

94. Dejerine, J.: Aphasie et cécité des mots. *Progr. Med., 8*:629, 1880.

95. Dejerine, J.: Étude sur l'aphasie. *Rev. de Méd., 5*:174–191, 1885.

96. Dejerine, J.: Sur un cas de cécité verbale avec agraphie, suivi d'autopsie. *Mem. Soc. Biol., 3*:197–201, 1891.

97. Dejerine, J.: Contribution à l'étude anatomopathologique et clinique des différentes variétés de cécité verbale. *Mem. Soc. Biol., 4*:61–90, 1892.

98. Dejerine, J.: Considerations sur la soi-disant "aphasie tactile." *Rev. Neurol., 13*:597–601, 1906.

99. Dejerine, J.: A propos de l'agnosie tactile. *Rev. Neurol., 15*:781–784, 1907.

100. Dejerine, J.: *Semiologie des Affections du Système Nerveux.* Masson, Paris, 1914.

101. Delmas-Marsalet, P.: Lobe frontale et equilibre. *Encephale, 31*:15–91, 1936.

102. Denny-Brown, D.: The nature of apraxia. *J. Nerv. Ment. Dis., 126*:9–32, 1938.

103. Denny-Brown, D.: The physiological basis of perception and speech, in *Problems of Dynamic Neurology,* L. Halpern (Ed.), Jerusalem, pp. 30–62, 1963.

104. De Renzi, E., Faglioni, P. and Spinnler, H.: The performance of patients with unilateral brain damage on face recognition tasks. *Cortex, 4*: 17–34, 1968.

105. De Renzi, E., Pieczuro, A. and Vignolo, L.: Oral apraxia and aphasia. *Cortex, 2*:50–73, 1966.

106. De Renzi, E., Pieczuro, A. and Vignolo, L.: Ideational apraxia: a quantitative study. *Neuropsychologia, 6*:41–52, 1968.

107. De Renzi, E. and Scotti, G.: Autotopagnosia: Fiction or reality. *Arch. Neurol., 23*:221–227, 1970.

108. De Renzi, E., Scotti, G. and Spinnler, H.: Perceptual and associative disorders of visual recognition. *Neurology, 19*:634–642, 1969.

109. Dubois, J., Hecaen, H., Angelergues, R., Maufras du Chatelier, A. and Marcie, P.: Étude neurolinguistique de l'aphasie de conduction. *Neuropsychologia, 2*:9–44, 1964.

110. Domarus, von E.: In *Language and Thought in Schizophrenia,* J. Kasanin (Ed.). Norton, New York, 1964.

111. Efron, R.: What is perception? in *Boston Studies in the Philosophy of Science,* R. Cohen and M. Wartofsky (Eds.), *4*:137–173, 1968.

112. Ettlinger, G.: Sensory deficits in visual agnosia. *J. Neurol. Neurosurg. Psychiat., 19*:297–307, 1956.

113. Ettlinger, G., Warrington, E. and Zangwill, O.: A further study of visual-spatial agnosia. *Brain, 80*:335–361, 1957.

114. Faglioni, P., Spinnler, H. and Vignolo, L.: Contrasting behavior of right and left hemisphere-damaged patients on a discriminative and a semantic task of auditory recognition. *Cortex, 5*:366–389, 1969.

115. Fant, G.: Auditory patterns of speech, in *Models for the Perception of Speech and Visual Form.* W. Wathen-Dunn (Ed.). M.I.T. Press, Cambridge, pp. 111–125, 1967.

116. Farnsworth, D.: *The Farnsworth-Munsell 100 Hue Test for the Examination of Color Discrimination.* Manual, Baltimore, 1949.

117. Faust, C.: In Hecaen, H. and Angelergues, R., *Arch. Neurol., 7*:92–100, 1947.

118. Feuchtwanger, E.: *Amusie.* Springer, Berlin, 1930.

119. Finkelnburg, F.: Ueber Aphasie und Asymbolie nebst Versuch einer Theorie der Sprachbildung. *Arch. f. Psychiat., 6,* 1876.

120. Flechsig, P.: Developmental (myelogenetic) localization in the cerebral cortex in the human subject. *Lancet, 2*:1027–1029, 1901.

121. Foerster, O.: Symptomatologie der Erkrankungen des Gehirns, in *Handb. der. Neurolog.,* O. Bumke and O. Foerster (Eds.). Springer, Berlin, 1936.

122. Freud, S.: On Aphasia. Transl. E. Stengel, 1891 ed., International Universities Press, New York, 1953.

123. Freund, C.: Uber optische Aphasie und Seelenblindheit. *Arch. Psychiat. Nervenkr., 20*:276–297, 371–416, 1889.

124. Froeschels, E.: A peculiar intermediary state between waking and sleep. *J. Clin. Psychopath., 7*:825–833, 1946.

125. Froeschels, E.: Transition phenomena. *Amer. J. Psychother., 7*:273–277, 1953.

126. Gainotti, G.: Les maniféstations de negligence et d'inattention pour l'hémispace. *Cortex, 4*:64–91, 1968.

127. Garcin, R., Varay, and Hadji-Demo: Document pour servir à l'étude des troubles du schema corporel. *Rev. Neurol., 69*:498–510, 1938.

128. Gazzaniga, M., Bogen, J. and Sperry, R.: Dyspraxia following division of the cerebral commissures. *Arch. Neurol., 16*:606–612, 1967.

129. Gazzaniga, M. and Sperry, R.: Language after section of the cerebral commissures. *Brain, 90*:131–148, 1967.

130. Gerstmann, J.: Fingeragnosie. *Wien. Klin. Wochenschr., 40*:1010–1012, 1924.

131. Gerstmann, J.: Fingeragnosie und isolierte Agraphie ein neues Syndrom. *Z. ges. Neurol. u. Psychiat., 108*:152–177, 1927.

132. Gerstmann, J.: Zur Symptomatologie der Hirnläsionen im Übergangsgebiet der unteren Parietal und mittleren Occipitalwendung. *Nervenarzt., 3*:691–695, 1930.

133. Gerstmann, J.: Problem of imperception of disease and of impaired body territories with organic lesions. *Arch. Neurol. Psychiat., 48*: 890–913, 1942.

134. Gerstmann, J. and Schilder, P.: Über eine besondere Gangstörung bei Stirnhirnerkrankung. *Wien. med. Wschr., 76*:97–102, 1926.

135. Geschwind, N.: Sympathetic dyspraxia. *Trans. Amer. Neurol. Ass., 88*: 219–220, 1963.

136 Geschwind, N.: Non-aphasic disorders of speech. *Int. J. Neurol., 4*:207–214, 1964.

137. Geschwind, N.: Disconnexion syndromes in animals and man. *Brain, 88*:237–294, 585–644, 1965.

138. Geschwind, N.: The varieties of naming errors. *Cortex, 3*:97–112, 1967.

139. Geschwind, N. and Fusillo, M.: Color-naming defects in association with alexia. *Arch. Neurol., 15*:137–146, 1966.

140. Geschwind, N. and Kaplan, E.: A human cerebral deconnection syndrome. *Neurology, 12*:675–685, 1962.

141. Geschwind, N., Quadfasel, F. and Segarra, J.: Isolation of the speech area. *Neuropsychologia, 6*:327–340, 1968.

142. Gloning, I., Gloning, K. and Hoff, H.: Aphasia-a-no-clinical syndrome, in *Problems of Dynamic Neurology*, L. Halpern (Ed.), Jerusalem, 1963.

143. Gloning, I., Gloning, K. and Hoff, H.: Neuropsychological symptoms and syndromes in lesions of the occipital lobes and the adjacent areas. Gauthiers-Villars, Paris, 1968.

144. Gloning, I., Gloning, K., Jellinger, K. and Quatember, R.: A case of "prosopagnosia" with necropsy findings. *Neuropsychologia, 8*:199–204, 1970.

145. Gogol: *Ein Beitrag zur Lehre von Aphasie.* Inaug. Diss., Breslau, 1873.

146. Goldstein, K.: Die transkortikalen Aphasien. *Ergbn. Neurol. u. Psychiat.*, G. Fischer, Jena, 1915.

147. Goldstein, K.: Das Wesen der amnestischen Aphasie. *Schweiz. Arch. f. Neur. u. Psychiat., 15*:163–175, 1924.

148. Goldstein, K.: Some remarks on Russell Brain's article concerning visual-object agnosia. *J. Nerv. Ment. Dis., 98*:148–153, 1943.

148a. Goldstein, K.: The significance of psychological research in schizophrenia. *J. Nerv. Ment. Dis., 97*:261–279, 1943.

149. Goldstein, K.: *Language and Language Disturbances.* Grune and Stratton, New York, 1948.

150. Goldstein, K. and Gelb, A.: Psychologische analysen hirnpathologischer Fälle auf Grund von Untersuchungen Hirnverletzter. *Z. Ges. Neurol. Psychiat., 41*:1–142, 1918.

151. Goldstein, K. and Marmor, J.: A case of aphasia, with special reference to the problems of repetition and word-finding. *J. Neurol. and Psychiat., 1*:329–339, 1938.

152. Goodglass, H.: Redefining the concept of agrammatism in aphasia. Proc. XII Internat. Sp. and Voice Ther. Conf., Padua, pp. 108–116, 1962.

153. Goodglass, H.: Psycholinguistic aspects of aphasia, Speech given at "Linguistic and Oral Communication Aspects of Rehabilitation of Adults with Aphasia." Adelphi Univ., New Jersey, 1967.

154. Goodglass, H.: Studies on the grammar of aphasics, in *Developments in Applied Psycholinguistic Research,* S. Rosenberg and J. Kaplan (Eds.). Macmillan, New York, 1968.

155. Goodglass, H., Barton, M. and Kaplan, E.: Sensory modality and object-naming in aphasia. *J. Speech and Hearing Res., 11*:488–496, 1968.

156. Halle, M. and Stevens, K.: Speech recognition: A model and a program for research. I.R.E., Trans. Info. Theory, IT–8, pp. 155–159, 1962.

157. Head, H.: *Aphasia and Kindred Disorders of Speech.* Macmillan, New York, 1926.

158. Hecaen, H.: Clinical symptomatology in right and left hemisphere lesions, in *Interhemispheric Relations and Cerebral Dominance,* V. Mountcastle (Ed.). Johns Hopkins Press, Baltimore, 1962.

159. Hecaen, H.: Aspects des troubles de la lecture (alexies) au cours des lésions cérébrales en foyer. *Word, 23*:265–287, 1967.

160. Hecaen, H.: Suggestions for a typology of the apraxias, in *The Reach of Mind: Essays in Memory of Kurt Goldstein,* M. Simmel (Ed.). Springer, New York, 1968.

161. Hecaen, H.: Essai de dissociation du syndrome de l'aphasie sénsorièlle. *Rev. Neurol., 120*:229–237, 1969.

162. Hecaen, H. and Ajuriaguerra, J.: L'apraxie de l'habillage. *Encephale, 35*:113–143, 1942–1945.

163. Hecaen, H. and Ajuriaguerra, J.: Le problème clinique et anatomique de l'apraxie de l'habillage. *Sist. Nerv., 3*:1–18, 1951.

164. Hecaen, H., Ajuriaguerra, J.de, Magis, C. and Angelergues, R.: Le problème de l'agnosie des physionomies. *Encephale, 4*:322–355, 1952.

165. Hecaen, H. and Angelergues, R.: Agnosia for faces (prosopagnosia). *Arch. Neurol., 7*:92–100, 1962.

166. Hecaen, H. and Angelergues, R.: *Pathologie du Langage.* Larousse, Paris, 1965.

167. Hecaen, H., Dell, M. and Roger, A.: L'aphasie de conduction. *Encephale, 44*:170–195, 1955.

168. Hecaen, H., Dubois, J. and Marcie, P.: Mecanismes de l'aphasie et rapport de la neurolinguistique a l'aphasiologie. *Acta Neurol. et Psychiat. (Belg.), 67*:959–987, 1967.

169. Heilbronner, K.: In Kleist, *Jahrb. f. Psychiat. u. Neurol., 28*:46–112, 1907.

170. Heilbronner, K.: Zur Symptomatologie der Aphasie. *Archiv. f. Psychiat. u. Nervenheilk., 43*:234–298, 1908.

171. Hemphill, R. and Klein, R.: Contribution to the dressing disability as a focal sign and to the imperception phenomena. *J. Ment. Sci., 94*: 611–622, 1948.

172. Hemphill, R. and Stengel, E.: A study on pure word-deafness. *J. Neurol. Psychiat., 3*:251–262, 1940.

173. Henschen, S.: On the hearing sphere. *Acta Oto-laryngol., 1*:423–486, 1919.

174. Henschen, S.: Clinical and anatomical contributions on brain pathology. *Arch. Neurol. and Psychiat., 13*:226–249, 1925.

174a. Hermann, K., Turner, J., Gillingham, F. and Gaze, R.: The effects of destructive lesions and stimulation of the basal ganglia on speech mechanisms. *Confin. Neurol., 27*:197–207, 1966.

175. Herrmann, G. and Pötzl, O.: *Ueber die Agraphie und ihre lokaldiagnostischen Beziehungen.* Karger, Berlin, 1926.

176. Hillman, J.: *Emotion: A Comprehensive Phenomenology of Theories and Their Meanings for Therapy.* Evanston, Northwestern Univ. Press, 1961.

177. Hinshelwood, J.: *Letter-, Word- and Mind-Blindness.* Lewis, London, 1900.

178. Hinshelwood, J.: *Congenital Word-Blindness.* Lewis, London, 1917.

180. Hoff, H. and Pötzl, O.: Experimentelle Nachbildung von Anosognosie. *Ztschr. f. d. ges. Neurol. u. Psychiat., 137*:722–734, 1937.

181. Holmes, G.: Pure word blindness. *Fol. Psychiat. Amst., 53*:279–288, 1950.

182. Howes, D. and Geschwind, N.: Quantitative studies of aphasic language. *Ass. Res. Nerv. Ment. Dis., 42*:229–244, 1964.

183. Hubel, D. and Wiesel, T.: Receptive fields and functional architecture in two nonstriate visual areas (18 and 19) of the cat. *J. Neurophysiol., 28*:229–289, 1965.

184. Humphrey, G.: *Thinking.* Wiley, New York, 1963.

185. Humphrey, M. and Zangwill, O.: Cessation of dreaming after brain injury. *J. Neurol. Neurosurg. Psychiat., 14*:322–326, 1951.

186. Inouye, T. and Shimizu, A.: The electromyographic study of verbal hallucination. *J. Nerv. Ment. Dis., 151*:415–422, 1970.

187. Isserlin, M.: Aphasie. In *Handb. der. Neurol.,* O. Bumke and O. Foerster (Eds.). Springer, Berlin, *6*:627–806, 1936.

188. Jackson, H.: In *Selected Writings of John Hughlings Jackson,* V. 2, J. Taylor (Ed.). Hodder and Stoughton, London, 1932.

189. Jakobsen, R.: *Child Language, Aphasia and Phonological Universals.* Mouton, The Hague, 1968.

190. Jerger, J., Weikers, N., Sharbrough, F. and Jerger, S.: Bilateral lesions of the temporal lobe. *Acta Oto-laryngol. Suppl., 258,* 1969.

191. Kahler, O. and Pick, A.: *Beiträge zur Pathologie und Pathologischen Anatomie des Centralnervensystems.* Hirschfeld, Leipzig, 1879.

192. Kaplan, E. and Werner, H.: The acquisition of word meanings: A developmental study. *Monogr. Soc. Res. Child Devel., 15,* Evanston, 1952.

193. Kasanin, J.: *Language and Thought in Schizophrenia.* Norton, New York, 1964.

194. Kertesz, A. and Benson, D.: Presentation at Academy of Aphasia. Boston, 1969.

195. Kimura, D.: Functional asymmetry of the brain in dichotic listening. *Cortex, 3:*163–178, 1967.

196. Kinsbourne, M. and Warrington, E.: Jargon aphasia. *Neuropsychologia, 1:*27–37, 1963.

197. Klein, R. and Harper, J.: The problem of agnosia in the light of a case of pure word deafness. *J. Ment. Sci., 102:*112–120, 1956.

198. Kleist, K.: Kortikale (innervatorische) Apraxie. *Jahrb. f. Psychiat. u. Neurol., 28:*46–112, 1907.

199. Kleist, K.: Der Gang und der gegenwärtige Stand der Apraxieforschung. *Ergbn. Neurol. Psychiat., 1:*342–452, 1911.

200. Kleist, K.: Aphasie und Geisteskrankheit. *München. Med. Wschr., 1:* 8–12, 1914.

201. Kleist, K.: Über Leitungsaphasie und grammatische Storungen. *Monatsschr. f. Psych. u. Neurol., 40:*118–121, 1916.

202. Kleist, K.: Konstruktive (optische) Apraxie, in *Handb. Ärtzlichen Erfahrungen im Weltkriege,* K. Bonhoeffer (Ed.). Barth, Leipzig, 1934.

203. Kleist, K.: *Gehirnpathologie.* Barth, Leipzig, 1934.

204. Kleist, K.: *Sensory Aphasia and Amusia.* Pergamon, Oxford, 1962.

205. Konorski, J., Kozniewska, H. and Stepien, L.: Analysis of symptoms and cerebral localization of the audio-verbal aphasia. Proc. VII *Int. Cong. Neurol., 2:*234–236, Rome, 1961.

206. Kraepelin, E.: Über Sprachstorungen im Traume, in *Psychol. Arb. (Leipzig), 5:*1, 1910.

207. Kramer: Alloästhesie und fehlende Fahrenhmung der gelähmten Körperhälfte bei subvertikalen Hirnherd. *Neurol. Centralbl., 34:*287, 1915.

208. Krayenbuhl, H., Siegfried, J., Kohenef, M. and Yasargil, M.: Is there a dominant thalamus? *Confin. Neurol., 26:*246–249, 1965.

209. Kreindler, A. and Ionasescu, V.: A case of "pure" word blindness. *J. Neurol. Neurosurg. Psychiat., 24:*275–280, 1961.

210. Kroll, M.: Beitrag zum Studium der Apraxie, *Ztschr. f. d. ges Neurol. u. Psychiat., 2:*315–345, 1910.

211. Kussmaul, A.: Disturbances of speech. *Cyclop. Pract. Med., 14:*581–875, 1877.

212. Lagrange, H., Bertrand, I. and Garcin, R.: Sur un cas de cécité corticale par ramollissèment des deux cunei. *Rev. Neurol., 1:*417–427, 1929.

213. Lange, J.: Fingeragnosie und Agraphie. *Mschr. f. Psychiat. u. Neurol.*, *76*:129–188, 1930.

214. Lange, J.: Agnosien u. Apraxien. *Handb. der Neurol.*, O. Bumke and O. Foerster (Eds.). Springer, Berlin, *6*:807–960, 1936.

215. Lashley, K.: The problem of serial order in behavior, in *Cerebral Mechanisms in Behavior* (Hixon Symposium). L. Jefress (Ed.). Wiley, New York, pp. 112–136, 1951.

216. Lewandowsky, M.: Ueber Apraxie des Lidschlusses. *Berl. klin. Wochenschr.*, *29*:921–923, 1907.

217. Lewandowsky, M.: Ueber Abspaltung des Farbensinnes. *Mschr. Psychiat. Neurol.*, *23*:488–510, 1908.

218. Lhermitte, J., de Massary, J. and Kyriaco, N.: Le role de la pensèe spatiale dans l'apraxie. *Rev. Neurol.*, *2*:895–903, 1928.

219. Liberman, A., Cooper, F. and Gerstmann, L.: An experimental study of the acoustic determinants of vowel quality. *Word*, *8*:195–210, 1952.

220. Lichtheim, L.: On aphasia. *Brain*, *7*:433–484, 1885.

221. Liepmann, H.: Das Krankheitsbild der Apraxie ("motorischen asymbolie"). *Mtschr. f. Psychiat. u. Neurol.*, *8*:15–44, 102–132, 181–197, 1900.

222. Liepmann, H.: Die linke Hemisphäre und das Handeln. *Münch. Med. Wochenschr.*, *2*:2375–2378, 1905.

223. Liepmann, H.: Ueber die agnostischen Störungen. *Neurol. Centralbl.*, *27*:609–617, 1908.

224. Liepmann, H.: Apraxie. *Ergbn. der ges. Med.*, *1*:516–543, 1920.

255. Liepmann, H. and Maas, O.: Fall von linksseitiger Agraphie und Apraxie bei rechtsseitiger Lähmung. *J. f. Psychol. u. Neurol.*, *10*:214–227, 1907.

226. Liepmann, H. and Pappenheim, M.: Über einen Fall von sogenannter Leitungsaphasie mit anatomischen Befund. *Z. Neurol. Psychiat.*, *27*:1–41, 1914.

227. Lissauer, H.: Ein Fall von Seelenblindheit nebst einem Beitrage zur Theorie derselben. *Arch. Psychiat. Nervenkr.*, *21*:222–270, 1889.

228. Lotmar, F.: Zur Kenntnis der erschwerten Wortfindung und ihrer Bedeutung für das Denken des Aphasischen. *Schweiz. Archiv. f. Neurol. u. Psychiat.*, *5*:206–239, 1919.

229. Lotmar, F.: Zur Pathophysiologie der erschwerten Wortfindung bei Aphasischen. *Schweiz. Arch. f. Neur. u. Psychiat.*, *30*:86–158, 322–379, 1933.

230. Low, A.: A case of agrammatism in the English language. *Arch. Neurol. Psychiat.*, *25*:556–597, 1931.

231. Luria, A.: Factors and forms of aphasia, in *Disorders of Language*. Churchill, London, 1964.

232. Luria, A.: *Human Brain and Psychological Processes*. Harper, New York, 1966.

233. Luria, A.: *Higher Cortical Functions in Man*. Basic Books, New York, 1966.

234. Marcuse, H.: Apraktische Symptome bei einem Fall von seniler Demenz. *Centralbl. f. Nervenheilk, u. Psychiat., 27*:737–751, 1904.

235. Marie, P.: Révision de la question de l'aphasie. *Sem. Méd., 21*:241–247, 493–500, 565–571, 1906.

236. Marie, P., Bouttier, H. and Bailey, P.: La planotopokinésie. *Rev. Neurol., 1*:505–512, 1922.

237. Marie, P. and Foix, C.: Les aphasies de guerre. *Rev. Neurol., 24*:53–87, 1917.

238. Marshall, J. and Newcombe, F.: Syntactic and semantic errors in paralexia. *Neuropsychologia, 6*:169–176, 1966.

239. Martin, J.: Pure word blindness considered as a disturbance of visual space perception. *Proc. Roy. Soc. Med., 47*:293–295, 1954.

240. Maspes, P.: Le syndrome expérimental chez l'homme de la section du splenium du corps calleux: alexie visuelle pure hémianopsique. *Rev. Neurol., 80*:100–113, 1948.

241. Mayer-Gross, W.: Some observations on apraxia. *Proc. Roy. Soc. Med., 28*:63–72, 1935.

242. McFie, J. and Zangwill, O.: Visual-constructive disabilities associated with lesions of the left cerebral hemisphere. *Brain, 83*:243–260, 1960.

243. Meyer, A.: The relation of the auditory center to aphasia. *J. f. Psychol. u. Neurol., 13*:203–213, 1908.

244. Meyer, J. and Barron, D.: Apraxia of gait: A clinical physiological study. *Brain, 83*:261–284, 1960.

245. Miller, G.: *The Psychology of Communication*. Basic Books, New York, 1967.

246. Milner, B.: Laterality effects in audition, in *Interhemispheric Relations and Cerebral Dominance*, V. Mountcastle, (Ed.). Johns Hopkins, Baltimore, pp. 177–195, 1962.

247. Milner, B.: Brain mechanisms suggested by studies of temporal lobes, in *Brain Mechanisms Underlying Speech and Language*, F. Darley (Ed.). Grune and Stratton, pp. 122–145, 1967.

248. Mintz, A.: Schizophrenic speech and sleepy speech. *J. Abnorm. Soc. Psychol., 43*:548–549, 1948.

249. Monakow, C. von: Experimentelle und pathologische-anatomische Unterschungen uber die Beziehungen der sogennanten Sehsphare zu den infrakortikalen Opticuscentren und zum N. opticus. *Archiv. f. Psychiat., 16*:151–199, 1885.

250. Monakow, C. von: *Gehirnpathologie*. Halder, Vienna, 1905.

251. Morax, P.: La cécité corticale, in *Les Grandés Activités du Lobe Occipital*, T. Alajouanine (Ed.). Paris, Masson, pp. 217–234, 1960.

252. Monakow, C. von: *Die Lokalisation im Grosshirn*. Bergmann, Wiesbaden, 1914.

253. Morel, F.: L'audition dans l'aphasie sénsorielle. *Encephale*, 2:533–553, 1935.

254. Morlaas, J:. Contribution à l'étude de l'apraxie. *Dissertation*, Paris, Legrand, 1928.

255. Morsier, G. de: Les troubles de la déglutition et des mouvements de la langue dans l'anarthrie (aphasie motrice). *Pract. Oto-Rhino-Laryngol.*, 11:125–133, 1949.

256. Mouren, P., Tatossian, A., Trupheme, R., Giudicelli, S. and Fresco, R.: L'alexie par déconnection visuo-verbale. *Encephale*, 2:112–137, 1967.

257. Munk, H.: Erfahrungen zu Gunsten der Localisation. *Verh. Physiol. ges. Berl., 16; Dtsch. med. Wschr.*, 13:31, 1877.

258. Neisser, U.: *Cognitive Psychology*. Appleton, New York, 1967.

259. Newcombe, F. and Russell, W.: Dissociated visual perceptual and spatial deficits in focal lesions of the right hemisphere. *J. Neurol. Neurosurg. Psychiat.*, 32:73–81, 1969.

260. Nielsen, J.: The possibility of pure motor aphasia. *Bull. Los Angeles Neurol. Soc.*, 1:11–14, 1936.

261. Nielsen, J.: Unilateral cerebral dominance as related to mind blindness. *Arch. Neurol. & Psychiat.*, 38:108–135, 1937.

262. Nielsen, J., Disturbances of the body scheme. *Bull. Los Angeles Neurol. Soc.*, 3:127–135, 1938.

263. Nielsen, J.: Agnosias and the body scheme. *Bull. Los Angeles Neurol. Soc.*, 4:69–76, 1939.

264. Nielsen, J.: The unsolved problems in aphasia I. Alexia in "motor" aphasia. *Bull. Los Angeles Neurol. Soc.*, 4:114–122, 1939.

265. Nielsen, J.: The unsolved problems in aphasia II. Alexia resulting from a temporal lesion. *Bull. Los Angeles Neurol. Soc.*, 4:168–183, 1939.

266. Nielsen, J.: The unsolved problems in aphasia III–amnesic aphasia. *Bull. Los Angeles Neurol. Soc.*, 5:78–84, 1940.

267. Nielsen, J.: The unsolved problems of apraxia and some solutions. *Bull. Los Angeles Neurol. Soc.*, 6:1–20, 1941.

268. Nielsen, J.: *Agnosia, Apraxia, Aphasia*. (Reprint 1946 ed.). Hafner, New York, 1965.

269. Nielsen, J.: Discussion in *Cerebral Mechanisms in Behavior* (Hixon Symposium). L. Jefress (Ed.). Wiley, New York, pp. 182–193, 1951.

270. Nielsen, J. and Friedman, A.: Kinetic apraxia of wrist extension. *Bull. Los Angeles Neurol. Soc.*, 6:48–52, 1941.

271. Niessl v. Mayendorf, E.: Die aphasischen Symptome und ihre kortikale Lokalisation. Barth, Leipzig, 1911.

272. Ojemann, G., Fedio, P. and Van Buren, J.: Anomia from pulvinar and subcortical parietal stimulation. *Brain, 91*:99–116, 1968.

273. Oldfield, R.: Things, words and the brain. *Quart. J. Exp. Psychol., 18*:340–353, 1966.

274. Ombredane, A.: Sur le mecanisme de l'anarthrie. *J. Psychol. Norm. Path., 23*:940–955, 1926.

298 — Aphasia, Apraxia and Agnosia

Aphasia, Apraxia and Agnosia

298 *Aphasia, Apraxia and Agnosia*

275. Oxbury, J., Oxbury, S. and Humphrey, N.: Varieties of colour anomia. *Brain, 92*:847–860, 1969.
276. Pallis, C.: Impaired identification of faces and places with agnosia for colours. *J. Neurol. Neurosurg. Psychiat., 18*:218–224, 1955.
277. Parisi, O. and Pizzamiglio, L.: Syntactic comprehension in aphasia. *Cortex, 6*:204–215, 1970.
278. Penfield, W., and Roberts, L.: *Speech and Brain Mechanisms.* Princeton, New Jersey, 1959.
279. Pershing, H.: A case of Wernicke's conduction aphasia with autopsy. *J. Nerv. Ment. Dis., 27*:369–374, 1900.
280. Petrovici, I.: Apraxia of gait and of trunk movements. *J. Neurol. Sci., 7*:229–243, 1968.
281. Pick, A.: Beiträge zur Lehre von den Storungen der Sprache. *Arch. f. Psychiat. u. Nervenkr., 23*:896–918, 1892.
282. Pick, A.: *Beiträge zur Pathologie und Pathologische Anatomie des Centralnervensystems.* Karger, Berlin, 1898.
283. Pick, A.: *Studien über motorische Apraxie und ihre nahestehende Erscheinungen.* Deuticke, Leipzig, 1905.
284. Pick, A.: *Die agrammatischen Sprachstörungen.* Springer, Berlin, 1913.
285. Pick, A.: Störung der Orientierung am eigenen Korper. *Psychol. Forsch., 1*:303–318, 1922.
286. Pick, A.: On the pathology of echographia. *Brain, 47*:417–429, 1924.
287. Pick, A.: Aphasie. *Handb. d. Norm. u. Path. Physiol., 15* (2) 1416–1524, (Engl. transl., Ed. J. Brown, in press), Springer, Berlin, 1931.
288. Piercy, M., Hecaen, H. and Ajuriaguerra, J.: Constructional apraxia associated with unilateral cerebral lesions, left and right sided cases compared. *Brain, 83*:225–242, 1960.
289. Piercy, M., and Smyth, V.: Right hemispheric dominance for certain non-verbal intellectual skills. *Brain, 85*:775–790, 1962.
290. Pitres, A.: L'aphasie amnésique et ses variétés cliniques. *L'Écho Méd., 24*:276–281, 289–294, 301–306, 313–317, 325–332, 337–342, 351–352, 373–378, 385–390, 397–405, 409–425, 433–437, 1898.
291. Poppelreuter, W.: *Die Psychischen Schädigungen durch Kopfschuss im Kriege.* 2 vol., Voss, Leipzig, 1914–1917.
292. Pötzl, O.: *Die optisch-agnostichen Störungen.* Deuticke, Leipzig, 1928.
293. Pötzl, O.: Zur agnosie des Physiognomiegedachtnisses. *Wien. Z. Nervenheilk, 6*:335–354, 1953.
294. Rapaport, D.: Consciousness: A psychopathological and psychodynamic view. In, *Problems of Consciousness.* H. Abramson (Ed.). Josiah Macy Fdn., New York, pp. 18–57, 1951.
295. Raymond, M. and Egger, M.: Un cas d'aphasie tactile. *Rev. Neurol., 12*:371–375, 1906.
296. Redlich, E. and Bonvicini, G.: Weitere klinische und anatomische Mitteilungen über das Fehlen der Wahrnehmung der eigenen Blindheit bei Hirnkrankheiten. *Neurol. Centralbl., 30*:227–301, 1911.

297. Redlich, F. and Dorsey, J.: Denial of blindness by patients with cerebral disease. *Arch. Neurol and Psychiat., 53*:407–417, 1945.
298. Riese, W.: The early history of aphasia. *Bull. Hist. Med., 21*:322–334, 1947.
299. Rochford, G. and Williams, M.: Studies in the development and breakdown of the use of names. *J. Neurol. Neurosurg. Psychiat., 25*:228–233, 1962.
300. Rubens, A. and Benson, D.: Associative visual agnosia, *Arch. Neurol.,* 1971.
301. Russell, B.: *The Analysis of Mind.* Allen and Unwin, London, 1921.
302. Sabouraud, O., Gagnepain, J. and Sabouraud, A.: Vers une approche linguistique des problèmes de l'aphasie (II). L'aphasie de Broca. *Rev. Neuropsychiat. de l'Ouest, 2*:3–38, 1963.
303. Salomon, E.: Motorische Aphasie mit Agrammatismus und sensorisch-agrammatischen Störungen. *Mschr. f. Psychiat. u. Neurol., 35*:181–275, 1914.
304. Scheerer, M.: Cognitive theory, in *Handbook of Social Psychology.* G. Lindsey (Ed.). Addison-Wesley Publ., Cambridge, pp. 91–142, 1954.
305. Schilder, P.: Localization of the body image (postural model of the body). *Assoc. Res. Nerv. Ment. Dis., 13*:466–484, 1932.
306. Schilder, P.: *The Image and Appearance of the Human Body.* Kegan, London, 1935.
307. Schilder, P.: On the development of thoughts, in *Organization and Pathology of Thought.* D. Rapaport (Ed.). Columbia University Press, New York, 1951.
308. Schilder, P.: *Brain and Personality.* International Universities Press, New York, 1951a.
309. Schilder, P. and Sugar: Zur Lehre von den schizophrenen Sprachstörungen. *Z. f. Neurol. u. Psychiat., 104*:689–714, 1926.
310. Schjelderup-Ebbe, T.: (1923) In Mintz, *J. Abnorm. Soc. Psychol., 43*:548–549, 1948.
311. Schneider, D.: The clinical syndrome of echolalia, echopraxia, grasping and sucking. *J. Nerv. Ment. Dis., 88*:18–35, 200–216, 1938.
312. Schuell, H.: Paraphasia and paralexia. *J. Speech Hearing Disorders, 15*:291–306, 1950.
313. Schuster, P. and Taterka, H.: Beitrag zur Anatomie und Klinik der reinen Worttaubheit. *Ztschr. Neurol. Psychiat., 105*:494–538, 1926.
314. Seelert, H.: Beitrag zur Kenntnis der Rückbildung von Apraxie. *Mschr. Psychiat. Neurol., 48*:125–149, 1920.
315. Serafetinides, E. and Falconer, M.: Speech disturbances in temporal lobe seizures. *Brain, 86*:333–346, 1963.
316. Shankweiler, D.: Effects of temporal-lobe lesions on recognition of dichotically-presented melodies. Presented at Eastern Psychol. Assoc., 1964.

317. Sittig, O.: Störungen im Verhalten gegenuber Farben bei Aphasischen. *Mschr. f. Psychiat. u. Neurol., 49*:63–88, 169–187, 1921.

318. Sittig, O.: Über Echographie. *Msschr. f. Psychiat. u. Neurol., 68*:574–604, 1928.

319. Sittig, O.: *Ueber Apraxie.* S. Karger, Berlin, 1931.

320. Smith, A. and Burklund, C.: Dominant hemispherectomy: Preliminary report on neuropsychological sequelae. *Science, 153*:1280–1282, 1966.

320a. Smyth, G. and Stern, K.: Tumours of the thalamus—A clinico-pathological study. *Brain, 61*:339–374, 1938.

321. Souques, A.: Quelques cas d'anarthrie de Pierre Marie. *Rev. Neurol., 2*:319–368, 1928.

322. Sparks, R. and Geschwind, N.: Dichotic listening in man after section of neocortical commissures. *Cortex, 4*:3–16, 1968.

323. Spreen, O., Benton, A. and Fincham, R.: Auditory agnosia without aphasia. *Arch. Neurol., 13*:84–92, 1965.

324. Spreen, O., Benton, A. and Van Allen, M.: Dissociation of visual and tactile naming in amnestic aphasia. *Neurology, 16*:807–814, 1966.

325. Stauffenberg, V.: *Ueber Seelenblindheit.* Arb. Hirnanat. Inst. Zurich, Wiesbaden, *8*:1–212, 1914.

326. Steinthal: *Abriss der Sprachwissenschaft.* Berlin, 1871.

327. Stengel, E.: Zur Lehre von der Leitungsaphasie. *Z. ges. Neurol. Psychiat., 149*:266–291, 1934.

328. Stengel, E.: A clinical and psychological study of echo-reactions. *J. Ment. Sci., 93*:598–612, 1947.

329. Stengel, E.: The syndrome of visual alexia with colour agnosia. *J. Ment. Sci., 94*:46–58, 1948.

330. Stengel, E. and Lodge Patch, I.: "Central" aphasia associated with parietal symptoms. *Brain, 78*:401–416, 1955.

331. Stengel, E. and Steele, G.: Unawareness of physical disability (anosognosia). *J. Ment. Sci., 92*:379–388, 1946.

332. Stertz, G.: Zum Verständnis der mangelnden Selbstwahrenhmung der eigenen Blindheit. *Z. ges. Neurol. Psychiat., 55*:327, 1920.

333. Strauss, H.: *Ueber konstruktive Apraxie. Mschr. Psychiat. Neurol., 56*:65–124, 1924.

334. Strauss, A. and Werner, H.: Deficiency in the finger schema in relation to arithmetic disability. *Amer. J. Orthopsychiat., 8*:719–725, 1938.

335. Strohmayer, W.: Über "subkortikale Alexie" mit Agraphie und Apraxie. *Dtsch. z. Nervenheilk., 24*:372–380, 1903.

336. Symonds, C.: Aphasia. *J. Neurol. Neurosurg. Psychiat., 16*:1–6, 1953.

337. Talland, G.: *Deranged Memory: A Psychonomic Study of the Amnesic Syndrome.* Academic Press, New York, 1965.

338. Teuber, H.: In *Analysis of Behavioral Change.* L. Weiskrantz (Ed.). Harper, New York, p. 287, 1968.

339. Trescher, J. and Ford, F.: Colloid cyst of the third ventricle. *Arch. Neurol. Psychiat., 37*:959–973, 1937.

340. Ustvedt, H.: Üeber die Untersuchung der musikalischen Funktionen bei Patienten mit Gehirnleiden, besonders bei Patienten mit Aphasie. *Acta Med. Scand., Suppl., 86*:1–737, 1937.

341. Van der Horst, L.: The psychology of constructive apraxia. *Psychiat. en Neurol. Bl., 36*:243–259, 1932.

342. Van Vleuten, C.: Linksseitige motorische Apraxie. *Allg. Zeitschr. f. Psychiat., 64*:203–239, 1907.

343. Vignolo, L.: Auditory agnosia: A review and report of recent evidence, in *Contributions to Clinical Neuropsychology.* A. Benton (Ed.). Aldine, Chicago, pp. 172–208, 1969.

344. Vygotsky, L.: *Thought and Language.* M.I.T. Press, Cambridge, 1962.

345. Wallaschek, V.: *Les troubles de l'expression musicale dans l'aphasie.* Vierteljahrschr. f. Musikwissenschaft., Leipzig, 1891.

346. Warren, R.: Perceptual restoration of missing speech sounds. *Science, 167*:392–393, 1970.

347. Warrington, E.: Constructional apraxia, in *Handbook of Clinical Neurology.* Vol. 4, P. Vinken and G. Bruyn (Eds.). Wiley, New York, pp. 67–83, 1969.

348. Warrington, E. and Zangwill, O.: A study of dyslexia. *J. Neurol. Neurosurg. Psychiat., 20*:208–215, 1957.

349. Weigl, E. and Bierwisch, M.: *Neuropsychology and Linguistics: Topics of Common Research,* 1969.

350. Weinstein, E. and Cole, M.: Concepts of anosognosia, in *Problems of Dynamic Neurology.* L. Halpern (Ed.). Jerusalem, 1963.

351. Weinstein, E. and Kahn, R.: *Denial of Illness: Symbolic and Physiological Aspects.* Springfield, Charles C Thomas, 1955.

352. Weinstein, E. and Keller, N.: Linguistic patterns of misnaming in brain injury. *Neuropsychologia, 1*:79–90, 1964.

353. Weinstein, E., Lyerly, O., Cole, M. and Ozer, M.: Meaning in jargon aphasia. *Cortex, 2*:165–187, 1966.

354. Weisenberg, T. and McBride, K.: *Aphasia: A Clinical and Psychological Study* (reprint of 1935 ed.). Hafner, New York, 1964.

355. Weiskrantz, L.: Experiments on the R.N.S. (real nervous system) and monkey memory. *Proc. Roy. Soc., 171*:335–352, 1968.

356. Werner, H.: Microgenesis and aphasia. *J. Abnorm. Soc. Psychol., 52*:347–353, 1956.

357. Wernicke, C.: *Der aphasische Symptomenkomplex.* Cohn & Weigart, Breslau, 1874.

358. Wernicke, C.: The symptom-complex of aphasia, in *Modern Clin. Med., Diseases of the Nervous System.* A. Church (Ed.). Appleton, New York, 1908.

359. Wertheim, N.: Disturbances of the musical functions, in *Problems of Dynamic Neurology.* L. Halpern (Ed.). Jerusalem, pp. 162–180, 1963.

360. Wertheim, N.: The amusias, in *Handb. Clin. Neurol.* P. Vinken and G. Bruyn (Eds.). Wiley, New York, pp. 195–206, 1969.

361. Westphal, C.: Ueber einen Fall von motorischen Apraxie. *Allg. Z. f. Psychiat., 64*:452–459, 1907.

362. Wilbrand, H.: *Ophthalmiatrische Beiträge zur Diagnostik der Gehirn-Kranheiten.* Wiesbaden, 1884.

363. Wilbrand, H.: *Die Seelenblindheit als Herderscheinung.* Wiesbaden, 1887.

364. Wingfield, A.: in Oldfield, R., *Quart. J. Exp. Psychol., 18*:340–353, 1966.

365. Woerkom, W. van: Uber Störungen im Denken bei Aphasiepatienten. *Mschr. Psychiat. u. Neurol., 59*:256–322, 1925.

366. Wortis, S. and Pfeffer, A.: Unilateral auditory-spatial agnosia. *J. Nerv. Ment. Dis., 108*:181–186, 1948.

367. Zangwill, O.: Le problème de l'apraxie ideatoire. *Rev. Neurol., 102*:595–603, 1960.

368. Ziegler, D.: Word deafness and Wernicke's aphasia. *Arch. Neurol. Psychiat., 67*:323–331, 1952.

AUTHOR INDEX

SUBJECT INDEX